SHRINK YOUR FEMALE FAT ZONES

SHRINK YOUR FEMALE FAT ZONES

Lose Pounds and Inches—*Fast!*—From Your Belly, Hips, Thighs, and More

DENISE AUSTIN

Star of *The Daily Workout* and *Fit & Lite*, Lifetime Television

RODALE®

Notice

This book is intended as a reference volume only, not as a medical manual. The information given here is designed to help you make informed decisions about your health, diet, fitness, and exercise program. It is not intended as a substitute for professional fitness and medical advice. If you suspect that you have a medical problem, we urge you to seek competent medical help. As with all exercise programs, you should seek your doctor's approval before you begin.

Mention of specific companies, organizations, or authorities in this book does not imply endorsement by the publisher, nor does mention of specific companies, organizations, or authorities imply that they endorse this book.

Printed in the United States of America
Rodale Inc. makes every effort to use acid-free ∞, recycled paper ♲.

Interior photographs © Mitch Mandel/Rodale Images, except: © Hilmar, pages v, viii, 34, 92, 242, and 380. Before and after photos on pages 10, 14, 24, 32, 142, 182, 250, and 256 were provided by the individuals.

Interior design by Patricia Field

Library of Congress Cataloging-in-Publication Data
Austin, Denise.
    Shrink your female fat zones : lose pounds and inches—fast!—from your belly, hips, thighs, and more / Denise Austin.
        p. cm.
Includes index.
    ISBN 1–57954–733–8 hardcover
    ISBN 1–57954–734–6 paperback
    1. Weight loss. 2. Women—Health and hygiene. 3. Reducing diets.
4. Physical fitness. 5. Exercise—Health aspects. I. Title.
    RM222.2.A923 2003
    613.7'045—dc21   2003005706

Distributed to the book trade by St. Martin's Press

    4 6 8 10 9 7 5   hardcover
        6 8 10 9 7 5   paperback

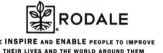

RODALE
WE **INSPIRE** AND **ENABLE** PEOPLE TO IMPROVE
THEIR LIVES AND THE WORLD AROUND THEM

FOR MORE OF OUR PRODUCTS
WWW.RODALESTORE.COM
(800) 848-4735

To my "honeybunny" Jeff
and our precious daughters,
Kelly and Katie.

I am so blessed to have such a wonderful family and great friends. All I truly hope is that everyone is healthy and happy.

I'm so thankful to my husband, Jeff, who lets me be *me*. We're celebrating our 20th wedding anniversary this year and couldn't be happier. I thank God every day for my sweet, little girls, Kelly and Katie, who are growing up way too fast.

I miss my mom so much. It's been 2 years since her passing, and a day doesn't go by without me thinking about her. My dad is 78 and still working full-time—thanks, Dad, for instilling in me a strong work ethic.

To my three sisters and my brother who have been amazingly supportive all these 25 years; they still get excited when I'm in a magazine or on a TV show.

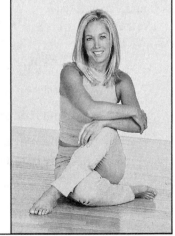

I want to thank all the wonderful people I work with at Rodale and *Prevention* magazine . . . plus extra thanks to Tami Booth and Mariska van Aalst.

A big thanks to Alisa Bauman and nutritionist Janis Jibrin who truly made this book happen . . . thank you.

Special thanks to Michael Broussard and Jan Miller, my literary agents. I love you guys.

CONTENTS

PART 1   FEMALE FAT ZONES DEFINED

Chapter 1: The "Genealogy" of Female Fat   3

Chapter 2: The Amazing Shrinking Fat Cell   18

PART 2   THE FAT ZONE WALKING AND STRETCHING PROGRAM

Chapter 3: Target Toning As You Walk   37

Chapter 4: Denise's Daily Stretch   73

PART 3   THE FAT ZONE WORKOUTS

Chapter 5: The Upper Body   95

Chapter 6: The Midsection   140

Chapter 7: The Lower Body   180

Chapter 8: Total-Body Shape-Ups   221

PART 4	THE SHRINK YOUR FEMALE FAT ZONES DIET	
	Chapter 9: The Shrink-Fat Eating Plan	245
	Chapter 10: Week 1: Go on Portion Patrol	260
	Chapter 11: Week 2: Fight Fat with Fiber	280
	Chapter 12: Week 3: Savor Good Fats	298
	Chapter 13: Week 4: Fill Up on Fruits and Vegetables	318
	Chapter 14: Week 5: Home In on Hunger	336
	Chapter 15: Week 6: Identify and Change Behaviors	356
PART 5	THE SHRINK YOUR FEMALE FAT ZONES TOOLS	
	Chapter 16: Recipes for Success	383
	Chapter 17: Your 6-Week Fat Zone Workbook	406
	Index	413

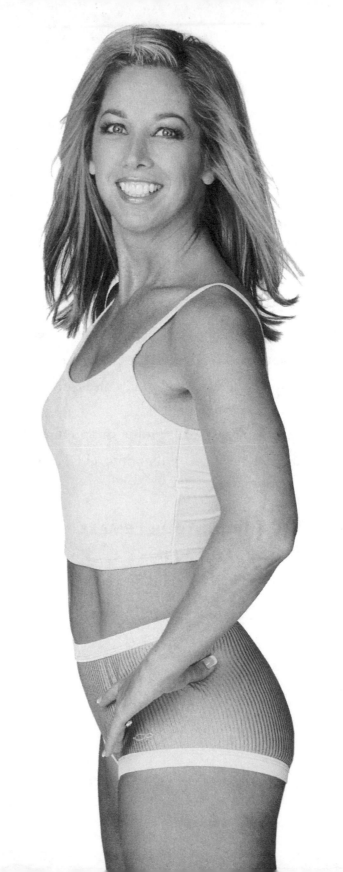

PART 1

Female Fat Zones Defined

CHAPTER 1

FEMALE FAT ZONES DEFINED

The "Genealogy" of Female Fat

Congratulations on making the commitment to shrink your female fat zones! I'm excited to bring you my newest body-slimming program, one designed specifically to help you maximize your results within a minimum amount of time. Think of it as a shortcut to your best body ever, a shortcut to a new you.

I truly believe that inside every out-of-shape woman lies a trim, well-proportioned body. The Shrink Your Female Fat Zones program will help you zero in on your personal trouble spots while you increase your metabolism and decrease your appetite. You'll reshape your body, losing fat from the areas you want to minimize—your waist, thighs, tummy, buttocks, hips, lower back, and upper arms—and not from the areas you want to accentuate.

Best of all, you'll look and feel fantastic!

Every day, women write to me, telling me that no matter how hard they try, they can't seem to shrink their waistlines or thighs, lift their buns, flatten their tummies, or tone their arms. They complain of stubborn fat deposits that just won't budge. They tell me that they eat less—but the fat doesn't shrink. Often, they're even exercising, seemingly doing everything right.

Yet, once I dig a little deeper, I usually find out that they are not doing the best types of exercise for shrinking fat and they're not eating the best foods for lowering appetite. I have great news! You *can* shrink your female fat zones without feeling hungry all the time, without craving foods, and without feeling tired. In fact, you will have *more* energy and eat delicious foods. You'll feel satisfied and fantastic! And you'll do so by spending only 15 to 60 minutes a day exercising. You'll never need to count calories. And you'll *never* feel hungry, deprived, guilty, or pressed for time.

What's my secret? The Shrink Your Female Fat Zones program works with the natural rhythms of the female body, encouraging your fat cells to release their cargo and your muscle cells to burn it up. (Of course, "cargo" is just a slang term that I use to describe the fatty acids that reside in your fat cells. You're going to release those fatty acids and burn them!)

I know it works because this is the same system I've used to shrink my personal fat zone: my thighs. Oh, you're surprised that I have a fat zone, too? As you'll soon find out, all women do. And, like me, most women tend to gain fat in the lower body first and lose it there last.

But thanks to the Shrink Your Female Fat Zones program, I've been able to keep my thighs trim and toned well into my forties. With this program you can do the same, whether you tend to gain fat in your lower body, your midsection, or your upper body.

This unique 6-week body-toning and weight-loss program incorporates the latest and most effective strategies for shrinking your waistline, slimming your thighs, lifting and toning your buns, flattening your tummy, shaping your shoulders, and firming your arms.

I'm happy to tell you that the Shrink Your Female Fat Zones program includes no diet gimmicks. Rather, I've based this four-pronged body-shaping plan on the latest discoveries in the science and origins of female fat.

You see, for the past 20 years, researchers have busily studied why women tend to gain fat in one of three predictable fat zones: the upper body, the midsection, or the lower body. They've also been unraveling why women tend to gain more fat than men—and why we have a harder time losing it.

Now, hundreds of studies later, researchers have revealed the secret formula

What's Your Body Type?

To GET THE BEST RESULTS on the Shrink Your Female Fat Zones program, first identify the area on your body where you tend to gain fat first and lose fat last.

For the vast majority of women, the answer is the lower-body fat zone: the hips, thighs, and buttocks. If you wear a smaller bikini top than bottom, this is your fat zone. If you've always been able to carve a flat tummy but always hated the size of your thighs, this is your personal fat zone.

Most other women claim the midsection fat zone as their personal fat zone. If you gain weight in your abdomen first and lose it there last, this is your fat zone. If you've always had skinny legs and a tiny butt but had to wear oversize shirts to cover up your tummy, this is your fat zone.

For a minority of women, the upper body may serve as a fat depot. If you have large breasts, with extra "pudge" pressing out around your bra straps along with heavy upper arms, this is your personal fat zone.

Knowing your personal fat zone will help you to best combine the most effective toning and cardiovascular exercise strategies for you.

needed to boost your metabolism, lower your appetite, and shrink the areas you want to shrink and not the areas you don't. This formula includes targeted toning workouts, regular walking and stretching, and six important eating strategies that will help fill you up on fewer calories.

Sometimes, it can seem as if I've spent my life battling my personal fat zone. Whenever I overindulge—by eating too many desserts, for example—I see the results on my thighs. As I age, I've found that keeping my thighs trim has required me to exercise in a very specific way and be more aware of what I eat. And thanks to recent discoveries in the science of female fat, I've learned that I can keep my thighs—as well as the rest of my body—toned and trim with mild but consistent cardiovascular and toning workouts and absolutely no dieting.

In fact, as you'll soon learn, overdoing it by cutting too many calories can actually make you gain weight! It's true.

But before I get to that, let's first look at the science of female fat to find out why women experience a tougher time than men losing weight and keeping it off. Once you understand this important science, you'll more easily understand my four-pronged attack on female fat.

Built for Survival

Have you ever wondered why men seem to lose weight faster and more easily than women? Perhaps you know men who were able to shrink a huge beer belly simply by drinking less beer. But when you tried the same strategy, it didn't work.

The answer lies in the unique genetics of the female body. When it comes to fat zones, men and women were not created equal. Women's bodies contain on average 10 percent more body fat than men. Our bodies burn fewer calories at any given time, and our hormones make it tougher to burn off fat.

To understand why our bodies resist fat loss, I'd like to take you on a journey back in time, to thousands of years ago when our ancient female cousins needed fat—and lots of it—to provide a regular source of calories during extended famines. These early ancestors survived by foraging for food. They lived off berries, seeds, and the occasional animal they could kill.

Sometimes they feasted. Other times, during a long drought, they ate little to no food.

Such famines could drag on for months or even a year. Women who survived were able to pass on their genes to their offspring. These genes contained a set of instructions that encouraged the female body to scrimp and save every excess calorie, channeling these calories into strategic fat depots in the thighs, buttocks, hips, breasts, tummy, and upper arms. These fat depots acted much like a food bank, one that encouraged regular deposits and few withdrawals. They allowed our ancient ancestors to survive for months on little to no food.

A woman who had many extra pounds of fat could survive 9 months or more of famine, long enough to deliver a baby, nurse it, and pass on her genes. Women whose bodies didn't store fat as efficiently would miscarry during a famine. Thus, the slender women's genes didn't get passed down the generations.

Thousands of years later, most of us have inherited the genes of our plumper cousins. These genes program our bodies to encourage fat storage and discourage fat burning. Of course, in modern times, our food is never farther than a trip to the grocery store. We no longer need this efficient genetic programming. Unfortunately, genetics takes a very long time to change.

Thanks to these built-for-survival genetics, our female fat cells are larger than our male counterparts. A woman's body contains roughly the same number of fat cells as a man's—about 30 billion—but our female fat cells contain more enzymes that help store fat, whereas the male fat cells contain more enzymes that help burn fat.

Here's the exciting part. You can trick your body into turning on your fat-burning enzymes and turning off your fat-storing enzymes. To shrink your female fat zones, you'll take advantage of your feminine genetic programming rather than work against it.

To understand how to do just that, let's take a look at how your hormones affect fat storage.

The Hormone Connection

So we know now that certain enzymes help fill fat cells up, whereas others help cells release their fat. Both kinds of enzymes act like fat transporters: The enzyme called lipoprotein lipase (LPL) escorts fat into your fat cells, and the enzyme called hormone-sensitive lipase (HSL) takes fat out of your cells and transports it to your muscle cells to get burned for energy.

Though you have the same total number of fat cells as your husband or other male friends, you have more LPL fat-storing enzymes and fewer HSL fat-burning enzymes. These fat-storing LPL enzymes get turned on and flourish with the help of the female hormone estrogen. Basically, estrogen encourages fat cells to hold on to fat for survival.

Throughout our lives, there are certain stages when almost all women experience a sudden increase in body fat. You probably first noticed this change during your teenage years, when that initial surge of estrogen started your menstrual cycle. This jolt of estrogen transforms rail-thin girls into women with hips and curves.

Later, in your twenties, if you were taking the older, higher-dose oral contraceptives, you may have put on more fat during that stage as well. At a high enough dose, supplemental estrogen makes fat cells even more efficient at storing fat. These changes could also reduce your metabolic rate (the rate at which you burn calories) by as much as 10 percent. If you didn't compensate by eating 10 percent fewer calories (150 to 200 fewer calories a day), you could have seen the results in expanding fat zones.

To make matters more unfair, you may also find that you tend to gain weight at the beginning of your menstrual cycle. At this time, estrogen is at its peak, attempting to store up extra fat to fuel a potential pregnancy.

And then there's pregnancy. (It's not *just* about those extra bowls of ice cream.) During pregnancy, estrogen doubles your fat-storing LPL enzymes in order to fill out your breasts for future milk production as well as the rest of your fat zones to cushion and support your growing fetus. The hormone progesterone also helps expand your fat zones by making you feel hungry, which helps drive you back to the freezer for the second dish of Rocky Road. (Progesterone also rises during the second half of your menstrual cycle, which is why you tend to grab for the ice cream scoop during that phase, too.)

After pregnancy, the hormone prolactin rises to start milk production. Like estrogen, this hormone encourages your fat-storing enzymes to stay busy—holding on to that extra calorie supply to fuel milk production and keep your baby well-fed while you're nursing.

The Age Connection

You may be wondering, if estrogen makes you gain fat, why do many women gain even more weight after menopause when estrogen levels drop?

That's a good question, one that I had wondered for many years. To find out the answer, I went straight to the experts. As a member of the President's Council on Physical Fitness and Sports, I have access to some of the most respected researchers and doctors in the country, the top experts in their fields.

They told me that the female body contains more than one type of estrogen. During menopause, you maintain levels of one type of estrogen, called estrone. This type of estrogen slows your metabolism and encourages fat storage.

At the same time, you rapidly lose a type of estrogen called 17-beta-estradiol, the most abundant type of estrogen made by your ovaries. Estradiol keeps energy up, regulates blood pressure, and helps make sure that insulin properly shuttles energy into your cells. So it's no wonder that you feel tired and moody when estradiol plummets.

In addition to changing hormone levels, a slowdown in activity causes many women to lose muscle as they get older, and this dramatically curbs their metabolism. Less muscle mass accounts for one of the reasons we burn fewer calories than men. A man's body contains nearly double the amount of muscle than a woman's—before menopause. Each muscle cell contains a calorie-burning hotbox called a mitochondrion. In this cell compartment, the mitochondrion burns fat and sugar to fuel the muscle's movements and overall maintenance.

Just 1 pound of muscle burns 35 to 50 calories a day. Consequently, the more muscle in your body, the higher your metabolism, and the more you can eat without gaining weight.

If they're not careful, most women lose 1 to 2 pounds of muscle during each decade after age 20. By age 75, many women have lost up to 40 percent of their muscle mass, slowing their metabolism by more than 200 calories a day. No wonder that daily handful of cookies is a lot more visible on the hips!

Muscle mass drops dramatically after menopause, thanks to a drop in the hormone testosterone. You may think of testosterone as a male hormone, but all women have small amounts that help fuel their sex drives and build their muscles. You lose about half of the levels of this hormone at menopause, which means you must work harder to build and preserve muscle in order to fuel your metabolism.

All of these reasons combined help to explain why many women gain 7 pounds during every decade. And it's also why, by age 75, most women have doubled their fat zones compared to when they were age 20.

But before you throw your hands up in despair—stop! Please don't worry. I won't let any of this discourage you, because I have great news: You don't *have* to gain fat as you age! I'm excited to tell you that a simple 15-minute muscle-building routine done 5 days a week can reverse the muscle loss typically seen with aging. The simple Shrink Your Female Fat Zones program will help you boost your metabolism permanently, for the rest of your life. Quite simply, it's the most effective 15 minutes you'll ever spend on your body!

I Shrunk My Female Fat Zones!

Switching to a morning exercise routine helped Candy Hammond to more effectively tone her trouble spots.

Before I started doing Denise's workout every day, I realized that I had been spending more and more time exercising and getting less out of it. I found that combining my 20- to 30-minute walk every morning with Denise's workout allowed me to tone up and target all of my body areas more effectively.

I love the diversity of working a different body area each day. I also love the convenience. I now walk from 7:00 to 7:30 A.M. and get home just in time to do Denise's workout. It makes it easy to commit to.

I work as a life coach, and walking my talk is important! I have turned on many clients to Denise. She is motivating, and being my age helps, too! (She's not a 20-something supermodel—she's my age and a mom, like me.)

Denise got me interested in Pilates, and I love her kickboxing moves.

Denise's exercise routines have helped me to lift my butt—not glamorous sounding, but true! My abs and arms are better, too! After two C-sections, I'll never have a perfectly flat stomach, but the Pilates ab exercises have helped a lot!

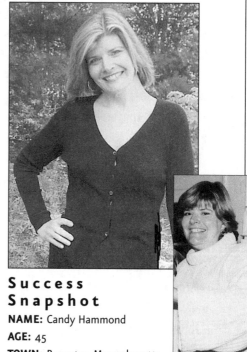

Success Snapshot

NAME: Candy Hammond

AGE: 45

TOWN: Brewster, Massachusetts

OCCUPATION: Life coach, writer

FITNESS GAINED: Toned her trouble spots

OTHER ACCOMPLISHMENTS: More energy and happiness

Candy's Secret to Success

"Set a time for exercise and make it a habit. Also, know that taking time for yourself is not a luxury, it's a necessity. Put yourself on the top of your 'to do' list and make taking care of yourself a priority. The better you feel about yourself, the more you will have to give to those you love. Self-care is self-love. Practice it every day."

Your Personal Fat Zone

It seems like one of those perverse laws of nature. When you go on a diet, you usually lose weight where you *don't* want to—such as your breasts—and not where you want to—your waistline, tummy, thighs, and butt.

In most women, the female hormone estrogen directs fat storage into the lower-body fat zone: the hips, thighs, and buttocks. This creates the body shape known as the pear shape. These are the areas where most women gain weight first—and lose it last. Of course, not every single woman is shaped like a pear. That's because we didn't all inherit the same genes from our ancestors. A small number of women have inverted triangle shapes and tend to gain fat primarily in the upper-body fat zone: the breasts and upper arms. Finally, some women are genetically prone to store fat in the midsection: the abdomen and lower back, creating a circular body shape also known as the apple.

All women's bodies store fat predominantly in one of these three fat zones. Your fat zones aren't set in stone, however. They can change with age, most notably after menopause.

After menopause, if you recall, estradiol drops to much lower levels than before. Because this type of estrogen directs fat storage into the lower-body fat zone, the drop in estradiol changes your body shape. Your body begins to store fat like a man—in the abdomen—rather than in the thighs, buttocks, and hips.

On the bright side, because abdominal fat cells are smaller and less resistant to releasing their cargo, you will experience an easier time losing extra tummy fat than you did losing extra thigh fat. Numerous studies show, however, that abdominal fat is far more dangerous to your health than lower body fat.

For example, researchers from the University of Minnesota measured the body mass index (BMI, a comparison of weight to height), waist circumference, and hip circumference of 31,702 women ages 55 to 69 and then followed them for 12 years in a large, groundbreaking research project known as the Iowa Women's Health Study. After crunching the data, researchers found that the women who had had the thickest waist circumferences at the start of the study were most likely to die early, regardless of their BMI. The scientists found that greater amounts of abdominal fat were also associated with heart disease, diabetes, and high blood pressure.

In a separate study of 6,296 men and women in Rotterdam, the Netherlands, researchers also found that those with the thickest waists were most likely to die early, regardless of their overall weight.

Abdominal fat poses such a high health risk in women that researchers have already dubbed it syndrome W. Women with syndrome W have the following characteristics in common.

- Gained more than 20 pounds after midlife

- Have been diagnosed with high blood pressure

- Have body cells that are resistant to the hormone insulin (a prediabetic condition)

- Have high blood cholesterol levels

Though researchers are not completely sure why abdominal fat raises the risk of premature death, they point out that this type of fat sits close to critical organs, like the heart, and contributes to clogged arteries. Abdominal fat may also be metabolized differently than other types of fat, contributing to higher cholesterol, blood fats, and blood pressure—which is all the more incentive to get out there and shrink that fat zone!

I'm happy to tell you that you can change your God-given body shape. Whether you're an apple or pear or inverted triangle, you can create balanced proportions. You can lose excess fat, and you can improve your health. Yes, you can! I'll teach you how throughout the pages of this book. No matter your life stage, your lifestyle, your age, or your individual genetics—you can reshape your body from head to toe.

Meet the Metabolism Busters

You really *can* shrink your fat zones! Do you know what is the most exciting discovery in the science of female fat? That you can work *with* your genetics to lose fat, gain muscle, and reshape your body. That's why I've written this book: to teach you how to work with—not against—your body's genetic tendencies.

Too many women try to lose weight by working against their natural genetic tendencies. For example, have you ever gone on a diet? If you did, you worked against your body, not with it.

When you diet, you certainly do lose fat and weight—but no one can stay on a diet forever. And when you start eating normally again, you may have noticed that the fat generally comes back—and then some. Here's what's going on. As you restrict calories during a diet, your fat cells send signals to your brain, saying, "Famine! Enter survival mode." Your brain responds by ordering your fat-storing enzymes to increase. Eventually, you hit a plateau in your efforts because these LPL enzymes make it more and more difficult for your body to release fat.

Numerous studies have documented this dieting-induced metabolic slowdown. One of the more notable ones, done at Cedars-Sinai Medical Center in Los Angeles, found that obese women who went on very low calorie diets experienced a surge in LPL fat-storing enzyme levels, which the researchers suspected would make future weight-loss attempts more difficult.

In addition to increasing your fat-storing enzymes, dieting also tends to cause your body to cannibalize muscle protein for fuel. Less muscle equals a slower metabolism. So when you break your diet, your body is burning fewer calories—as much as 250 fewer calories a day—and has a higher amount of fat-storing enzymes.

Your metabolism also slows for another reason. When you restrict calories, your body lowers the activation of your thyroid hormone. Your thyroid hormone regulates your metabolism. Your body is actually trying to slow your metabolism in order to protect you from starvation.

Before your diet, you may have been able to eat 1,800 calories a day and not gain weight. Now, with your slower metabolism, you might only be able to eat 1,550. Indeed, a study from the Netherlands found that those who dieted most often were also more likely to regain lost weight.

So you end up on a dieting roller coaster, a never-ending process of cutting calories, losing fat, slowing your metabolism, and gaining back even more

I Shrunk My Female Fat Zones!

Changing her lifestyle in small baby steps helped Danielle Koerber lose her baby weight.

I have done Denise's program three to five times a week since my daughter was born. It has increased my energy and decreased my stress. Thanks to her program, I got back to my prepregnancy weight of 125 pounds within 6 months.

I started slowly, especially since that was all I could do after giving birth. My transformation was gradual, and I didn't allow myself to obsess about my weight on the scale. Before I knew it, the weight came off and people began telling me how great I looked.

Denise's routines all take less than 30 minutes, and that has made it easy for me to fit exercise in and not find excuses to skip my workouts.

Denise has also helped me to change my diet. I now eat at least five fruits and vegetables a day, drink eight glasses of water a day, and never eat after 8:00 P.M. Putting a curfew on the kitchen has certainly helped me to lose weight a little faster.

I have to say that the most important thing is to value yourself enough to make exercise a part of your life. Focus on how you feel—not on how you look—and you can't go wrong.

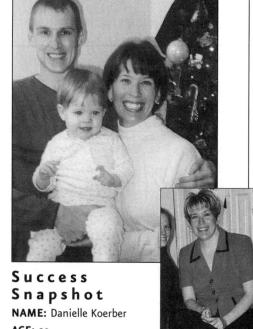

Success Snapshot

NAME: Danielle Koerber

AGE: 29

TOWN: Allen Park, Michigan

OCCUPATION: Customer service representative

WEIGHT LOST: 15 pounds

OTHER ACCOMPLISHMENTS: Increased energy, lowered stress, and has more motivation to move

Danielle's Secret to Success

"Make exercise a part of your routine, like brushing your teeth. I get up with my husband, even though he gets up for work earlier than I have to, and I get my workout done. At a certain point, it just becomes a habit, and you miss that part of your day if you don't do it."

fat. Each time that you try to lose weight, your goal weight will feel even more difficult to reach. This is why some women complain that they have virtually no metabolism.

Besides hampering your future weight-loss efforts, chronic dieting also hurts your health. When you lose weight on a diet, at least a quarter of that weight comes from water, muscle, and bone. Yes, bone. The faster you lose weight, the more bone you lose. In fact, doctors have found anorexic teens with bones as porous and brittle as women in their seventies or eighties—all a result of crash dieting.

Besides dieting, the chronic stress of trying to be a "supermom" can also encourage fat storage. Research done by Pamela Peeke, M.P.H., M.D., at the National Institutes of Health shows that the stress hormones cortisol and adrenaline rise when you are under stress. Cortisol and adrenaline work to take sugar out of your liver and shuttle it into your blood, making energy readily available for fight or flight.

Most of us, however, don't experience the type of stress that extra calories will help solve, the way our ancient female cousins might have. Most of us experience mental rather than physical stress, but our bodies don't know the difference. So once we no longer feel stressed, our bodies want to replace the sugar it took from our livers. To do so, stress hormones make us crave sweets and feel hungry, even though our bodies don't actually need calories. This causes us to overeat.

For example, a study of more than 5,000 women and men found that stress eaters were more likely to reach for sausage, hamburgers, pizza, chocolate, and alcohol. They also were most likely to be overweight.

Too much stress also makes you tired, which causes you to skip your best-intentioned plans to exercise. (It's much more difficult to get up and at 'em in the morning if your body doesn't feel as though it has recuperated from the day before yet.)

If you experience chronic stress on a daily basis, you expose your body to high levels of cortisol constantly. This can eventually lower your immunity, encourage your body to store abdominal fat for easy burning during stress, disturb your sleep, and make you constantly hungry.

Finally, stress also brings down estrogen levels to abnormally low levels.

Seeing Yourself Shrink

AS YOU PROGRESS on the Shrink Your Female Fat Zones program, I want you to keep track of and celebrate your successes.

To track your results, a scale may be just one way to measure up. On my program, you'll perform toning exercises that will build metabolism-boosting muscle. Because muscle is more compact than fat, it also weighs more. So you may not lose as much weight on the scale as you expect, but you'll still shrink in size. Research shows that women who begin a strength-training program can expect to drop as many as three dress sizes, even if their weight remains the same.

If you'd like to use your scale, go for it. In fact, stepping on the scale once a week can help keep some women motivated. But in addition to the scale, I'd like you to use one of the following methods to track your progress.

YOUR MEASUREMENTS. Use a flexible tape measure to find out the circumference of your waist, hips, thighs, and upper arms. (Although it may be tempting, try not to suck in your belly when you're doing it! Take a deep breath, let it out, and then take your measurement.) Write down these numbers. Notice particularly if your waist measurement is larger than your hip measurement. If so, try to work specifically on reversing those numbers, as a thick waist increases your risk of disease.

If you can control your curiosity, it's best to wait the full 6 weeks to see how much your measurements can shrink, but if it's too much temptation, a once-a-week check-in can help keep you motivated.

YOUR CLOTHING SIZE. You probably know which clothes in your closet feel a little too snug or don't fit at all. Pick one garment, perhaps a pair of jeans or a slinky black dress and use it as your gauge. At the 6-week mark, you'll really see how much you've shrunk!

YOUR BODY-FAT PERCENTAGE. Not long ago, the only way to find out your body-fat percentage—the percentage of your fat tissue compared to your lean tissue such as muscle and bone—was at a doctor's office or health club. Now, you can buy an inexpensive scale such as the one made by Healthometer to take your body-fat percentage at home. (Because this number can vary depending on a lot of variables, try to wait the full 6 weeks for maximum accuracy—and shrinkage!)

Note your beginning measurements in Day 1 of your daily planner. You'll notice a place to mark your progress, as well as to track your walking, toning, and stretching programs and to plan your shopping, cooking, and meals for each day of the 6 weeks that you're on the Shrink Your Female Fat Zones program.

Too little estrogen is just as bad as too much. Low estrogen levels put women at risk for premature heart disease.

So now you know what *not* to do—eat too little or feel stressed too much—in order to shape up and slim down. Now let's move on to what *works*.

Meet the Metabolism Boosters

So if you can't diet and you can't get stressed-out, what can you do to shrink your female fat zones?

A lot.

You'll learn in chapter 2 about a powerful combination of eating and exercising strategies that will work with your body to boost your metabolism and encourage your fat cells to release their cargo. This four-pronged attack on flab includes walking, stretching, toning, and healthful eating. Put it all together, and the fat comes off. Yet you'll never feel hungry.

This four-step program is designed to outsmart your body's natural genetic tendency to hold on to fat. It breaks the starvation/fat-sparing cycle, giving your body the signal it needs to release fat for good. You won't ever feel hungry because you'll be eating healthful fats that turn off your appetite. You'll also fill up on high-fiber foods that take up a lot of room in your stomach, making you feel fuller on fewer calories. Fiber also helps regulate your insulin and blood sugar levels. This, too, will help control your appetite.

You'll eat the right foods in the right combinations. You'll follow a balanced diet. That's what *Shrink Your Female Fat Zones* is all about—balance.

I don't want you to aspire to be a skinny mini. I want you to aspire to create balanced body proportions. My goal for you is to shrink fat and keep it off for life.

This program works. I know because it's the approach I've personally used to keep off fat and remain lean and toned well into my forties. I've seen it work for hundreds of women—including me!—and I know it will work for you.

CHAPTER 2

The Amazing Shrinking Fat Cell

Now that you understand the inner workings of the female fat zones, you're ready to arm yourself with the four most effective strategies to shrink fat and keep it off for good!

The Shrink Your Female Fat Zones program will work with your body's natural tendencies, coaxing fat out of your cells, boosting your metabolism, increasing your energy, and decreasing your hunger. You'll shrink your fat cells and keep them that way for life. You'll redistribute your fat-to-muscle ratio, increasing the number and size of your muscle cells as you decrease the size of your fat cells.

The program includes two important types of exercise—cardio and toning—that will encourage your fat cells to release their cargo, helping you burn fat during your workouts as well as afterward and revving up your metabolism so that you burn more calories all day long, even while you sleep. These exercises will also change your brain chemistry, allowing you to naturally control your eating without counting calories. You'll feel hungry when you need to eat, and you'll stop eating once your body no longer needs calories.

In addition to cardio and toning, you'll also incorporate regular stretching into your daily routine, allowing you to melt away the stress that can sometimes lead to overeating and weight gain, especially in your tummy. Finally, you'll learn proven eating strategies designed to fill you up on fewer calories. Don't worry—you'll still be able to eat all the foods you love. You'll just learn how to treat those foods with the respect they deserve and reserve them for the times you'll really savor and enjoy them.

To begin, let's learn about the first part of your four-pronged Shrink Your Female Fat Zones workouts and eating plan, your opening weapon in the fight against female fat: cardiovascular exercise.

Move It to Lose It

On the Shrink Your Female Fat Zones plan, you'll walk or do some other form of cardiovascular exercise four times a week, starting with as little as 25 minutes per session.

Cardiovascular exercise, such as walking, tricks your body into burning more fat as fuel.

Normally, your body burns a combination of carbohydrate (stored in your muscles) and fat (stored in your liver and fat cells) during everyday tasks. As you boost your cardiovascular fitness, however, your body switches to burning more fat and less carbohydrate during both rest and exercise. End result: You lose fat and gain muscle. Because muscle is more compact than fat, your body size shrinks.

As I mentioned in chapter 1, your muscle-to-fat ratio is extremely important when it comes to shrinking your fat zones. The more muscle you have, the more calories you burn all day long. Regular walking will help you preserve muscle, particularly as you age. For example, researchers from the University of Colorado in Boulder compared sedentary and active postmenopausal women with younger women in their twenties and thirties. The older women who didn't exercise had lower resting metabolic rates—meaning, they burned fewer calories at rest. But the older active women had maintained the metabolisms of their youth.

And when researchers at the University of North Carolina in Charlotte looked at all the available studies on exercise and metabolism, they concluded

(continued on page 22)

Your Personal Shrink
Your Female Fat Zones Schedule

WHEN FITTING EXERCISE into your routine, do what works best for your schedule and personal interests. I prefer to exercise in the morning, when I feel most energetic and before the hustle and bustle of the day has begun. I get up, stretch, head out for my walk, and return to do my chosen 15-minute fat zone toning routine for that day.

Here are some sample routines for you to follow, based on your personal fat zone. Just keep in mind that these are sample routines. You can feel free to mix up your walking and toning workouts based on your personal schedule. Just follow four important rules.

- Always walk four times a week.
- Never work the same fat zone 2 days in a row.
- Always work your personal fat zone three times a week and your "nonfat" zones one time each or more often.
- No matter what your fat zone, stretch three times a day.

Here are some sample workout schedules for the three different fat zones.

FAT ZONE: UPPER BODY

Weeks 1 and 2

MONDAY: 25-minute walk, 15-minute lower body routine

TUESDAY: 15-minute upper body routine

WEDNESDAY: 25-minute walk, 15-minute abdominal routine

THURSDAY: 15-minute upper body routine

FRIDAY: 25-minute walk

SATURDAY: Day off

SUNDAY: 25-minute walk, 15-minute upper body routine

Weeks 3 and 4

MONDAY: 35-minute walk, 15-minute lower body routine

TUESDAY: 15-minute upper body routine

WEDNESDAY: 35-minute walk, 15-minute abdominal routine

THURSDAY: 15-minute upper body routine

FRIDAY: 35-minute walk

SATURDAY: Day off

SUNDAY: 35-minute walk, 15-minute upper body routine

Weeks 5 and 6

MONDAY: 45-minute walk, 15-minute lower body routine

TUESDAY: 15-minute upper body routine

WEDNESDAY: 45-minute walk, 15-minute abdominal routine

THURSDAY: 15-minute upper body routine

FRIDAY: 45-minute walk

SATURDAY: Day off

SUNDAY: 45-minute walk, 15-minute upper body routine

FAT ZONE: MIDSECTION

Weeks 1 and 2

MONDAY: 25-minute walk, 15-minute abdominal routine

TUESDAY: 15-minute lower body routine

WEDNESDAY: 25-minute walk, 15-minute upper body routine

THURSDAY: 15-minute abdominal routine

FRIDAY: 25-minute walk

SATURDAY: 15-minute abdominal routine

SUNDAY: 25-minute walk

Weeks 3 and 4

MONDAY: 35-minute walk, 15-minute abdominal routine

TUESDAY: 15-minute lower body routine

WEDNESDAY: 35-minute walk, 15-minute upper body routine

THURSDAY: 15-minute abdominal routine

FRIDAY: 35-minute walk

SATURDAY: 15-minute abdominal routine

SUNDAY: 35-minute walk

Weeks 5 and 6

MONDAY: 45-minute walk, 15-minute abdominal routine

TUESDAY: 15-minute lower body routine

WEDNESDAY: 45-minute walk, 15-minute upper body routine

THURSDAY: 15-minute abdominal routine

FRIDAY: 45-minute walk

SATURDAY: 15-minute abdominal routine

SUNDAY: 45-minute walk

FAT ZONE: LOWER BODY

Weeks 1 and 2

MONDAY: 25-minute walk, 15-minute upper body routine

TUESDAY: 15-minute lower body routine

WEDNESDAY: 25-minute walk, 15-minute abdominal routine

THURSDAY: 15-minute lower body routine

FRIDAY: 25-minute walk

SATURDAY: Day off

SUNDAY: 25-minute walk, 15-minute lower body routine

Weeks 3 and 4

MONDAY: 35-minute walk, 15-minute upper body routine

TUESDAY: 15-minute lower body routine

WEDNESDAY: 35-minute walk, 15-minute abdominal routine

THURSDAY: 15-minute lower body routine

FRIDAY: 35-minute walk

SATURDAY: Day off

SUNDAY: 35-minute walk, 15-minute lower body routine

Weeks 5 and 6

MONDAY: 45-minute walk, 15-minute upper body routine

TUESDAY: 15-minute lower body routine

WEDNESDAY: 45-minute walk, 15-minute abdominal routine

THURSDAY: 15-minute lower body routine

FRIDAY: 45-minute walk

SATURDAY: Day off

SUNDAY: 45-minute walk, 15-minute lower body routine

that aerobic exercise can help offset the decrease in resting metabolic rate typically seen with dieting.

Here's another exciting reason to walk regularly. Remember those fat-storing and fat-burning enzymes I mentioned in chapter 1? Over time, walking will increase your number of fat-burning enzymes and decrease the fat-storing ones. That means your body will burn fat more easily.

This wonderful bonus is seen most clearly when we look at it from the opposite perspective, as in the case of fit people who *stop* exercising. Researchers at Cedars-Sinai Medical Center in Los Angeles asked 16 active runners to stop running for 2 weeks. During that time, the researchers measured lipoprotein lipase (LPL) activity (a fat-storing enzyme) in muscle and fat cells. When they stopped exercising, LPL activity rose in the fat cells and dropped in the muscle cells, indicating a shift to storing fat rather than burning it.

That's why you need to always keep it up. This is a lifetime program. When you realize how much fun it is and how much you get out of it, you'll start walking and keep walking for life! In fact, I want you to commit yourself right now to making fitness a part of your lifestyle. That commitment will help to cement your success on the Shrink Your Female Fat Zones program.

Here's another important reason to walk. Your fat distribution also changes when you begin cardiovascular exercise, with some fat now stored in your muscles for easier access. Again, this enables easier fat burning—making weight loss easier. But don't get me wrong—fat and muscle are two different tissues. When you lose weight, your fat doesn't turn into muscle; and when you gain weight, your muscles don't turn back into fat. As you become more fit, however, your muscles will grow and burn more fat for fuel, which in turn will shrink your fat cells.

Why does cardiovascular exercise help your body burn fat? Think back to your ancient female cousins from thousands of years ago. During times of feasting, these women walked a lot to gather berries and seeds and other foods. Their bodies sensed this movement and learned to attribute daily cardiovascular exercise with feasting rather than famine. In turn, their bodies switched from the fat-conservation mode into a fat-burning mode.

These days we move little during the normal course of our lives. We drive to the grocery store to "forage" for food. We spend the vast majority of our days sitting rather than walking. This lack of activity signals our fat cells to fill up, making weight loss difficult—that is, unless we trick our bodies by walking on a regular basis.

Besides increasing your ability to burn fat, walking also keeps your heart fit—fit enough to pump fresh oxygen throughout your body. That oxygen reaches all of your cells, from your head to your toes, energizing your entire body.

Regular cardiovascular exercise may also change the subtle biochemistry of the brain, which in turn changes your set point, the point at which your body starts to resist weight loss. Without exercise, you usually feel hungry when you cut back on calories. But exercise lowers levels of a brain chemical called neuropeptide Y, which stimulates appetite. Lower levels of this chemical equals a smaller appetite.

My Shrink Your Female Fat Zones walking plan will help you burn more than 640 calories a week as you exercise. But when you're not walking, you'll burn even more calories than you normally do as your metabolism kicks into high gear and your renewed energy fuels move movement all day long!

Release Tension, Release Fat

Stretching—along with cardio—is essential when it comes to shrinking your fat zones. On the Shrink Your Female Fat Zones plan, you'll stretch for just 3 to 5 minutes, three times a day: first thing in the morning, at midday, and just before bedtime.

Remember when I mentioned in chapter 1 about how stress can encourage your body to store abdominal fat? Well, stretching helps counteract stress by helping you take a time-out. During that 5-minute stretch break, your frenzied thoughts slow down and order themselves, helping you to calm down and reexamine your feelings and emotions.

Also, when we feel stressed, we tend to tense up our muscles. Stretching soothes away that muscle tension, which in turn helps us to automatically calm down.

Stretching also helps you shrink your fat zones in other important ways. For one, it lengthens your muscles, creating a long, lean appearance. When you

I Shrunk My Female Fat Zones!

Total-body workouts provided Lori Gilbert's fat-shrinking answer.

Denise's workouts have helped me to shrink every trouble spot on my body! I've been doing her routines for 5 years. Every morning I wake up, put on my shoes, turn on Denise's program on the TV, and start my day.

One of my favorite exercises is the lunge. My trouble spot is my legs, so I try to work lunges in as much as I can. When I do that exercise, I can see and feel my legs become more toned and lean.

I love Denise's style of exercise, too. Her Shrink Your Female Fat Zones program is more effective than the other workouts that I have tried in the past. Rather than working only one area, Denise targets every part of the body during the week. I get to target all of my body spots and feel great doing it!

I eat what I want, but watch my amounts and portion sizes. I don't eat after 8:00 P.M., and I try not to eat out too often or get a fast-food lunch. To avoid feeling tempted by McDonald's and other chain restaurants, I go home and eat lunch every day.

Overall I've lost 80 pounds and shrunk from a size 20 to a size 10! I feel better about myself, and I have more energy. I reached a goal that I've been longing for, and it feels good!

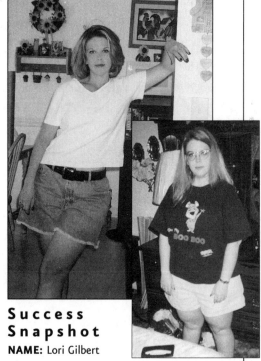

Success Snapshot

NAME: Lori Gilbert

AGE: 24

TOWN: Raeford, North Carolina

OCCUPATION: Bank teller

WEIGHT LOST: 80 pounds

OTHER ACCOMPLISHMENTS: More self-confidence, energy, and focus at work

Lori's Secret to Success

"Commit yourself to making a difference in your life. Don't wait for weight loss and fitness to happen. Make it happen. Eat what you want, but watch how much of it you are eating. Don't think of it as a diet; think of it as making your lifestyle better."

stretch, you extend the ends of your muscles, creating space for oxygen to flow more freely. For example, when you bend forward, your hip joints move upward, but your knee joints stay put. This elongates the ends of your hamstring muscles, which run from your back to your knees. Bend over often enough, and the muscles permanently lengthen, creating the longer, leaner appearance of a ballerina.

Regular stretching also increases your energy and strength. As your muscles grow longer, they'll hold less tension and move more fluidly with less tightness. One of the best ways that stretching works in tandem with your walking program is that it makes you want to move. Also, stretching pumps blood into your muscles and releases tension from them, which generally makes you feel good. This circulation helps to heal your body, patching up any injuries and soothing away aches and pains.

With stretching, you not only feel better, you look better, too! This better circulation can also directly improve your appearance by preventing both cellulite and varicose veins. Cellulite is a type of fat that pushes through weak spots in your connective tissue, creating a dimpled appearance. Stretching boosts circulation to these areas, helping your body mobilize and burn this fat during your workouts.

Varicose veins form when the muscles in your leg veins fail to push blood against gravity up to your heart. Instead blood flows backward, enlarging the vein. Stretching helps encourage proper blood circulation, helping your blood flow in the right direction.

Finally, stretching before bedtime can help you to release any remaining muscle tension, empty your busy mind, and deeply relax your entire body. I always look forward to this part of my day, the time-out just for me. I know that when I stretch right before bed, I'll fall asleep faster, sleep more deeply, and wake in the morning feeling more refreshed.

Build Muscle and Rev Up Your Metabolism

On the Shrink Your Female Fat Zones plan, you'll tone up for just 15 minutes, 5 days a week, working your personal fat zone three times a week and your two "nonfat" zones once a week each.

For example, my personal fat zone is my lower body. So I do the Shrink Your

Female Fat Zones lower body workout three times a week. I follow up with an upper body routine once a week and the midsection routine once a week.

If your midsection is your fat zone, you'll do the midsection routine three times a week and the other two routines one time each. If your upper body is your fat zone, you'll do the upper body workout three times and the other fat zone workouts one time each. This 5-day-a-week muscle-toning program provides the secret for your changing the shape of your body.

What sets this program apart from others that you've tried? Rather than work your entire body in just 2 or 3 days a week, I've shortened your workouts to just 15 minutes and allowed you to target a specific fat zone during each session. You'll spread these workouts over 5 days to kick your metabolism into high gear.

Here's how it works: When you do a toning workout, you burn a number of calories during your routine. More important, you continue to burn calories at a higher-than-normal rate *after* your workout as your body busily synthesizes muscle protein.

This afterburn lasts for as long as 2 hours, according to research done at Johns Hopkins and Arizona State Universities. Researchers at these institutions studied women who did a series of resistance exercises and measured their resting energy expenditure for many hours afterward. Most women continued to burn calories at a higher rate for at least 2 hours after the workout.

In other words, for only 15 minutes of exercise, you gain up to 2 hours of an elevated metabolism! When else can you get such a great return on an investment? In fact, if you wanted to experience results faster, you could add two more workouts to your schedule, working your nonfat zones one more time each and kicking your metabolism into high gear every single day.

The increased calorie burning doesn't stop there. You may wonder why you must work your nonfat zones in addition to your personal fat zone. After all, why not tone only your thighs, buns, and hips? In this program, you'll train your entire body in order to create a permanent metabolism boost.

The average woman loses ½ pound of muscle each year starting in her midtwenties. Because every pound of muscle burns 35 to 50 calories a day, you can see how this muscle loss could slow your metabolism dramatically as you age.

Also, many of us are constantly on diets. But as I mentioned in chapter 1, when you eat too few calories, your metabolism slows down to conserve calories. Then you lose muscle tissue as well as fat, which lowers your metabolism even more.

That's where strength training comes in. My Shrink Your Female Fat Zones workouts will help you build lean muscle throughout your entire body to reverse this metabolism slowdown.

In one study from the University of Rhode Island, weight lifting made the difference in whether women dropped 2½ percent body fat or lost no body fat at all. In another study, done at Tufts University by noted strength-training expert Miriam E. Nelson, Ph.D., women either dieted or dieted and strength-trained. Both groups lost the same average number of pounds, but the dieters lost muscle tissue whereas the strength trainers lost fat and gained muscle—and *still* saw a drop in the numbers on the scale!

All totaled, your 15-minute workouts will help you burn an extra 300 calories a day. You're accomplishing a lot in just 15 minutes! According to research done by the widely respected fitness expert Wayne Westcott, Ph.D., at the South Shore YMCA in Quincy, Massachusetts, you can expect to lose 3½ pounds of fat for every 1¾ pounds of muscle you build. This muscle is more compact than fat, too. So even if you replace each pound of fat you lose with a pound of muscle, you'll still shrink in size.

Strength training also increases your overall strength by 30 to 50 percent, which helps you to increase the number of calories you burn in many other ways. More strength means that you're more able to carry groceries, play with your kids, garden, and do housework. You feel more energetic and accomplish much more as a result. You may even burn extra calories without intending to: Dr. Nelson found that women who strength-trained increased their amount of cardiovascular exercise automatically by climbing more steps and walking more often.

This newfound strength has a way of making you want to move. When you find yourself sitting for long periods of time, you won't be able to help tapping your foot and adjusting your body position. And these subtle fidgeting motions add up to a stunning amount of extra burned calories. In fact, a study done at the Mayo Clinic in Rochester, Minnesota, found that small, habitual movements such as tapping your feet, adjusting your posture, and fidgeting can burn up to 700 calories *a day*.

Strength training also does wonders for your health. Most important, it will increase bone mineral density by as much as 13 percent, which helps prevent osteoporosis and bone fractures. You'll decrease your risk for diabetes, improve your cholesterol levels, and alleviate aches and pains. Some research shows that strength training works as well as counseling at alleviating symptoms of depression. Talk about letting your body heal your mind!

Best of all, you'll build sleek, compact muscle that will act like a girdle to shrink and define your waist, thighs, buns, and the rest of your body. You'll firm up your entire body. No more jiggly arms or thighs. No more flab pressing out from your bra straps. No more love handles. No more saddlebags. Just firm, feminine curves.

Design Your New Body

The only way to change your body shape is by training your muscles. Muscles are really like modeling clay. If you do nothing, they will sit there in the shape of a big blob. If you add shape to them with the fat zone toning exercises, you can work them into the shape and structure you desire.

On the Shrink Your Female Fat Zones program, you'll design a new body. Of course, you can't change your bone structure. You can't change the places where you tend to carry fat. You can't spot-tone by only working one muscle group over and over.

You *can* spot-train, however, by filling out one part of your body and minimizing another. That's exactly how we're going to reshape your body, by resizing those thighs, hips, tummy, and arms to the perfect size.

You can *reshape* your body by accentuating some areas and minimizing others. For example, the upper-body fat zone routine will help women with large breasts and arms increase their upper back strength. This helps you to pull back your shoulders and stand taller. Better posture makes you appear slimmer.

If you tend to gain fat in your tummy, you'll tone that area in addition to sculpting your already lean legs, providing a beautiful set of long, shapely gams

Before You Start

FOR OPTIMAL SUCCESS on the Shrink Your Female Fat Zones program, you'll need a good pair of walking shoes and three sets of dumbbells—weighing 3, 5, and 8 pounds—available at most sporting goods stores.

Though optional, the following items will help optimize your success.

- A cushioned exercise mat

- A large, air-filled stability ball, available at most sporting goods stores
- A towel
- A pillow, an aerobics step, or a weight bench
- A sturdy chair
- A pair of walking shoes
- A water bottle

to take the attention away from your midsection. The upper-body fat zone workout will help to improve your posture, which will lengthen your midsection and make it appear slimmer.

If you tend to gain fat in your thighs, the upper-body fat zone routine will add shape to your upper back and shoulders, which will make your lower body appear slimmer. Working your midsection will help you to carve a beautifully flat tummy—that way you can show off your flat midriff to take the emphasis off your legs. The net result will be beautiful proportions!

Throughout the fat zone workouts, I've chosen my favorite exercises from my vast experience with weight training, Pilates, Power Yoga, and ballet. I've included only the most effective exercises that are proven to zero in on the specific muscles that I want you to target. Trust me, you will experience amazing results.

Every other week on your program, you'll switch routines, taking on a new set of exercises. Each exercise in each routine works your muscles in a slightly different way. For example, some of the Pilates moves work your muscles primarily as they lengthen, whereas many dumbbell exercises work them as they contract. Some other exercises work your muscles isometrically as you hold an exercise whereas others work them dynamically.

One common reason we experience weight-loss plateaus is that we've been following the same routines for too long. By nature, your body adapts to exercise and learns how to do it efficiently, so your muscles don't have to work as hard to do the same moves—and you end up burning fewer calories. This constant variety will help keep your body guessing and that metabolism burning.

Healthful Eating Habits

With the Shrink-Fat Eating Plan, you'll stay just under your body's "dieting" radar. You'll never cut enough calories to make you feel hungry or slow your metabolism.

This is not a "diet" in the traditional sense of the word. Most women define a diet as something they go on and eventually go off. The Shrink-Fat Eating Plan helps you make changes that will give you such energy and make you feel so sharp that you'll want to keep them up for the rest of your life. You are embarking on a wonderful new way to eat healthy yet delicious foods and shrink fat in the process.

It's the same eating plan I follow—that's how I know for certain that you'll never feel deprived. My life philosophy: Life is too short and food is too fabulous to diet.

The best thing of all is that you'll make subtle dietary changes that will help you eat fewer calories automatically. You won't miss your favorite foods or ever feel hungry. You'll succeed by making six effective shifts in your eating habits. But don't feel overwhelmed—you won't have to make all the changes at once. I've taken all the guesswork out of it—just follow my delicious, easy eating plan, and you'll slowly incorporate the following six dietary strategies. You'll never feel pressured to do too much too soon.

- **Week 1.** In this week, you'll learn how to eyeball a *real* portion size. Your Shrink-Fat Eating Plan begins by teaching you simple ways to dish up foods in the right amounts with absolutely no calorie counting involved. If you spend this one week measuring, portion control will become automatic. You'll know just by looking how much cereal or pasta or meat you should eat.

- **Week 2.** You'll embrace fiber as your best Shrink Your Fat Zones friend! Learn how to maximize your fiber intake to help stabilize blood sugar levels, which in turn suppresses your appetite. Fiber also keeps the hormone insulin in check, encouraging your body to burn fat as fuel. Fiber feels heavy in your stomach, and it fills you up faster on fewer calories. It also sucks a small amount of calories out of your intestine before your body can absorb them.

▪ **Week 3.** Eating certain fats can actually help you shed fat! This week, you'll learn to enjoy right amounts of the right types of fat. My food plan gets 24 percent of its calories from fat, which allows you to cook foods that taste delicious, helps you feel fuller longer, and helps eliminate deprivation. You'll also maximize healthful sources of fat, such as the fat found in fish. Fish in particular has been shown to make the body more responsive to leptin, a hormone responsible in satiety. That means you're more likely to stop eating when you've consumed enough calories.

▪ **Week 4.** Pile on the veggies and fruits! This week, you'll maximize your consumption of fruits and vegetables. These gems help to fill you up on very few calories. They also come packed with satisfying fiber, and they're great for your health. You'll be eating five to seven servings a day on my food plans and loving every minute of it. They'll give you the nutrition you need to feel more energetic for your Shrink Your Female Fat Zones workouts.

▪ **Week 5.** Most of us consider hunger a foe, but in the quest to shrink your fat zones, you really need to make it a friend. This week, you'll learn how to eat only when you feel truly hungry. This is key as many of us eat for all sorts of other reasons, such as out of habit, for celebration, for energy, or for comfort. You'll get in touch with your body and learn to nourish it with the foods it needs to help you feel happy and satisfied.

▪ **Week 6.** Finally, you'll learn to tackle what can be the greatest saboteur of any new eating plan: cravings. These simple yet effective strategies will teach you to substitute other activities to help you overcome cravings, filling yourself up on noncalorie, nonfood, soul-satisfying options.

This eating plan won't disrupt your life. It's designed to make your life *easier*, not harder. That's why I've included a shopping list, quick-and-easy

I Shrunk My Female Fat Zones!

Regular exercise helped Silorn Pang find the energy she needed for her studies.

When I started doing Denise's workouts a couple of years ago, I weighed about 175 pounds. She helped me to lose 55 pounds in about 6 months! I've been able to keep the weight off for a little over a year so far.

I began with cardio workouts only, doing 20 minutes a day. After a few months, I added Denise's strength-training routines to the mix. As soon as I did so, I surged through a weight-loss plateau. After just a few weeks, I also noticed toner muscles, especially in my legs.

I also experienced a dramatic increase in my energy. I don't crave naps like I used to in the afternoons, and I easily fall asleep at night. I feel better about myself, too, especially because I know that I'm taking time to do something good for myself. Every time I feel a little stressed or burnt out, I go for a jog, and it always helps!

Denise always says to drink plenty of water, and I do. Staying hydrated helps me perform better when I'm working out and even when I'm not. She encourages a good night of rest, which I try to obtain as best as I can, with my full student schedule and part-time job. It's a great feeling to wake up refreshed and ready to take on the world!

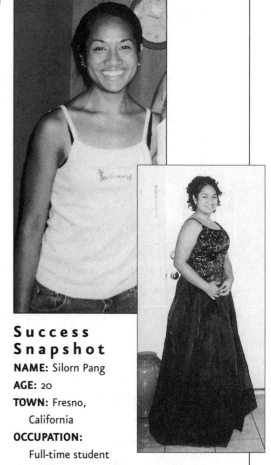

Success Snapshot

NAME: Silorn Pang

AGE: 20

TOWN: Fresno, California

OCCUPATION: Full-time student

WEIGHT LOST: 55 pounds

OTHER ACCOMPLISHMENTS: More energy, less stress, better sleep habits

Silorn's Secret to Success

"Patience! Never give up. My positive attitude is what drives me to exercise and eat well. Just knowing that I'm doing something good for myself provides enough motivation to get me up and going."

recipes, and loads of tips to help you with the plan. I'm a busy mom. I know convenience is important.

Healthful eating has never been easier.

Putting It All Together

There you have it. Your Shrink Your Female Fat Zones fat-fighting formula includes:

- Walking for 25 to 45 minutes, 4 days a week

- Stretching for 3 to 5 minutes, three times a day

- Toning for 15 minutes, 5 days a week

- Making one simple dietary change a week for 6 weeks

Each little baby step takes you closer to major body change. It's all about progression. Just as in your eating plan, in which you'll incorporate one small change each week, your exercise plans will also build in intensity. For example, the walking and toning programs change every other week. During weeks 1 and 2, you'll start at a beginner level, walking for just 25 minutes at a time and doing simple toning exercises. By weeks 3 and 4, you'll add time and more intensity to your daily walks. You'll also step up your toning workouts, taking on a new, slightly more challenging workout series. During weeks 5 and 6, you'll again increase the challenge of your walking and toning workouts.

Small changes add up to big transformations. By the end of the 6-week program, your fat zones will certainly appear smaller. You'll be able to cinch your belt a few notches tighter. Your jeans will feel roomier. You'll have lost inches from your thighs, hips, arms, and waist. You'll look and feel fantastic.

Even more important, you'll have tricked your body into releasing fat for good. No more yo-yo dieting. Keep up with the program, and you will see results. You'll never have to say "diet" again!

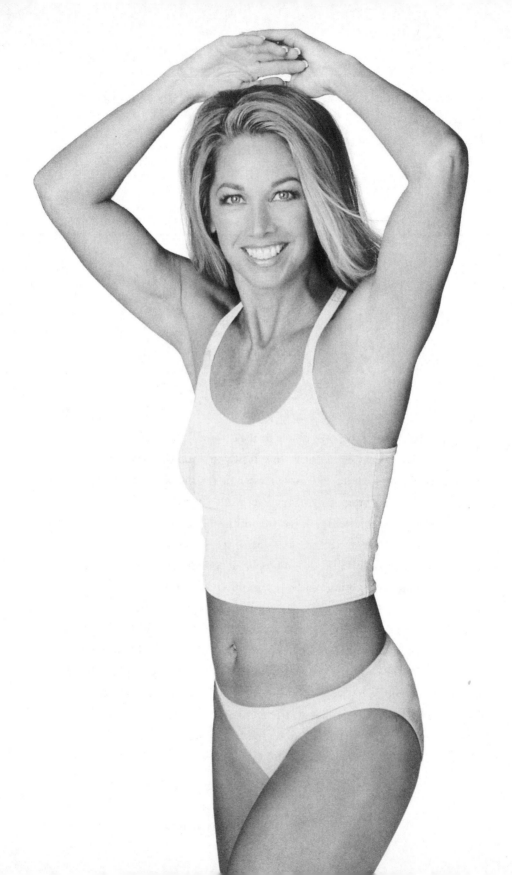

PART 2

The Fat Zone **Walking** and **Stretching** Program

CHAPTER 3

THE FAT ZONE WALKING AND STRETCHING PROGRAM

Target Toning As You Walk

I love to walk. It's such a great way to work out. It boosts your metabolism and puts you in a fabulous mood. After I walk, I feel invigorated and have a wonderful sense of self-accomplishment. I've found that it's one of the best tools for permanent weight loss.

Walking burns 50 to 100 calories during 10 minutes—the faster you walk, the more you burn. Plus, walking helps you shrink your fat zones in many ways beyond the calories you burn during your actual workout.

For example, in a recent study of 40 overweight women, a walking program combined with modest calorie restriction resulted in an average 8 percent drop in body weight, 17 percent drop in fat mass, and 20 percent drop in tummy fat. Overall, the women lost much more weight than you would expect from dietary restriction alone.

Researchers attribute the extra fat loss to the calories burned during each walking session coupled with a walking-induced boost in aerobic capacity. Your aerobic capacity refers to how efficiently your muscles use oxygen and convert fat into fuel. The better your aerobic capacity, the more efficiently your body burns fat, both during your walk and during the rest of your day.

In addition to bolstering your aerobic capacity, walking also lowers your

Getting Over the Hill

MY GIRLFRIEND SUSAN SHAW, who lives down the street, often meets me for a morning power walk. She usually powers her way right up the hill from her house to mine. Recently, she began complaining of shin-splints. I suggested that she first warm up on a flat street by walking around the block, which provided flat terrain, before walking up the hill to my house. This simple change in her routine eliminated her shinsplints.

Hills provide a great workout, particularly to firm up your buttocks. But you don't want to tackle them first thing during a walk. Hills place your foot in a flexed position, over-stressing your anterior tibials, your shin muscle, and overextending your calf muscles if you're not properly warmed up.

Try to avoid hills until after 5 minutes of flat-surface walking. That way, your legs will be ready.

levels of an enzyme called lipoprotein lipase (LPL). This enzyme tells the fat cells in your hips, thighs, butt, and abdomen to fill up. The lower the number of your LPL enzymes, the more likely your body will burn fat in these areas rather than store it. Not surprisingly, a reduction in this enzyme has also been associated with lowered risk for heart disease.

Regular walking will also help you to eat fewer calories and more easily stick to the Shrink-Fat Eating Plan. Research shows that regular cardiovascular exercise (any type of exercise that increases your heart and breathing rates) helps to regulate your appetite, making you less likely to overeat. In addition, numerous surveys show that women who begin a fitness program automatically choose healthier foods. Aerobic exercise may help by altering numerous body signals involved in hunger and satiety, helping you to feel satisfied on fewer calories.

Regular walking also strengthens your heart, expands your lung capacity, and improves blood circulation. All of this gives you the energy and stamina you need for everyday life. Simply put, when you feel better, you move more often, which helps you to burn more calories all day long.

In my experience, walking works for just about any woman of any age. Though other fitness pursuits such as running or cycling also burn fat and help to regulate your appetite, they, unfortunately, can take a toll on your joints, your knees, and your back. I love to run and still do a couple of times a week. I know

I can't run every day, however, especially now that I'm in my forties—but I'll be able to walk for the rest of my life.

Walking for Life

Besides burning fat, walking also performs wonders for your health.

Walking is a form of cardiovascular exercise, or cardio—a type of exercise that strengthens your heart muscle and lowers blood pressure and cholesterol buildup, reducing your heart disease risk by 40 percent.

Regular walking also stimulates the natural rhythm of your intestines, helping to enhance digestion and bowel regularity. Walking also normalizes blood sugar levels, helping to prevent diabetes and insulin resistance.

Walking can also lift depression and boost your mood. As you walk, your brain secretes opiate-like chemicals that soothe away aches and pains and create a feeling of euphoria. It's no wonder that a brisk walk can clear your head and soothe your nerves. Whenever you feel anxious, tense, sad, or depressed, head outdoors for a walk and leave your troubles behind. Walking can be addictive—in a good way.

Best of all, walking works for everybody. On a nice day, you can walk outdoors and take in the sunlight, fresh air, and beautiful scenery. On a very hot or rainy day, you can walk indoors on a treadmill or at a local mall. When you're feeling overextended, you can take a soulful, meditative walk by yourself. When you want to catch up with your friends, you can take a social walk and talk while you're burning calories.

I've had some of the deepest, most thoughtful—and most spirited!—conversations with my sisters and girlfriends during our walks. The movement seems to lubricate our brains as well as our joints, allowing us to spill out everything and anything as we move, move, move. I also love to walk with my

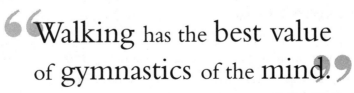

"Walking has the best value of gymnastics of the mind."

—*Ralph Waldo Emerson*

husband, Jeff. We strengthen our marital bond as we simultaneously do something healthy for both of us.

Once you feel the walker's high (it's not just for runners!) and see your results (a slimmer waistline, toned legs), you'll just love it.

Your Program

You can easily tailor walking to your schedule, personality, and lifestyle. You can walk practically anytime, anywhere. You need only a good pair of shoes and socks to walk your way to slimmer fat zones.

This Shrink Your Female Fat Zones walking program includes four specific types of walks—a basic endurance walk, a fat zone walk, a fat-burning walk, and a combined fat zone and fat-burning walk. Why so many different kinds of walks? The more variety in your walking repertoire, the more motivated you will feel. Variety also keeps your muscles constantly challenged, which helps you burn more calories during every workout. Plus, when you "change it up," you'll also keep your metabolism up, preventing a weight-loss plateau.

For each of your walking workouts (on pages 47 and 50), you'll work up to a total time of 45 minutes, starting with 25 minutes during weeks 1 and 2 and adding 10 minutes every other week. Your goal is to walk four times a week.

Though you can certainly walk at any time of day that fits best into your schedule, I encourage you to try it first thing in the morning. Research shows that you're more likely to fit in exercise in the morning rather than later in the day. Get out of bed, put on your walking clothes, do your morning and pre-walk stretches, and get on your way. Do what works best for you, but just do it.

To ensure that I squeeze in my four walks each week, I call my friends every Sunday to check their schedules for the coming days. Then I set up walking dates with various friends and mark those dates on my calendar, along with all the other important "stuff" in my life.

Besides your scheduled 25- to 45-minute walks four times a week, I encourage you to fit in as much walking as you can throughout each day. Make walking a regular habit. For example, I walk with my girls to school every

ARCH MUSCLES IN OUR FEET tend to deteriorate with age, making us more prone to shinsplints—that tender pain along the shinbone—when we walk. If you have a falling arch or flat feet, you can tone up your arches as well as your calves with this towel pull exercise.

While in your bare feet, sit in a chair. Place a rolled-up towel just in front of your toes. Grab the towel between your toes and your forefeet and unroll it, flexing the arches of your feet as you do so. This prevents shin pain by developing your tibials, arch, and shin muscles. Try it for 15 to 30 seconds every other day.

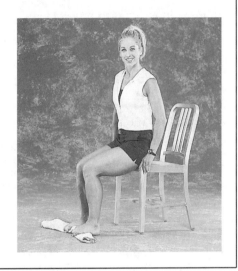

morning and then walk them home every afternoon. Though their school is only a few blocks away from our house, every little bit counts. My girls, husband, and I also walk our dog, Madonna, almost every night after dinner. I look forward to these precious nightly walks to fully reconnect with my family.

Looking for other ways to make your walking habitual? Decrease your dependence on your car—take care of errands by walking to the bank, the convenience store, or the post office. Pretend that elevators, escalators, and moving walkways don't exist, opting to use the power of your own two feet over the power of electricity and cables. Walk to your neighbor's house rather than call. Take mini walk breaks at work rather than coffee or snack breaks. I even walk around my house while I talk on the phone.

Eventually, such mini walks will become a natural part of your day.

Where to Walk

You can do your walking workouts just about anywhere. I love to walk outdoors when I can because I love to smell the fresh air and experience Mother Nature firsthand. Plus, I feel refreshed just to be outside.

But sometimes I can't walk outside. So my treadmill provides a nice backup. And that's the true beauty of walking. You can do it in so many places, from malls to gyms to parks. Here, you'll find a list of the different locations and benefits of all walking areas. No more excuses. You can walk anywhere.

- **The treadmill.** I love walking on my treadmill. It's always there, waiting for me, so I can walk at 5:00 A.M. or at night, when it's dark outdoors. It also allows me to walk during heavy rain or snowy weather, when it would be too uncomfortable or unsafe to walk outdoors. I've positioned my treadmill to face out the window of a second-story room in our house. Through the window I can see our entire backyard, allowing me to watch my girls playing outside. I've also placed a TV in front of my treadmill so I can watch the news or my favorite TV shows while I burn fat.

- **The mall.** If you don't own a treadmill or have access to one at a gym, the mall provides your next best option for walking indoors during bad weather or just for the fun of it. Many malls open early for walkers. Call your local mall to see if they offer mall walking hours. An added bonus: You'll meet other walkers, making it a social activity that you'll look forward to. Plus, you can window-shop!

- **The beach.** If you vacation at the shore or are lucky enough to live near a beach, take advantage of the beautiful scenery, sea breeze, and great-smelling ocean air by walking on the beach. Walking on sand burns more calories than walking on a paved surface because you must work harder to push off during each foot strike. It will also help to tone your calves and ankles. I wear shoes when I walk on the beach and like to walk right along the edge of the water,

“Bad weather isn't an excuse to skip a walking workout. Fat cells don't take crummy weather into account.”

The Power of Mini Workouts

I'M NOT AN EXERCISE FANATIC—I CAN'T BE. I have a full-time career and two children. I do only 30 to 45 minutes of "official" exercise a day. But I make every minute count by sprinkling mini workouts throughout my day.

Fidgeting works. There's research to prove it. In a study done at the Mayo Clinic in Rochester, Minnesota, a group of volunteers ages 20 to 35 ate 1,000 extra calories a day for 8 weeks. At the end of the study, some participants had gained as much as 16 pounds whereas others gained as little as 2 pounds. The people who gained the least weight tended to be restless—constantly standing up and stretching, shifting around in their chairs, or tapping their toes. Even small movements burn calories that might otherwise be stored as fat.

By getting up and moving, you also improve your circulation especially throughout your lower body and legs, where blood tends to stagnate. This can give you an instant energy boost, combating sluggishness and making you more alert.

I never miss an opportunity to move around. Here are some strategies that I personally use to burn extra calories throughout the day.

1. I power-walk when I walk through my house. Rather than dawdle down a hall, I lengthen my stride and pump my arms, even if I'm just walking from the kitchen to my office.

2. I walk as I talk on my cordless phone. I try not to talk on the phone while sitting down.

3. When I take the stairs, I go up two steps at a time, strengthening the muscles in my legs.

4. Whenever I find a spare 5 minutes, I fit in a toning exercise, such as abdominal crunches. Or I simply mimic an exercise by doing biceps curls or triceps extensions without using the weight. I also do some stretching during these spare moments, which gives me focus and energy.

5. Whenever I'm stuck in traffic or standing in a line, I do butt squeezes and tummy tucks. I pull my abs in and up, zipping them up like a corset and then holding the isometric contraction for about 5 seconds.

6. I walk every chance that I get, using my own two feet to take me to the store, to pick my daughters up from school, you name it.

You can find your own ways to "fidget-cize." You may not feel like it comes naturally. That's okay—it didn't for me either. I had to train myself. But the more movement I did, the more I moved. It eventually becomes second nature.

The Anatomy of a **Walking Shoe**

Walking shoes allow you to roll smoothly from heel to toe, and most offer cushioned insoles, which ease impact on your joints. Every woman has a different foot shape and type, so the right shoe for you largely depends on your individual foot. There's no one best brand—the best shoe for you is one that feels comfortable.

Start by getting the right size. Have your foot measured while you're standing, since your feet expand when you place weight on them. Also, shop in the afternoon, when feet are widest and longest. Try on the shoes and walk in them. If one foot is longer than the other, buy for the larger foot. Since your feet may grow a size after pregnancy, make sure to remeasure them periodically. Here are some tips for buying the perfect shoe for you.

UPPER: Look for a shoe that you can lace tightly, but not too tightly. If the laces are too short, you will have to pull them too tightly to tie the shoe, creating pressure along the top of your foot. If they are too long, you may tie them too loosely in an effort to keep them from dragging on the ground. Loosely tied shoes aren't snug enough to hold your heel in place.

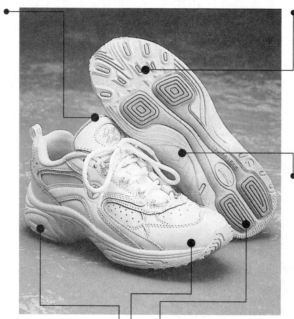

SOLE: When buying shoes, always take them for a test walk. Make sure that the sole of the shoe bends with the natural bend in your foot, allowing you to roll effortlessly from heel to toe.

ARCH SUPPORT: Our arches tend to flatten with age, allowing us to roll our feet inward as we walk and creating more stress on our shins and knees. A good arch support will help prevent this inward roll. Feel inside the shoe with your hand for an arch support. If the shoe doesn't have one, don't even bother trying it on. When you place your foot in the shoe, make sure that the support actually does support your arch—and not some other part of your foot.

HEEL: Make sure that the heel area of the shoe hugs your foot as you walk, not allowing your heel to slide as you move. If your foot slides in and out of the shoe, it creates friction—a sure recipe for heel blisters.

TOEBOX: Shoes that allow too little room in the toebox tend to mangle your toenails and make your feet hurt. Make sure that the widest part of your foot has plenty of room. It shouldn't feel mashed against the shoe. Also, make sure that your toes have enough room to wiggle.

CUSHIONING: You want shoes with enough cushioning to feel comfortable when you walk. You should not be able to feel the pavement. Most new shoes provide the right amount of cushioning. Cushioning in most shoes wears down over time, so replace your shoes at least twice a year if you walk three times a week.

where the sand is a little wet. The harder, wet sand makes it easier to move at a faster clip.

- **The trails.** I love walking on the trails at local parks and hiking trails near my house. I often do these walks alone, without the distraction of music or chatter, because I want to immerse myself in everything nature has to present to me. As I walk along the soft terrain, I'll reflect on my day and free my mind as I look at the flowers, bushes, and trees. These nature walks always lift my mood because I see things that I wouldn't notice when driving by the same park in a car. Sometimes my girlfriends and I drive to a great trail and make a morning of it, hiking for as long as 2 hours. I especially love these hikes during autumn, when I can take in all the beautiful, vibrant colors.

The winding nature of these park paths makes our walks more down to earth and interesting. The softness of the ground helps to absorb the pounding on our feet, knees, and back. (Note: If you have weak ankles, avoid rougher trails with lots of roots and rocks to prevent turning your ankle.)

- **The neighborhood.** If your neighborhood offers sidewalks, you've got a wonderfully safe and car-free walking route. I love to walk in my neighborhood with my girlfriends who live nearby. These walks help us get to know other neighbors that we pass. We always talk about the houses and neighbors' gardens that we admire, a great way to get ideas for garden projects at home. Plus, it's fun to know who's moving in and out or who's adding an addition to their house.

- **The school track.** Sometimes when I want to motivate myself to walk faster or do walk/run intervals, I head to the school track and time myself. I walk at a moderate pace for 1 mile (4 laps) and then try to walk or jog my fastest pace for the next mile. Then I slow down for the last mile, completing 12 total laps. If you have children, the track offers a fantastic place for you to walk while your kids play safely in the infield, under your watchful eye. My girls love it. Sometimes we bring their bikes, lacrosse sticks, or soccer ball to keep them active while we all burn off a big lunch!

Your **Schedule**

Walk at least four times a week. Pick the days that work best for you. I like to walk every Monday, Wednesday, and Friday. Then, depending on my family's schedule, I complete my fourth walk on a Saturday or Sunday. Sometimes I walk both weekend days. Unlike weight training, which you should only do every other day, you can walk back-to-back days and still recover easily for your next walk. Try to walk in the morning, since you'll be more likely to fit it in then.

Weeks 1 and 2

Walk 1	Endurance walk: 25 minutes	**TIP:** Drive around your neighborhood and use the odometer in your car to clock the distance to various places. Clock out a 1-mile route, but know other distances in case you want to add on.
Walk 2	Endurance walk: 25 minutes	**TIP:** If you walk the same route day after day, your motivation will begin to wane pretty quickly. Try to walk different routes as much as possible, even if you simply walk your normal route backward.
Walk 3	Endurance walk: 25 minutes	**TIP:** Walk with a friend, family member, or coworker. Talking as you walk helps to pass the time and keeps you from looking at your watch. Multitasking—by catching up with your friends as you fit in a workout—will save you time in the long run. Also, when you make a commitment to a walking buddy, you're less likely to cancel.
Walk 4	Endurance walk: 25 minutes	**TIP:** Keep your head up and look at the scenery. It's beautiful out there! Check out the gardens, absorb the different colors, listen to the birds, and feel the breeze.

Weeks 3 and 4

Walk 1	Endurance walk: 35 minutes	**TIP:** Stay hydrated. Dehydration lowers your blood volume, making your blood viscous and slow moving. This, in turn, zaps your energy. I keep water bottles everywhere in my house to encourage myself to take sips of water all day long to keep my energy level high.
Walk 2	Fat zone walk: 35 minutes	**TIP:** Congratulate yourself for every achievement. If you focus on your successes and not your failures, you'll maintain more motivation to stick with your walks.
Walk 3	Endurance walk: 35 minutes	**TIP:** Shorter, quicker steps will help you pick up your pace. Alternate these with longer ones to tone your butt and thighs, as well as to keep your walk interesting.
Walk 4	Fat-burning walk: 35 minutes	**TIP:** Don't walk in just any old outfit. Buy a brightly colored outfit just for walking. On the days when your motivation wanes, that sexy outfit will beg you to wear it and take it for a walk!

Weeks 5 and 6		
Walk 1	Endurance walk: 45 minutes	**TIP:** Keep track of your consistency by marking a calendar when you walk. Then you'll easily be able to see how often you've walked and congratulate yourself on your successes.
Walk 2	Fat zone fat-burning blast: 45 minutes	**TIP:** Breathe deeply when you walk, taking full breaths by using your tummy to draw the air in and out. These deep breaths will give you more energy, helping you to pick up your pace.
Walk 3	Fat-burning walk: 45 minutes	**TIP:** Try to notice one new thing on your walk that you didn't notice last time. You'll smell the flowers, hear the rustle of the leaves, and feel the wind or sunlight against your skin, making your walk fly by.
Walk 4	Fat zone fat-burning blast: 45 minutes	**TIP:** Turn your car into a walking-wardrobe closet. Keep spare walking shoes and socks in it—and even a water bottle and outfit—just in case you find yourself with spare time to take a walk.

Your Fabulous Four Walking Workouts

For the next 6 weeks, you'll walk four times a week, building up to a total of 45 minutes per walk. Before each workout, don't forget to stretch (see "Stretching: Don't Leave Home without It" on page 52). If you're a beginner or extremely out of shape, start with four 10-minute walks for your first week. For your second week, add 10 minutes, making each of your four walks last 20 minutes. By the third week, you will be ready to start week 1 of this walking program.

If you're a runner, you can follow the same workouts below at a running pace rather than a walking pace. Just add only 10 minutes a session.

Can't do 25 to 45 minutes at once? On busy days, break up your walking time into 10- or 15-minute bursts, two or three times a day. But try to fit it all in at once, as that's when you'll achieve optimal mental benefits. Continuous walking is also better for your heart, helping to more effectively fight heart disease.

During the next 6 weeks, you'll take on the following four workouts.

▪ **Basic endurance walk.** Warm up for 5 minutes by walking slowly at a comfortable pace. If you're on a treadmill, set the speed at 2.5 to 3.2 miles per hour. This will warm up your muscles, loosen your joints, and ready your

(continued on page 50)

People Ask Me . . .

"HOW MANY CALORIES WILL I BURN AS I WALK?" Many of us want to know the number of calories we're burning as we move. It gives us the little push we need to add an extra block to the route or to pick up the pace.

To find out how many calories you burn during your walking workouts, use this handy, detailed grid. It shows the number of calories burned based on your weight, walking time (based on time periods), and speed (intensity). In general, when you walk at a brisk pace, you burn about 4 calories per minute. That equals about 120 calories per walk during weeks 1 and 2 of your program,

140 during weeks 3 and 4, and 160 by weeks 5 and 6. Precisely how many calories you burn during these walks, however, depends on your weight and pace. The faster you walk, the higher your calorie burn.

Also, the more you weigh, the higher your calorie burn as your muscles must work harder to move a heavier body through space.

(Note: 2 mph equals a very slow pace; 3 mph equals a slow to moderate pace; 3.5 equals a moderate pace; 4, a brisk pace; and 4.5 mph is the equivalent of walking extremely briskly—at almost a jog—or walking moderately to briskly uphill or up stairs.)

WEIGHT: 120 POUNDS

TIME WALKED	2 MPH	3 MPH	3.5 MPH	4 MPH	4.5 MPH
25 min.	75	81	99	126	141
35 min.	105	113	139	176	197
45 min.	135	146	178	227	233

WEIGHT: 140 POUNDS

TIME WALKED	2 MPH	3 MPH	3.5 MPH	4 MPH	4.5 MPH
25 min.	87	95	116	146	165
35 min.	122	132	162	205	230
45 min.	157	169	208	265	296

WEIGHT: 160 POUNDS

TIME WALKED	2 MPH	3 MPH	3.5 MPH	4 MPH	4.5 MPH
25 min.	93	108	132	168	188
35 min.	129	151	185	235	263
45 min.	166	194	238	302	338

WEIGHT: 180 POUNDS

TIME WALKED	2 MPH	3 MPH	3.5 MPH	4 MPH	4.5 MPH
25 min.	112	122	149	189	211
35 min.	157	170	208	245	296
45 min.	202	219	266	340	381

WEIGHT: 200 POUNDS

TIME WALKED	2 MPH	3 MPH	3.5 MPH	4 MPH	4.5 MPH
25 min.	125	135	165	210	235
35 min.	175	189	231	294	329
45 min.	225	243	297	378	423

WEIGHT: 220 POUNDS

TIME WALKED	2 MPH	3 MPH	3.5 MPH	4 MPH	4.5 MPH
25 min.	137	149	181	231	259
35 min.	192	208	254	323	362
45 min.	247	267	327	416	465

WEIGHT: 240 POUNDS

TIME WALKED	2 MPH	3 MPH	3.5 MPH	4 MPH	4.5 MPH
25 min.	150	162	198	252	282
35 min.	210	227	277	353	395
45 min.	270	292	356	454	508

WEIGHT: 260+ POUNDS

TIME WALKED	2 MPH	3 MPH	3.5 MPH	4 MPH	4.5 MPH
25 min.	162	175	214	273	305
35 min.	227	246	300	382	428
45 min.	292	316	386	491	550

heart for exercise. Then pick up the pace by pumping your arms and using your butt muscles to power your body forward. Maintain a pace that you can keep for the next 15 to 35 minutes (depending on the designated length of that day's walk). Then cool down by walking more slowly for 5 minutes.

- **Fat zone workout.** Warm up for 5 minutes by walking slowly at a comfortable pace. If you're on a treadmill, set the speed for 2.5 to 3.2 miles per hour. This will warm up your muscles, loosen your joints, and ready your heart for exercise. Then speed up, maintaining a pace that you can keep for the next 15 to 20 minutes (depending on the designated length of that day's walk). During the next 10 minutes, do exercises that target your personal fat zones (see pages 60 to 72). If you're on a treadmill, slow the speed to 1.5 miles per hour. Work in walking lunges, punches, or abdominal squeezes. You can even do these moves in the privacy of your home or backyard. Cool down after your exercises with 5 minutes of slow walking.

- **Fat-burning workout.** Warm up for 5 minutes by walking slowly at a comfortable pace. If you're on a treadmill, set the speed at 2.5 to 3.2 miles per hour. This will warm up your muscles, loosen your joints, and ready your heart for exercise. Then pick up the pace. If you feel up to it, you can even jog. Keep this up for 5 minutes. Then slow down and recover for 5 minutes. Pick up the pace again for 5 minutes, then slow down and recover. Continue alternating between 5 minutes of fast walking and 5 minutes of moderate walking for a total of 25 to 35 minutes (depending on the length of that day's walk) and then cool down with 5 minutes of slower walking.

- **Combined fat zone and fat-burning blast.** Warm up for 5 minutes by walking slowly at a comfortable pace. If you're on a treadmill set the speed at 2.5 to 3.2 miles per hour. This will warm up your muscles, loosen your joints, and ready your heart for exercise. Then pick up the pace. If you feel up to it, you can even jog. Keep this up for 5 minutes. Then slow down and do your fat zone exercises for 10 minutes. (If you're on a treadmill, slow the speed to 1.5 miles per hour before doing the exercises.) Pick up the pace again for 5. Then slow down and do your exercises for 10 minutes. Speed up for one last 5-minute blast and then slow down for a 5-minute cooldown.

What to **Wear**

What you wear can make a huge difference between walking in comfort and feeling hot, sticky, and dreadful, so suit up with the following essential items before heading out for that walk.

A JACKET: You may feel a little cold and chilly when you start off, but as you move, you'll quickly warm up. I like to layer, wearing a tank top, short- or long-sleeved shirt, and then a jacket. As I walk, I peel off the layers, tying them around my waist. On a rainy day, consider a rain slicker or a performance waterproof jacket made of Gore-Tex. Some offer heat vents that you can unzip under your arms and elsewhere to allow body heat to escape while still keeping rainwater out.

SYNTHETIC CLOTHING: Cotton clothes absorb water, making you feel sticky during muggy summer days. Opt for synthetic fabrics made from Lycra, CoolMax, and other brands. These fabrics wick away sweat and dry quickly, helping you to feel cool and dry.

A WATER BOTTLE: Always take water with you, aiming to drink a cup of water during every 30 minutes of walking. The water will help keep you energized, as dehydration causes your blood to thicken, making your heart beat harder to push the blood through your body. Just breathing through your mouth causes water loss! I also drink water before I go for a walk and a glass when I arrive home.

A PORTABLE STEREO: If I'm not walking with my girlfriends, I take a portable radio or tape player and listen to my favorite music as I walk. There's nothing like a catchy tune to help me pick up the pace. More than one neighbor has caught me singing out loud as I walk by! I really get into it.

SUNSCREEN: Use a waterproof SPF 30 sunscreen gel on your face to prevent wrinkles and sun damage. Gels absorb faster than creams or lotions, so they'll sting your eyes less when you sweat. They

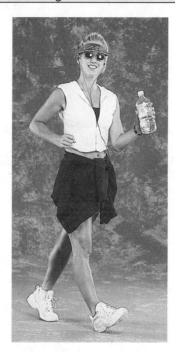

also generally are less likely to cause acne breakouts.

A HAT OR VISOR: I always wear a hat or visor for any outdoor activity to protect my face and forehead from wrinkles. A full hat will protect your hair from sun damage.

SUNGLASSES: Direct sunlight damages your eyes, increasing your risk of cataracts and macular degeneration, the leading cause of blindness. Plus, it makes you squint. Wear sunglasses with 100 percent UV protection. As an added bonus, the glasses will help keep your contact lenses from drying out on a windy day as well as keep bugs away from your eyes on a muggy day.

SOCKS: Steer clear of cotton, particularly on a hot day. Cotton soaks up water, loses its shape after repeated washings, and bunches up, increasing your risk of hot spots and blisters. Look for synthetic socks and make sure that they fit snugly.

SHOES: Don't wear any old shoes you find in the back of your closet. Shoes specifically designed for walking will encourage your feet to smoothly roll from heel to toe with complete comfort. Replace your walking shoes every 6 months, as your shoes will offer less cushioning and support over time. Consider buying a pair of separate insoles for extra cushioning and arch support.

A WATCH: If you walk for time, you'll need a sports watch with a chronograph function to time your walks.

A PEDOMETER: This is optional, of course, but these inexpensive devices will help you track how many steps you take during an entire day. I was amazed to learn that I took 10,000 steps in a day!

Stretching: Don't Leave Home without It

All your walking workouts should begin with a few targeted stretches. As I wait for my girlfriends to meet me for our morning walks, I do the following stretches to get my body ready to move.

Stretching your calves in your lower legs will help prevent shinsplints, discomfort along the shinbone. Stretching will also help lengthen the muscles in your thighs, back, and torso, allowing you to walk with better posture. Plus, stretching feels oh-so-good and improves your circulation, helping to warm up your body for your walk.

This stretching sequence takes me only 3 minutes but helps me feel so much better on my walk.

> ➤ Stretches the backs of your lower legs ➤ Stretches your Achilles tendons

Calf Stretch

Stand facing a wall with your left foot about 12 inches from the wall and your right foot about 2 to 3 feet behind your left. Place your hands on the wall at shoulder height. Inhale and then exhale and lean forward, bending your left knee and keeping both heels on the floor, as shown. You should feel the stretch along the calf of your right leg. Hold for 20 seconds. Then move on to the Achilles stretch.

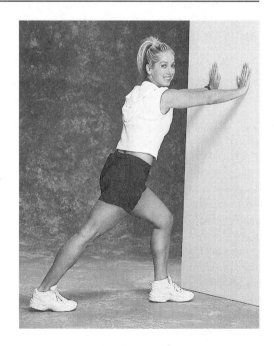

Achilles Stretch

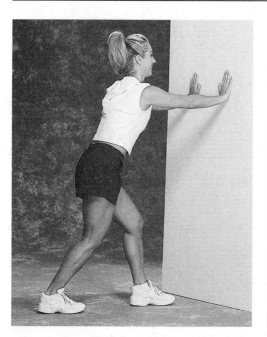

From the calf stretch, now bend your right knee. This will move the stretch down to your Achilles tendon. Hold for 20 seconds. Then switch legs and repeat both stretches.

MAXIMUM RESULTS	Minimum Time
You can stretch more of your calf muscle by pressing back through your rear heel in different directions. For example, try placing more of your body weight toward the left corner of your heel, then toward the right corner. You'll feel the stretch move from the left to the right side of your calf. Breathe normally as you hold the stretch.	

"It's proven. Walking is an easy way to lose weight."

Quad Stretch

Stand with your left hand against a wall for balance and with your feet aligned under your hips. Inhale and then exhale as you bend your right leg, lifting your right foot toward the right buttock. Grab your right foot with your right hand and gently pull your heel closer to your buttock, as shown, with your right knee pointed toward the floor. Breathe normally as you hold the stretch.

Hold for 20 seconds. Then face the opposite direction and repeat with the other leg.

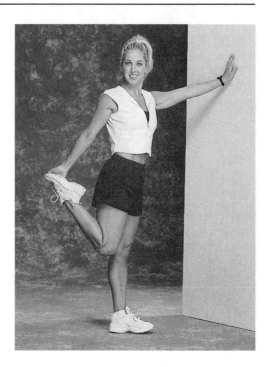

MAXIMUM RESULTS	Minimum Time

To gain a deeper stretch, press down through your thigh as you simultaneously tighten your lower abs. This will tilt back your pelvis slightly, lengthening your quadriceps muscles.

Waist Twist

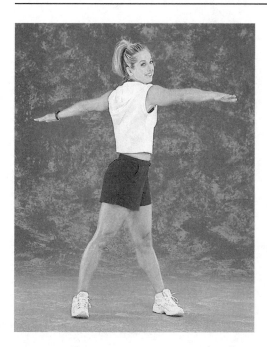

Stand with your feet slightly wider than shoulder-width apart. Raise your arms out to your sides at shoulder height.

Twist your torso to the right as you exhale. Then twist to the left, as shown. Continue to twist from right to left for 20 seconds, moving with your breath.

MAXIMUM RESULTS	Minimum Time
Try to keep both hipbones level and pointing forward as you twist, isolating the movement in your tummy, sides, and back.	

Butt and Thigh Stretch

Stand facing a wall. Place your hands against the wall for balance. Shift your body weight to your left foot and bend your left knee slightly. Raise your right foot and place your right ankle just above your left knee, letting your right knee open to your right side.

Inhale and then exhale as you bend your left knee more, as shown, leaning forward from your waist and keeping your right knee open to the side. You should feel this in the right side of your butt and your right thigh. Hold for 20 seconds and then repeat on the other side.

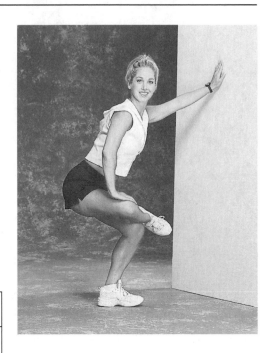

MAXIMUM RESULTS	Minimum Time
As you bend forward from the waist, keep your back long and straight. Try not to allow your spine to curve.	

➤ WARMS UP YOUR LOWER BACK

Leg and Back Stretch

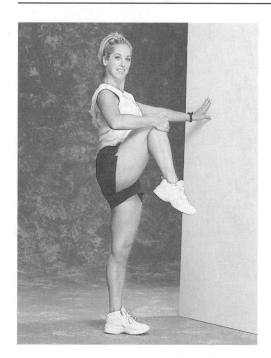

Stand near a wall or a chair, using it for balance. Shift your body weight to your left foot as you raise your right, bringing your right thigh and knee toward your chest. Inhale and then exhale as you grasp your right knee with your right hand, gently pulling your thigh toward your abdomen and chest a little more. Hold for 20 seconds and then release. Repeat with your left leg.

MAXIMUM RESULTS	Minimum Time
Focus on your lower back as you hold this stretch. Imagine it opening and lengthening as the muscles warm. Feel your tailbone drop as your pelvis relaxes.	

Hamstring Stretch

Extend your left leg in front of you and place your left foot on the seat of a chair. Keeping your right leg straight, inhale and then exhale as you bend forward from the waist and reach out for your left foot, as shown. Hold for 20 seconds and then repeat with your right leg.

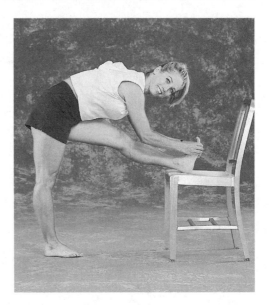

MAXIMUM RESULTS	Minimum Time

As you bend forward from the waist, keep your back long and straight. Try not to allow your spine to curve, as this will move the stretch into your lower back and out of your thighs.

"I like to do this stretch even after I get home from my walk."

Walk This Way

Once you do your pre-walk stretches, you're ready to roll—literally. Although you've probably been walking since you were in diapers, your technique might need a little tweaking to help you burn more calories, eliminate discomfort, and naturally speed up your pace. Use these tips to make your walks more effective.

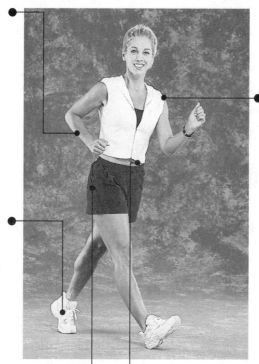

ARMS: Hold your arms at 90-degree angles and pump them as you walk. This will help tone muscles in your upper body, increase your calorie burn, and speed up your gait. It also helps to prevent swelling in your hands. Pump those arms as you walk. The more muscles you use, the more calories you burn.

FEET: As you walk, try to roll your foot from heel to toe, with your feet and toes pointed straight ahead. If you hear a slapping sound when you walk, you're not rolling. Rather, you're walking with a flat foot. You want to feel light on your feet. If you experience trouble rolling from heel to toe, you may need new shoes—your shoes may not be providing enough give in the sole where your foot naturally bends.

BUTT: Squeeze your buttocks periodically, as if you were trying to hold a dime between them. (Remember, if you don't squeeze it, nobody else will!) Squeezing the backs of your upper thighs and buttocks as you walk will help burn more calories with every step as well as help lift and tone your butt and thighs.

SHOULDERS: Relax those shoulders. Don't allow them to hunch up toward your ears. Periodically check by tensing your shoulders—raising them as high as you can and then releasing them with a vigorous exhale. Roll them back and down, opening your chest. This will help you take fuller breaths, bringing in more oxygen and consequently more energy. Plus, you'll eliminate neck and shoulder tension.

TUMMY: Zip up that tummy. Don't allow it to protrude forward. Pull it in and keep it tight. Imagine that you're zipping up a corset, pulling your tummy in and up to lengthen and lift your torso. This will help keep your pelvis in a neutral position, eliminating any strain to your lower back. It also will help you walk with more power and better overall posture. Plus you'll help develop rock-hard abs and a flat tummy.

The more muscles you use as you walk, the more calories you burn. The following exercises will help you tone those specific trouble spots as well as help keep you entertained as you walk.

Two of the four walks in your program include these exercises. Pick the moves that target your personal fat zone and do them during the last 10 minutes of your fat zone walk (see page 50).

Pick a section of your walk where few people are around. I like to do them toward the end of my walk—particularly the leg exercises—as a last push just before my cooldown. If you own a treadmill, these are ideal exercises to do indoors. Though they may seem difficult to do on a moving surface, I've found that I easily mastered the motions on my treadmill, so I'm confident that you can do it, too! Just slow down the treadmill speed to 1.5 miles per hour before you try them. Because your heart rate will already be elevated, just breathe as naturally as possible when you do these exercises. Whatever you do, don't hold your breath.

➤ UPPER BODY: TARGETS YOUR UPPER ARMS

Triceps Toner

A. As you walk, raise your arms overhead so that your upper arms are on either side of your head with your fingers reaching toward the sky, palms facing each other.

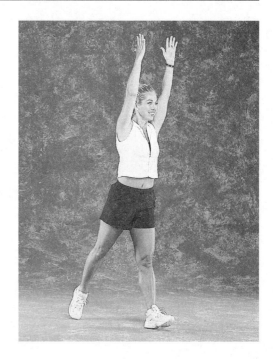

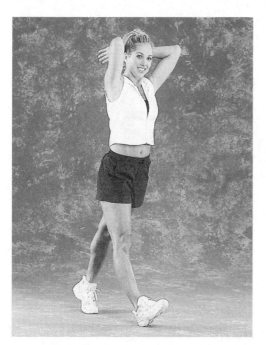

B. Bend your elbows, lowering your hands behind your head while keeping your upper arms stationary and elbows pointed upward. Extend your arms again. Continue to lower and extend for 2 minutes.

MAXIMUM RESULTS	Minimum Time
This is where your music can really help. Do your triceps toners to the beat of your favorite song.	

"Walk for energy. Walk for lower blood pressure. Walk for stress release. Walk for you."

Scissors

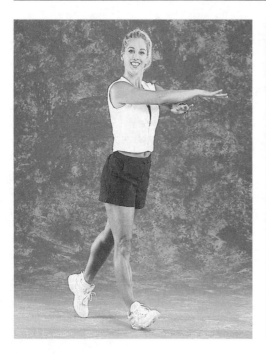

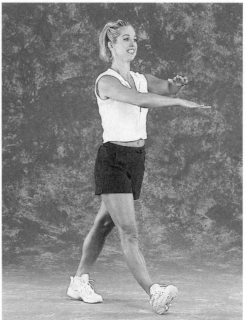

A. As you walk, extend your arms in front of your chest, palms down, so that your arms are parallel to the ground.

Bring your arms toward each other, allowing your left arm to pass underneath your right in a scissor motion.

B. Return to the starting position and then repeat, this time allowing your right arm to pass underneath your left. Continue to alternate your scissor motion for 2 minutes, but change the angle, doing it with your arms extended at eye level, at chest height, at rib height, and at navel height.

Back-of-Arm Scissors

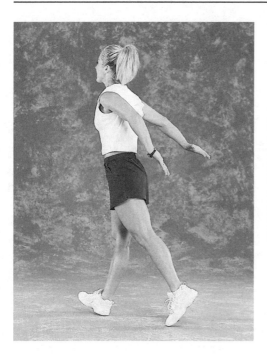

Extend your arms behind your body, scissoring your left under your right and then your right under your left. Continue to scissor, moving through the different motions, for 2 minutes.

MAXIMUM RESULTS	Minimum Time
Don't allow your shoulders to hunch up toward your ears as you do your scissors. Keep your neck long and relaxed and your shoulder blades low on your back.	

"Before you know it, the weight and inches will come right off."

Arm Circles

As you walk, raise your arms out to your sides at shoulder height. Draw small circles with your hands, palms down, circling them forward, down, back, and up. Continue to circle for 1 minute.

Reverse the direction, now circling back, down, and then back up. Continue to circle for 1 minute.

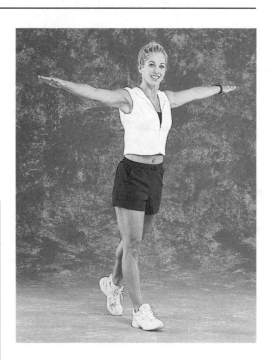

MAXIMUM RESULTS	Minimum Time

To keep your shoulders relaxed as you tone them, bend your elbows slightly and imagine the weight of your arms resting on your shoulder blades rather than on the tops of your shoulders. This simple visualization will help you to continue to circle your arms for a longer period of time before feeling fatigued.

" Walk your way to fitness and a lifetime of health. "

Punches

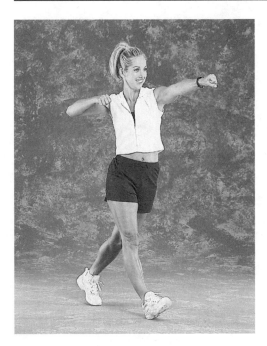

As you walk, bend your arms, bringing your fists just above chest level in a fighter stance. Punch straight out from your chest with your left arm, as shown. Recoil your fist back toward your shoulder at chest height and then punch out with your right.

Then change the angle, punching to chin height then eye height then back down to chin, chest, rib, and then navel height. Continue to alternate through the different punches for 2 minutes.

MAXIMUM RESULTS	Minimum Time

As you punch, try not to hyperextend your elbow, which can eventually cause discomfort and pain. Keep your elbow slightly bent at all times. To punch correctly at first, you may have to hold back a little, doing the movement slowly. Eventually, however, proper punching technique will become automatic, and you'll be able to speed up your cadence.

Biceps Curl

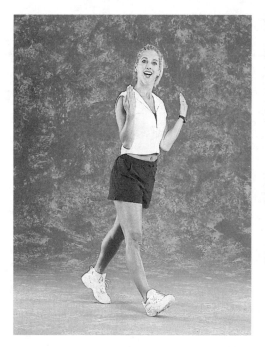 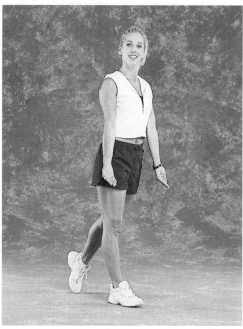

A. As you walk, bend your arms, bringing your lower arms and hands toward your upper arms, with your upper arms close to your sides and your hands open with palms facing upward.

B. Then lower your hands. Once your arms are fully extended, raise your hands back toward your shoulders, repeating for 2 minutes.

MAXIMUM RESULTS	Minimum Time
It's easy to get sloppy with this move. Pay attention to your movement, making sure to keep your elbows close to your sides throughout and slowly and methodically raising and lowering your hands.	

Ab Twist

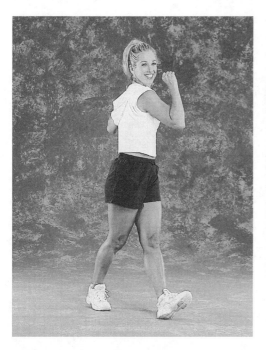 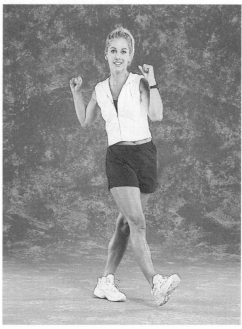

A. As you walk, tighten your abs, pull your navel in, and extend up through your crown to lengthen your spine. Then twist to the left, keeping your arms bent upward at 90-degree angles.

B. In quick but controlled succession, twist to the right. Continue alternating left and right for 2 minutes.

MAXIMUM RESULTS	Minimum Time
Try not to slouch as you twist, as this can put some pressure on your lower back. Imagine a string pulling your crown upward, helping you to lengthen from your hips all the way up to your head.	

Ab Tightener

As you walk, extend up through your crown to lengthen your spine, and then tighten your abs, pressing them in and up, as if someone were zipping an imaginary corset up your tummy, squeezing it in and upward.

Hold this isometric contraction for up to 5 seconds, releasing when you need to rest, then retightening your abs.

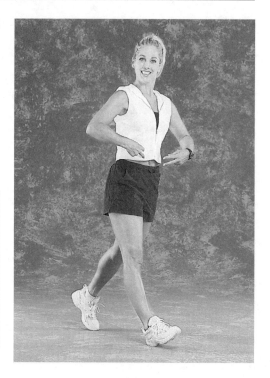

MAXIMUM RESULTS	Minimum Time
As you hold the contraction in your abdomen, you should still be able to breathe. Imagine the breath coming into your mouth and expanding your ribs and upper back. This will help you to take fuller breaths as you walk.	

"Turn that walk into a fat-blasting workout!"

Tush Tightener

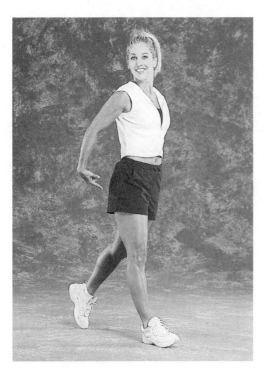

Periodically squeeze your butt muscles. Remember, the more muscles you use, the more calories you burn. Keep them tight for 5 seconds. Release then retighten your tush.

MAXIMUM RESULTS	Minimum Time
It's easy to get distracted and lose the squeeze. When I'm walking with my friends or sisters, I often say out loud, "Squeeze that tush," to remind us all to maintain the movement. You might say those words silently to yourself, sort of as a mantra to encourage yourself to keep your buns tight.	

" No one will know you're doing this move, but it's so effective. "

Walking Lunge

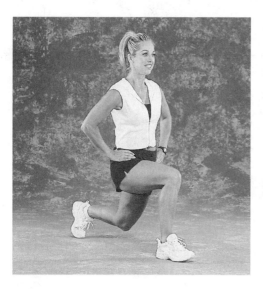 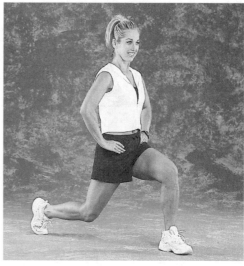

A. Take a giant step forward with your right foot, planting it about 2½ to 3 feet in front of your body. Bend your right knee as much as 90 degrees and let your left knee nearly touch the ground.

B. Then without a pause, press up through your right foot, bringing your left foot forward and planting it 2½ to 3 feet in front of your body and lunging with that leg. Continue walking forward as you lunge for 2 minutes.

MAXIMUM RESULTS	Minimum Time
Walking lunges are a great, fun exercise to do with small children. Rather than lunges, just call them "giant steps." You and your toddler will have fun taking these giant steps all over your backyard after your walk.	

➤ LOWER BODY: TONES THE FRONTS OF YOUR THIGHS

Walking Kickout

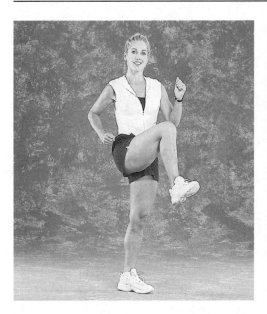 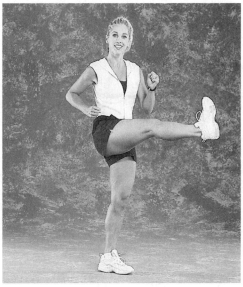

A. As you walk, lift your right knee to abdomen level.

B. Then kick out your foot and extend your leg straight out, as if you were a Canadian Mountie marching during the changing of the guards. Bend and lower your leg and repeat with your left leg, alternating back and forth for 2 minutes.

MAXIMUM RESULTS	Minimum Time
Though this move may feel awkward at first, you'll eventually find a smooth rhythm that allows you to feel as graceful as a ballerina.	

Rear Leg Press

As you walk, sweep your extended right leg back behind your body, using the back of your thigh and buttock to lift your right thigh back and up.

Lower your leg, take a few steps forward, and then repeat with your left leg. Continue alternating right and left for 2 minutes, interspersing each leg press with as many steps as you need to maintain your balance.

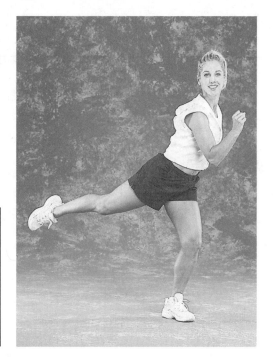

MAXIMUM RESULTS	Minimum Time
I find that I can better maintain a smooth rhythm on these if I count my steps as I walk. For example, I silently say to myself, "One, two, three, lift. One, two, three, lift."	

"The more **muscles** you **use**, the **more calories** you **burn**."

CHAPTER 4

THE FAT ZONE WALKING AND STRETCHING PROGRAM

Denise's Daily Stretch

I feel wonderful when I stretch, even if I stretch for only 1 minute. As my blood circulation increases, I almost instantly feel my energy level rise and any muscle tightness melt away.

Stretching—along with cardio and toning—is essential when it comes to shrinking your fat zones. Yes, it may not burn as many calories as a walk, but it does help shrink fat by:

■ **Changing your body shape.** Think of your muscles as rubber bands. When you stretch a rubber band, you make it longer. Once you stop stretching it, the rubber band resumes its former shape. If you stretch the band often enough, however, the band will eventually lose some of its tension and permanently lengthen.

The same principle applies to your muscles. When you stretch, you pull the ends of your muscles farther apart. For example, when you bend over, your hip joints move upward, but your knee joints stay put. This pulls the ends of your hamstring muscles, which run from your hips to your knees, farther apart, lengthening the muscles. Bend over often enough, and the muscles permanently lengthen, creating the longer, leaner appearance of a ballerina or gymnast.

■ **Increasing your energy and strength.** As your muscles grow longer, they'll hold less tension and move more fluidly with less tightness. Flexible muscles use oxygen more efficiently than shortened, tight muscles. This increased efficiency helps you pump up your walking workouts without feeling winded. Flexible muscles are also more able to contract than tight muscles, which creates more strength.

Also, the actual act of stretching pumps blood into your muscles and releases tension from them, which generally makes you feel good. Any time you need a natural energy boost, just take a stretch break. That's one reason why I like to stretch first thing in the morning. I *always* feel like working out when I'm done.

■ **Boosting productivity.** Have you ever had one of those days when 20 or more thoughts crowded your brain, and those thoughts made you feel so frenzied that you accomplished little more than worrying away your energy? It's on those days—those very same days when you think that you don't have time—that you need to stretch more than ever. Stretching helps you take a time-out. During that 5-minute time-out, your thoughts slow down and order themselves, helping you to accomplish more after your stretch break. When you accomplish more at work, you free up more time to work out.

Stretching also makes you *feel* better, which helps you to work harder. For example, one of my sisters, a dental hygienist, recently complained of

"Deep breathing provides a
natural high. Take **breathing breaks**
instead of coffee breaks!"

"When you stretch and relax, you elongate your muscles, which will make you appear up to 5 pounds thinner and an inch taller in just a few minutes!"

neck and shoulder discomfort from bending over most of the day as she did her job. I suggested that she try my midday stretching routine. She began taking stretch breaks between clients, and her aches and tension faded. She felt better all day long and more energetic when she got home at night. Every once in a while, she neglects to stretch, and not only does the tension return, it also intensifies into a headache.

▪ **Improving circulation.** Stretching improves blood circulation to your muscles. This circulation is what helps to heal your body, patching up any injuries and soothing away aches and pains. Fewer aches and pains equal more energetic walking and toning workouts.

Better circulation can also directly improve your appearance by preventing both cellulite and varicose veins. Cellulite is a type of fat that pushes through weak spots in your connective tissue, creating a dimpled appearance. Stretching boosts circulation to these areas, helping your body mobilize and burn this fat during your workouts.

Varicose veins form when the muscles in your leg veins fail to push blood up against gravity to your heart. Instead blood flows backward, enlarging the vein. When one of my sisters was beginning to develop these knotty veins, I suggested that she try my nighttime stretching routine, which contains a series of stretches that encourage bloodflow back to the heart. After a few weeks with the new stretching routine, she told me that her veins were subsiding.

- **Enhancing sleep.** Stretching before bedtime can help you to make the transition from go-go-go to slow-slow-slow. It helps you to release any remaining muscle tension, empty your mind, and deeply relax your entire body. Stretch right before bed, and you'll fall asleep faster, sleep more deeply, and wake in the morning feeling more refreshed.

Denise's Stretching Do's and Don'ts

For optimal energy, flexibility, sleep, and overall results, try to stretch at least three times a day. Start your first stretching session as soon as you wake in the morning. Get out of bed and begin your day by energizing your body and mind with my 5-minute Morning Wake-Up Stretch. Take your next stretch break during the workday with my Midday Tension Tamers, designed to relieve tightness and aches in your neck, shoulders, and back. Then cap off the day with my Evening Wind-Down Routine, designed to calm your body and mind for a restful and peaceful slumber.

When stretching, keep the following do's and don'ts in mind.

DO . . .

- **Stretch every day, many times a day.** The more often you stretch, the better. I often stretch whenever I need a break. It helps me collect my thoughts and release any built-up tension, allowing me to return to work or my kids invigorated.

- **Hold each stretch for about 20 seconds.** The longer you hold a stretch, the more your muscles relax.

- **Repeat as needed.** If you're really tense, you may need to run through your stretching routine more than once before you feel relaxed and

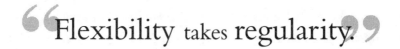
"Flexibility takes regularity."

"As you lengthen and stretch your muscles, you improve circulation and whisk tension away."

rejuvenated. I often flow through my morning and midday stretches numerous times, moving fluidly from one stretch into the next and repeating the entire sequence until I feel focused and relaxed.

■ **Breathe.** Try to breathe slowly and deeply, moving with your breath. This will help to make your stretching practice more mindful, allowing you to relax your mind with your body. It will also infuse your body with energizing oxygen. Never hold your breath while stretching. You need oxygen to get to the area you're stretching. So breathe naturally, as naturally as possible.

DON'T . . .

■ **Rush.** If you feel tempted to go through the motions because you have too much to do, remember that stretching *creates* time. When you stretch, you take an important time-out that helps to rejuvenate your mind, readying you to face the day.

■ **Bounce.** Move into each stretch slowly and then hold it once you reach your maximum stretch. Don't try to increase the stretch by bouncing or jerking your body. This could inflict small tears in your muscles, causing you to feel worse, not better.

■ **Strain.** Stretching should feel good. You should be able to feel your muscles warming, lengthening, and relaxing. You shouldn't feel pain, however, particularly around your joints. If you do, you're probably overstretching.

MORNING WAKE-UP STRETCH

The second I get out of bed, I stretch. It helps me wake up, get in the right frame of mind, and work out any early-morning kinks. It's a great gift that takes less than 5 minutes.

The stretching routine on the following pages is exactly what I do each morning. Flow through this sequence as many times as you need to feel warm, relaxed, and fluid.

It will wake up your spine and warm up your brain and muscles. It will rev up your circulation, helping you move more all day long and burn more calories as a result. It's a great morning jump start, a perfect way to begin the day.

Here's another tip. I try to put on my athletic shoes and clothes as soon as I get up and do these stretches. That way, I'm mentally ready to exercise. Your exercise clothes and your stretches will get you motivated, so plan to follow up with your walk or fat zone toning routine.

> ➤ WARMS UP YOUR BACK AND SPINE ➤ LENGTHENS YOUR SPINE

Reach-for-the-Sky Stretch

Stand with your feet aligned under your hips and your hands by your sides. Take a deep breath and raise your arms out to the sides, with your palms facing up. Press your hands as far apart as you can to open your chest and upper back.

Exhale and continue to raise your arms overhead, as shown, reaching for the sky as you rise onto the balls of your feet. Breathe deeply as you stretch out your entire body, holding until you feel your spine lengthen and warm. Then come to center and move on to the healthy back stretch.

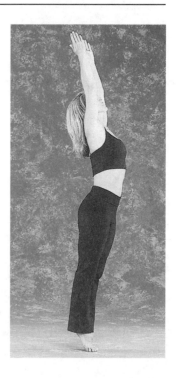

MAXIMUM RESULTS Minimum Time

As you reach your hands toward the sky, keep your neck long and your shoulder blades down. Try not to hunch your shoulders toward your ears.

Healthy Back Stretch

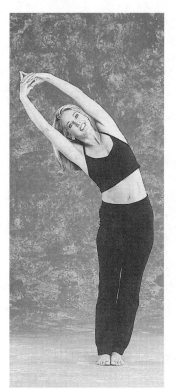

Lower your heels to the floor from the reach-for-the-sky stretch, but keep your arms outstretched overhead with your palms facing each other. Clasp your hands together overhead and press your index fingers together into a temple shape.

Take a deep breath and then exhale as you reach your hands toward the right, bending your entire torso to the right, as shown, and feeling a deep stretch all along your left side. Inhale as you return to center and then repeat to the other side, holding until you've fully exhaled. Alternate from side to side four times, then return to center for your shoulder rolls.

MAXIMUM RESULTS	Minimum Time

Many women round their backs forward during this stretch, which compresses the chest and makes it hard to breathe. As you stretch to the side, keep your shoulder blades pressed back, opening your chest toward the ceiling. It may help to turn your head to look up. Gazing upward will automatically encourage your upper torso to remain in the correct position.

❝Let's wake up the spine.❞

Shoulder Roll

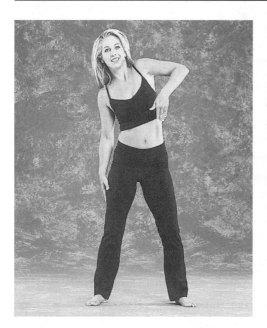 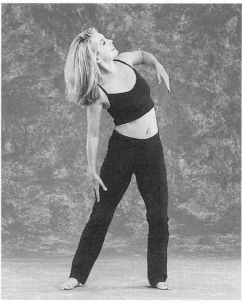

A. Return to center from the healthy back stretch and lower your arms to your sides. Widen your stance so that your feet are positioned a few inches wider than your hips. Take a deep breath. Exhale as you bend your left arm and lift your left elbow and forearm, as shown.

B. Continue to exhale as you bring your left elbow up and back in a large semicircle, letting your left hand hang down. Inhale when you need to, bringing your arm full circle. Repeat with your right elbow, continuing to breathe deeply and alternating back and forth five times on each side. Then move on to the standing cat stretch.

MAXIMUM RESULTS	Minimum Time
Taking full, deep breaths as you move will help to fully oxygenate your lungs, providing an extra surge of energy. Do it whenever you feel tired or sleepy.	

Standing Cat Stretch

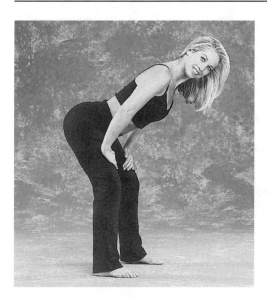
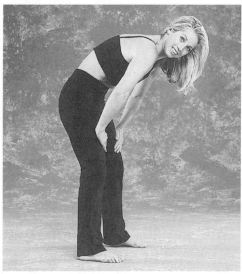

A. Bend your knees slightly. Bow forward from the waist and place your palms on your thighs just above your knees. Gently press into your thighs to lengthen your spine, bringing your tailbone and your crown farther apart. Inhale as you slowly look up toward the ceiling, raise your tailbone, and lower your navel, forming a concave shape with your spine, as shown.

B. Exhale as you reverse the stretch by pulling your navel up toward your spine as you curl your crown and tailbone down and toward one another, arching your back into a cat stretch. Alternate between the two stretches five times, moving with your breath.

MAXIMUM RESULTS	Minimum Time

Have you ever seen a cat arch its back? You want to achieve the same arch, stretching between every single vertebra of your spine. Tuck your chin to lengthen your neck and pull that tailbone down to stretch every single joint from your tailbone to your head.

Forward Bend

From the standing cat stretch, inhale and then exhale as you bend forward, using your hands against your knees to lower yourself slowly. You should feel the backs of your thighs and your lower back lengthen. Allow your head and shoulders to relax and surrender to gravity.

Hold for 20 seconds, breathing normally, and then slowly roll back up one vertebra at a time as you use your hands against your thighs for balance.

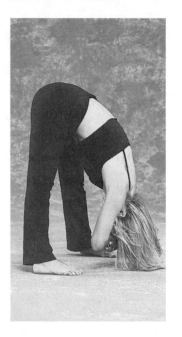

MAXIMUM RESULTS Minimum Time

If you have low blood pressure, you may not be able to do a full forward bend first thing in the morning without feeling light-headed. In that case, use your hands against your thighs as a safety prop and only bend as far forward as you feel comfortable.

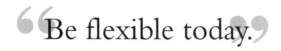

" Be flexible today. "

Most of us subconsciously hold tension, often in our necks and shoulders, whenever we're concentrating, nervous, scared, or anxious.

Tension may also build up simply from sitting at a desk most of the day. Even if you sit with the best posture, the pressure of your chair seat against your derriere and the lack of bloodflow from your lower body to your upper body will impede good blood circulation. Couple that with the common desk slump and phone cradling that most of us do, and you have a tight chest, neck, and hips.

That's where stretching comes in. It encourages tense muscles to relax. It also improves blood circulation, helping you to feel more energized at work and after. It counteracts any tightening that may result from poor posture and tired muscles. Though I call these midday stretches, you can do them at any time of day, particularly if you feel tired, irritable, tense, or achy.

> ➤ RELEASES TENSION IN YOUR NECK AND SHOULDERS ➤ LENGTHENS NECK MUSCLES
> TIGHTENED FROM CRADLING THE PHONE OR SLUMPING AT A DESK

Neck and Shoulder Release

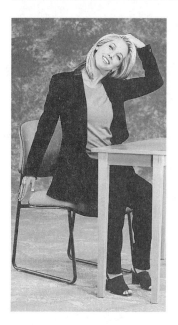

Sit up straight with your shoulders relaxed and your neck extended. Lower both arms, allowing them to hang toward the floor. Take a deep breath. Exhale and lower your left ear to your left shoulder. Raise your left hand and use it to apply gentle pressure against your head, as shown, to increase the stretch. Breathe deeply, feeling your neck relax on each exhale. Hold for 20 seconds. Repeat by returning to center and then bringing your right ear toward your right shoulder.

MAXIMUM RESULTS | Minimum Time

If you talk on the phone a lot, one side of your neck is probably tighter than the other. On your tighter side, hold the stretch twice as long. Also, try to alternate the ears you cradle the phone against or switch to a speakerphone or headset.

Shoulder and Chest Relaxer

A. Clasp your fingers behind the bottom of your skull. Take a deep breath as you open your elbows back behind your head as far as you can. Lift your sternum, look up, and feel your chest open.

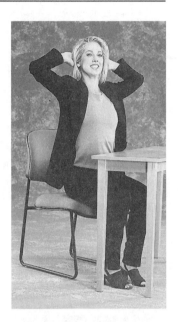

MAXIMUM RESULTS	Minimum Time

As you stretch your chest, imagine that someone is gently pulling your elbows back behind your torso, allowing you to feel the stretch all the way from your sternum to your armpits and even your upper arms.

B. Exhale and fold your elbows toward each other as you drop your sternum, curl your upper back, and contract your chest, folding your upper body into a tight ball and stretching your upper back. Release and then alternate between the two stretches five times.

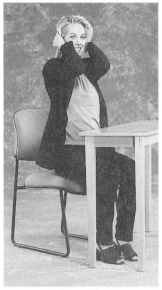

➤ STRETCHES YOUR SHOULDERS AND UPPER BACK

One-Arm Reach

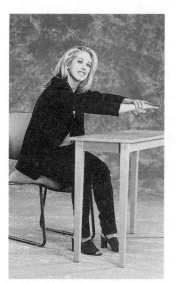

Sit tall with your hands by your sides. Inhale as you raise your right arm to the side to shoulder height. Slowly exhale as you bring your right arm forward and slightly down to the left in a large arcing motion, as if you were hugging a beach ball. Curl your upper back as you do so, allowing your right shoulder blade to open. Then gently pull against your right wrist with your left hand, as shown, to deepen the stretch. Hold for 20 seconds and then relax. Repeat with your left arm.

MAXIMUM RESULTS	Minimum Time

The secret to this stretch is in your shoulder blade. Keep it pressed back, and you'll feel a wonderful stretch right in that area of your back where you constantly ask your friends or hubby for a back rub. Also, try lifting the shoulder on the side of your body that you are stretching and lowering the opposite shoulder to further open your rib cage and deepen the stretch.

❝ I often **feel tension** between my **shoulder blades,** and this **stretch** really **hits** the **spot.** ❞

Hip Opener

A. Sit on the edge of your desk chair. Inhale as you lift your right knee and rest your right ankle on the top of your left thigh, just above the knee. Gently press your right knee down with your right hand so that your bent right leg is parallel to the floor.

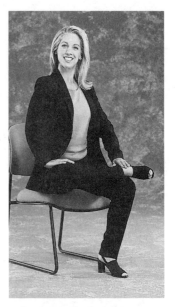

B. Exhale as you bend forward from the waist, keeping your back flat and feeling a wonderful stretch in your lower back and hips. Hold for 20 seconds and then repeat on the other side.

MAXIMUM RESULTS	Minimum Time

Keep your knee pressed down as you bend forward. This will open your hip and increase the stretch. Also, extend through your crown as you bend, lengthening your back from your tailbone all the way up to your crown.

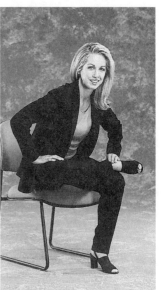

EVENING WIND-DOWN ROUTINE

I love to stretch right before bedtime. It helps me unwind and put aside my mental "to do" list, so I can smoothly make the transition from go-go-go to ah-h-h . . . rest. I've found that it's a great way to end the day peacefully and calmly and that it helps me to sleep deeply and wake up feeling refreshed.

The following stretches help prepare your body for sleep. Among my favorite stretches is the leg circulation series—it helps drain the fluid from your legs that tends to accumulate during a long day of standing or sitting. It also has a way of helping you to deeply relax.

You'll need a wall for many of these stretches, so find one in your house free of pictures and other hindrances. Also, make sure that your feet are clean. You don't want to mark up your walls! Breathe deeply as you stretch. Try exhaling with an audible sigh, exhaling out any mind chatter, anxiety, or unrestful thoughts.

➤ OPENS YOUR CHEST ➤ STRETCHES YOUR SHOULDERS, BACK, AND LEGS

Wall Hang

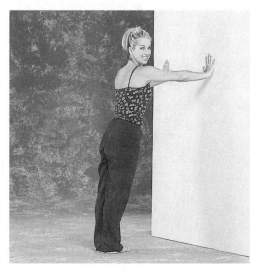

A. Stand an arm's distance from a wall. Raise your arms to chest level, palms facing the wall.

—continued

➤ OPENS YOUR CHEST ➤ STRETCHES YOUR SHOULDERS, BACK, AND LEGS

Wall Hang—*continued*

B. Bend forward as you exhale, reaching for the wall with your palms. Place your palms against the wall and sink into the stretch, as shown, allowing your chest and armpits to open. Step back if you need to, keeping your feet aligned under your hips. Extend and press back through your hips. Breathe deeply as you relax, holding the stretch for 20 seconds.

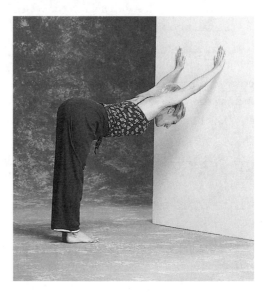

MAXIMUM RESULTS	Minimum Time
Lengthen your spine, bringing your tailbone back away from the wall. Also, feel your chest stretching forward through your arms as your armpits open.	

➤ STRETCHES YOUR HIPS AND BUTTOCKS

Hip Opener on Wall

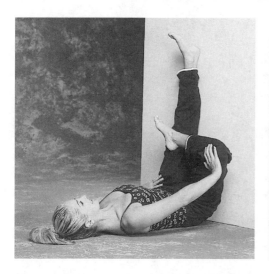
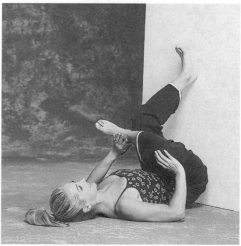

A. Sit on the floor and scoot your buttocks toward the wall. Inhale and extend your left leg up the wall as you bend your right leg, placing your right ankle against your lower left thigh and opening your right knee toward the wall.

B. Exhale and slowly bend your left leg, feeling a deep stretch in your hips. Hold for 20 seconds, then release and switch legs.

MAXIMUM RESULTS	Minimum Time
You probably won't have to bend your leg very far to feel this stretch. Use one hand to gently press against the knee of the leg you are stretching, pushing that knee toward the wall. This will open your hip and deepen the stretch.	

Leg Circulation Series

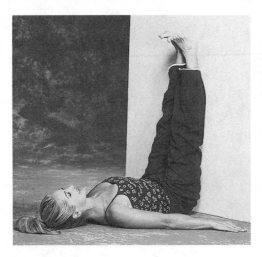 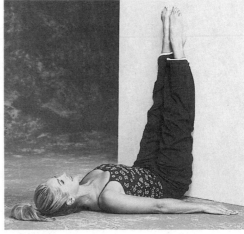

A. From the hip opener, raise both legs, and rotate your body so that the backs of both thighs rest against the wall, forming a 90-degree angle with your torso.

B. Breathe normally as you flex and then point your toes for 20 seconds, alternating between flexed and pointed.

MAXIMUM RESULTS	Minimum Time
Allow your body to surrender to these stretches. Let the weight of your legs sink into your hips. Feel your body press into the floor.	

"Breathe deeply, relaxing more and more with every exhale."

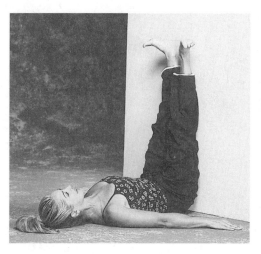

C. Draw circles with your big toes, stretching your ankles in all directions. Circle in both directions, clockwise and counterclockwise, for 20 seconds.

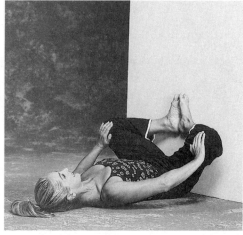

D. Exhale as you slide your feet down the wall toward your pelvis and open your knees out toward the wall, bringing the soles of your feet together. Hold for 20 seconds, breathing deeply.

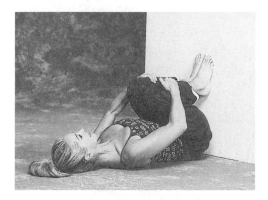

E. Inhale and draw your ankles back together. Bend your knees toward your chest, placing your feet flat on the wall. Exhale and hold for 20 seconds, breathing normally.

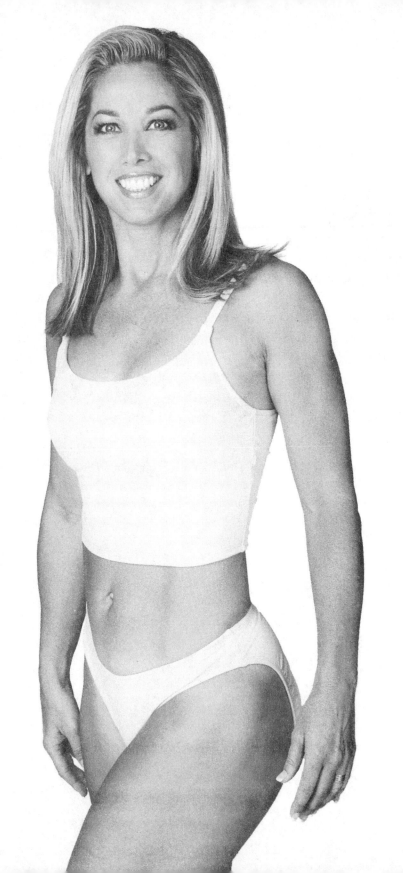

PART 3

The Fat Zone
Workouts

CHAPTER 5

THE FAT ZONE WORKOUTS

The Upper Body

Some women ignore upper body toning. They sometimes tell me that they want to focus solely on their trouble spots—their tummies and thighs. Or they tell me that they don't want to look big and muscular.

The thing is, these excuses are misguided reasons to skip upper body conditioning. Weight training can do amazing things to improve your appearance, and it is an integral part of shrinking your fat zones. Toning your upper body, especially with the exercises that I've included in my Upper-Body Fat Zone routines, will help you firm and shape your muscles.

But your muscles *won't* become large and bulky. Not many women possess the genetic potential to build the huge arm muscles and shoulders of a football player or a body builder. We just don't have the high levels of the hormone testosterone that men have.

So don't worry. Because muscle takes up less space than fat, you're most likely to shrink in size as you put on more muscle. Weight training will firm, tone, and sculpt your muscles, making them appear sleeker and more defined.

As a second benefit, doing exercises that firm and tone your upper body will help you to minimize your trouble spots down below. For example, weak, sloping shoulders can make your lower body appear wider. If, however, you firm and fill out your shoulders and upper body with my Upper-Body Fat Zone routines, you'll help create the shape of an upside-down triangle, allowing your shoulders to taper down to a thin waist and hips. Upper body toning helps you create better body proportions.

I think the most convincing reason to include upper body work in your routine is that it makes the rest of your life easier. You'll develop the arm, chest, shoulder, and back strength that you need to lift your children, carry your groceries, and lug suitcases with ease. Keeping my upper body toned and strong has allowed me, at age 46, to continue to do all of the things I used to do in high school. When my daughters want to do cartwheels at the park, I can do them, too. When they want to climb on the monkey bars, I'm right there. We even do handstand contests—and I usually win!

This improved strength will take the pressure off your neck and shoulders, preventing any tension that tends to accumulate in those areas and making you feel better all day long!

The Anatomy of a Firm Upper Body

My Upper-Body Fat Zone routines will shape and contour all of the muscles in your upper body and shrink any excess flab, making you look beautiful and slender in a backless dress or bikini. No part of you will "spill out."

You'll firm any flab under your arms that may jiggle when you wave your hand. You'll tone up and lift your breasts and help create muscle for sexy cleavage. Strengthening your upper back and shoulders helps you to stand upright automatically. The better your posture, the slimmer, taller, and more confident you appear. Also, as you firm your upper back, you'll notice that you no longer have that bra overhang, the fat that tends to press outward around your bra straps!

The three 20-minute routines will work the following:

- **Upper back.** You'll work your trapezius muscle—a large diamond-shaped muscle that begins at the base of your skull, fans out to your shoulders, and extends halfway down your back—and smaller upper back muscles including the teres minor and infraspinatus. You'll also work your latissimus dorsi (often called lats) slightly lower on your back. Together, these muscles hold you upright, helping you to stop slouching automatically. Working this area also helps to create the illusion of a smaller waist and slimmer hips.

▪ **Arms.** You'll target your biceps, along the front of your upper arms, as well as your triceps, along the back of your upper arms. Your triceps are the most underused muscles in your body. You use your biceps to carry groceries, but hardly ever use your triceps, which are helpful in pushing movements.

▪ **Chest.** You'll work your pectoralis major. This muscle lifts and gives shape to your breasts. Developing your chest helps you create a line of cleavage because the two sides of your pectoralis muscles meet just above your breasts. Your pectoralis major sits underneath your breast tissue, so it will lift your breasts, helping to counteract the pull of gravity.

▪ **Shoulders.** Working your deltoid muscles along the front, top, and back of your shoulders will help eliminate sloping shoulders, making you look more confident, youthful, and energetic. You'll give yourself natural shoulder pads, creating a strong sexy look.

Denise's Upper Body Do's and Don'ts

The exercises in my Upper-Body Fat Zone routines will target your upper body muscles from every angle, helping to fully shape your upper body. You're embarking on a 6-week toning plan that steps up the challenge every other week. You'll do the first routine during weeks 1 and 2, the second routine during weeks 3 and 4, and the last routine during weeks 5 and 6. Each routine demands more from you—and, in turn, gives you great results. During weeks 1 and 2, you'll learn the beginner modifications for some standard exercises, such as the pushup. In the weeks thereafter, you'll take on the tougher version of those same exercises—and you'll master them, too!

Also, during weeks 1 and 2, you'll do many exercises that work just one side of your body at a time. This will help you to concentrate on doing the move correctly. In coming weeks, however, you'll learn to exercise your right and left sides together, allowing you to complete more moves in less time.

If your upper body is your personal fat zone, do these routines three times a week along with your other fat zone workouts, regular stretching, and walking.

DO . . .

- **Use dumbbells.** Use a weight light enough for you to do the exercise with proper form in a fluid, smooth motion, yet heavy enough to allow you to reach muscle fatigue within 15 repetitions. You may need to use a different-size weight for some muscle groups than others, as larger muscles such as your chest and back are stronger than those in your arms and shoulders. My guide in "Repeat As Needed" will help you find the right weight for you.

- **Push yourself.** You should increase your dumbbell weight when you can do 15 reps and the last 2 or 3 feel easy. If you can do the entire routine without feeling fatigued, you need to add more weight. On your last 2 or 3 reps, you should feel the challenge.

- **Go slowly.** Try not to use momentum. Research shows that the slower you lift, the more muscle you incorporate, making the exercise more effective.

- **Breathe.** Exhale as you contract your muscles (usually the hard part of the exercise) and inhale as you release. Breathing helps you to focus on the movement. It also gives you more energy.

DON'T . . .

- **Develop white knuckles.** Hold your weights firmly enough that you won't drop them. But don't squeeze them so tightly that your hands begin to hurt.

Repeat As Needed

THE THREE UPPER-BODY Fat Zone routines include the most effective exercises for firming and toning your chest, back, shoulders, and arms. Every 2 weeks, you'll take on a new set of exercises, helping you to fully strengthen, shape, and contour your entire upper body.

Your current fitness level will determine how many repetitions you can perform for each exercise. Tune in to your body. Whether you are working your triceps, chest, or shoulders, pay attention to how those muscles feel as you move. When they start to burn and feel fatigued, do two more repetitions and then move on to the next exercise.

Here are a few handy rules of thumb for the right number of repetitions and weight as you progress on this 6-week toning program.

WEEKS 1 AND 2. Most women can start with 2- to 3-pound weights. If in doubt, go lighter rather than heavier. It's safer on your joints and allows you to do more reps, which helps add shape and tone to your muscles rather than size and bulk. Aim for 10 to 15 repetitions of each exercise.

WEEKS 3 AND 4. You can probably move up to 5-pound weights, completing 15 repetitions of each exercise.

WEEKS 5 AND 6. Try moving up to 8-pound weights, completing 15 reps of each exercise.

- **Tense your neck and shoulders.** Keep these muscles relaxed as you raise and lower your arms during different exercises. Always keep your neck nice and long, with your shoulders low and away from your ears.

- **Strain.** I've included stretch breaks through the routines. But any time you need an additional break, take it, especially to stretch your neck.

- **Ignore stretching.** These routines all take 20 minutes or less. Don't try to shorten them even more by skipping the suggested stretches. These stretches let you make the most of your upper body work by allowing you to recover between exercises, helping you to work each movement to your fullest potential.

- **Lock your joints.** Even when your arms are extended during an exercise, always keep your elbows soft and slightly bent to prevent any pressure on your elbow joints.

WEEKS 1 & 2

During your first 2 weeks of Upper-Body Fat Zone exercises, you'll learn many strength-training moves that you will build upon in the coming weeks. For example, you'll begin doing pushups—don't let that scare you. I've modified the standard pushup so that any beginner can do it, including you!

In these first 2 weeks, you'll also do many exercises that work just one side of your upper body at a time. While this may take a little longer, it allows you to concentrate more on the muscle you are working, ensuring that you use proper form.

> ➤ FIRMS THE SIDES OF YOUR CHEST
> ➤ PREVENTS FAT FROM BULGING FROM THE SIDE OF YOUR BIKINI TOP

Chest Fly

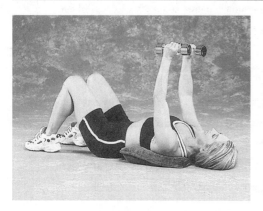

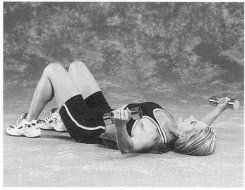

A. Lie with your back on a pillow. Bend your knees and keep your feet flat on the floor. Hold the dumbbells in your hands with your arms slightly bent and extended above your chest.

B. Slowly lower your arms out to the sides as you inhale, keeping them slightly bent at the same angle throughout. Slowly exhale and squeeze your chest muscles together as you bring the weights back to the starting position, as if you were hugging a large beach ball. Keep your tummy tight and your lower back flat throughout. Do 10 to 15 repetitions. (For extra fat-burning power, do two sets of 10 to 15 repetitions.)

> ➤ SHRINKS THE FLAB THAT HANGS OVER YOUR BRA STRAP
> ➤ TONES YOUR UPPER BACK ➤ MAKES YOUR WAIST APPEAR SMALLER

Lat Pullover

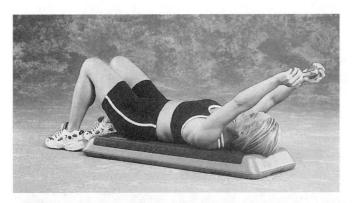

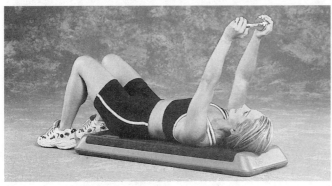

A. Lie on your back on an aerobics step, weight bench, pillow, or stability ball. Bend your knees, placing your feet flat on the ground, and hold a dumbbell with both hands, your arms extended above your eyes. Inhale as you bring the dumbbell back about 1 foot behind your head.

B. Imagine that someone is pressing down on your dumbbell, causing your shoulder blades to retract and press against the surface you're lying upon. Keep your shoulders pressed down as you exhale and bring your hands forward to eye level. Don't allow your back to rise—keep your ribs down. Inhale as you lower the weight back to the starting position. Do 10 to 15 repetitions. (For extra fat-burning power, do two sets of 10 to 15 repetitions.)

MAXIMUM RESULTS Minimum Time

If you do this exercise correctly, you'll probably be able to complete only 5 to 10 repetitions before fatigue. I shake from doing these! If, however, you do the exercise incorrectly, you won't feel it at all. To make the move most effective, keep your shoulder blades pressed down, as if magnets were pulling them toward the center of the earth. Also, imagine that the dumbbell is attached to a pulley and that you must pull against this pulley to raise the dumbbell.

Modified Beginner Pushup

A. Kneel on your mat and place your hands on an aerobics step or stair step. Your hands should be under your shoulders. Lift your feet and shins so that you are balanced on your hands and knees, with a long, straight torso.

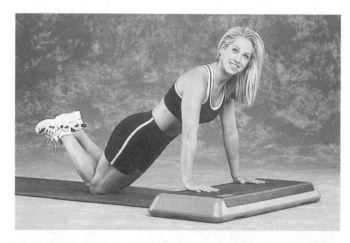

B. With a straight back and tight tummy, slowly bend your elbows as you inhale and lower your chest toward the mat. Lower yourself as far as you can while still being able to press up to the starting position. Exhale as you straighten your elbows and press up, keeping your neck long and relaxed. Repeat until fatigue. Do 10 to 15 repetitions. (For extra fat-burning power, do two sets of 10 to 15 repetitions.)

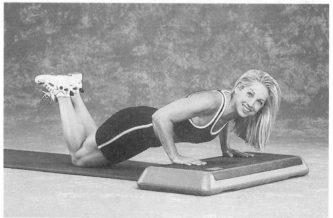

MAXIMUM RESULTS | Minimum Time

Don't let the pushup scare you. You may be able to complete only 1 repetition on your first try. Just do your best and focus on those chest muscles, using them to press up.

STRETCH BREAK

Chest Expansion

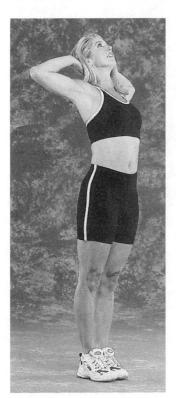

Stand with your feet aligned under your hips and your arms at your sides. Place your hands behind your head with your elbows open to the sides. Inhale and extend through your crown to lengthen your spine and straighten your back. Exhale as you bring your elbows back as far as you can, as shown, to open your chest. Hold for 20 seconds, breathing normally, relax, and repeat one time.

MAXIMUM RESULTS | Minimum Time

If you've spent years working at a desk job, you probably have a very tight chest and rounded shoulders, so you may not be able to pull your elbows back very far. That's okay. The secret to this stretch is keeping your shoulders low, away from your ears, and letting your sternum rise.

"Do this stretch every day to improve your posture and increase your oxygen and lung capacity. More oxygen equals more energy!"

Standing Biceps Curl

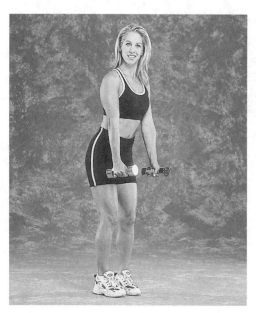

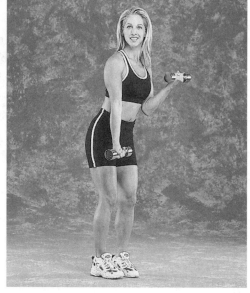

A. Stand while holding a pair of dumbbells at your sides, palms facing each other, and with your feet slightly wider than hip-width apart. Extend through the crown of your head, relax your shoulders, tighten your abs, and straighten your back.

B. Exhale as you slowly curl your left hand toward your left shoulder, keeping your elbow in close to your torso. Rotate your palm inward as you curl your hand toward your shoulder, squeezing your biceps muscle. Inhale as you lower, then repeat with your right hand. Continue to alternate sides until you've done 10 to 15 repetitions on each side. (For extra fat-burning power, do two sets of 10 to 15 repetitions.)

MAXIMUM RESULTS	Minimum Time

You can do curls almost anywhere, even during your walking workouts. I sometimes do them while I'm on the phone or while cooking to help fit in part of my workout while I'm doing something else.

SEATED BICEPS CURL (VARIATION)

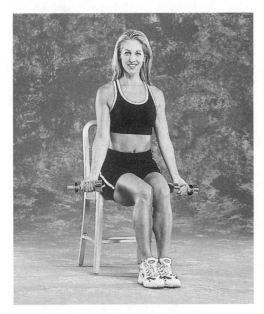

If you experience lower back discomfort, do the biceps curls while seated.

Sit on the edge of a sturdy chair, as shown. Extend through the crown of your head, relax your shoulders, tighten your abs, and straighten your back. Exhale as you slowly curl your left hand toward your left shoulder, keeping your elbow in close to your torso. Rotate your palm toward you as you curl your hand toward your shoulder, squeezing your biceps muscle. Inhale as you lower, then repeat with your right hand. Continue to alternate sides until you've done 10 to 15 repetitions on each side. (For extra fat-burning power, do two sets of 10 to 15 repetitions.)

"It's never too late to start working out with weights."

One-Arm Row

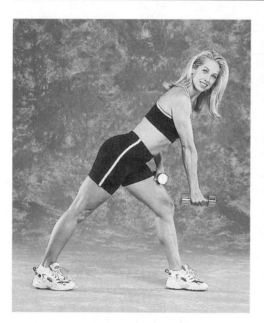
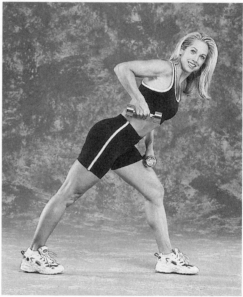

A. Stand with your feet slightly wider than shoulder-width apart and with a slight bend in your knees. Hold a dumbbell in your right hand. Take a step forward with your left foot, bend your left knee, and lean forward from your waist about 45 degrees. Place your left hand on your left thigh to support your back. Extend your right arm down toward the floor, as shown.

B. Keep your abs tight and back flat as you exhale and pull the weight up toward your armpit, as if you were tugging on the starter to a lawn mower. Inhale and lower. Do 10 to 15 repetitions and then switch sides. (For extra fat-burning power, do two sets of 10 to 15 repetitions.)

MAXIMUM RESULTS	Minimum Time

To pinpoint the correct back muscle, retract your shoulder blades as you keep your elbow close to your body throughout the movement. You should feel the inside of your upper arm brush lightly against your ribs as you raise and lower the weight.

One-Arm Row with Chair (variation)

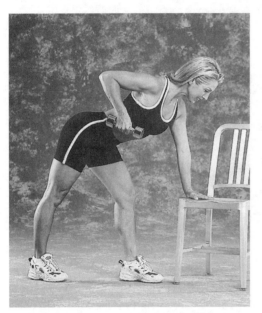

If you experience back discomfort, lean against a chair to release any pressure from your lower back.

Stand with your left palm against the seat of the chair, with your left leg forward and right leg back. Hold a weight in your right hand. Keep your abs tight and back flat as you exhale and pull the weight up toward your armpit, as shown, as if you were tugging on the starter to a lawn mower. Inhale and lower. Do 10 to 15 repetitions and then switch sides. (For extra fat-burning power, do two sets of 10 to 15 repetitions.)

"I love this exercise. It's so effective that I incorporate it into just about all of my workouts!"

➤ FIRMS THE FLAB BEHIND YOUR ARMS
➤ LETS YOU WAVE YOUR HAND WITH CONFIDENCE, WITHOUT JIGGLING

Standing Triceps Kickback

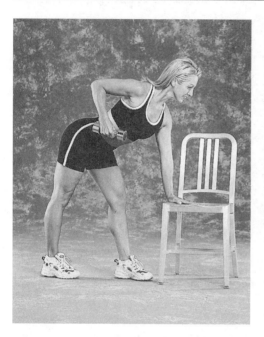
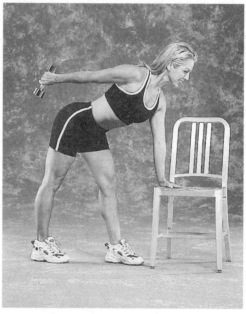

A. Stand with your feet slightly wider than shoulder-width apart and with a slight bend in your knees. Hold a dumbbell in your right hand. Take a step forward with your left foot, bend your left knee, and lean forward from your waist about 45 degrees. Place your left palm on the seat of a chair for balance. Bend your right arm, as shown, so that your right elbow and shoulder form a parallel line with the floor and your knuckles face the floor.

B. Slowly exhale and extend your right hand up past your thigh and behind your torso. Hold for 1 second, then inhale and lower. Do 10 to 15 repetitions, then switch arm and leg positions and repeat on the other side. (For extra fat-burning power, do two sets of 10 to 15 repetitions.)

MAXIMUM RESULTS	Minimum Time
Keep your elbow close to your body as you extend and lower your arm. Don't allow your elbow to move. This will focus the work in your triceps muscle.	

Standing Triceps Toner

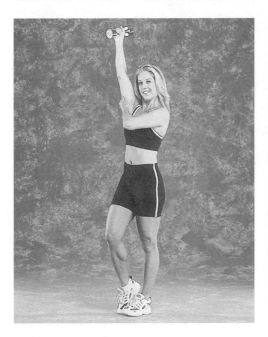

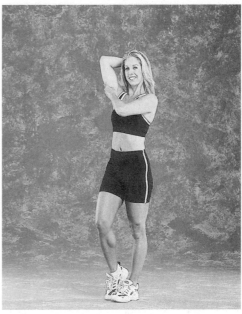

A. Stand with your feet aligned under your hips. Tighten your abs and straighten your back. Hold a weight in your right hand and extend your right arm overhead. Use your other hand to support your right arm and "feel" the muscle work.

B. As you slowly inhale, bend your right elbow and lower the weight behind your head toward your right shoulder. Raise the weight as you exhale. Do 10 to 15 repetitions and then switch arms. (For extra fat-burning power, do two sets of 10 to 15 repetitions.)

MAXIMUM RESULTS	Minimum Time
Keep your elbow as close to your head as possible to isolate the work in your triceps muscle. If you experience lower back discomfort, do this exercise in a seated position.	

STRETCH BREAK

Triceps Stretch

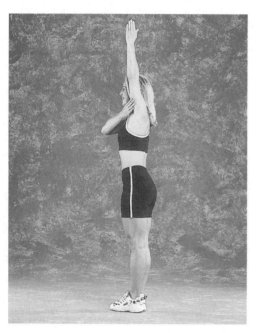

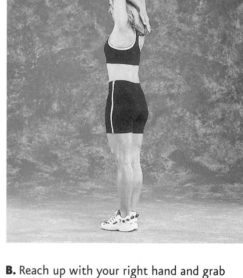

A. Stand with your feet aligned under your hips. Tighten your abs and straighten your back. Inhale as you raise your left arm overhead, as shown, and then exhale and bend it, bringing your left hand toward your right shoulder blade and giving yourself a pat on the back.

B. Reach up with your right hand and grab your left elbow, using gentle pressure with your right hand to pull your left elbow back and increase the stretch. Hold for 20 seconds, breathing normally, and then repeat on the other side.

MAXIMUM RESULTS	Minimum Time
Try not to allow your arm to press your head forward. Doing so may hurt your neck and decrease the effectiveness of the stretch.	

Standing Front Raise

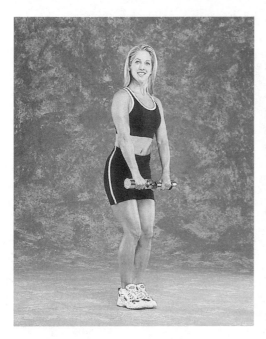
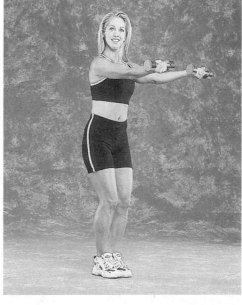

A. Stand with your abs tight, your back flat, and your knees slightly bent. Hold a pair of dumbbells in front of your thighs, with your palms facing your thighs.

B. Exhale as you raise your arms in front of your torso, bringing the dumbbells to shoulder level. Then rotate your arms slowly until your palms face up, as shown.

—continued

" There's nothing **more attractive** than **toned arms.** "

➤ TARGETS THE FRONTS OF YOUR SHOULDERS
➤ FIRMS THE AREA UNDER YOUR ARMS SO NOTHING PRESSES OUT OF A TANK TOP

Standing Front Raise—*continued*

C. Rotate them back until your arms face downward, and then inhale as you lower the weights to the starting position. Repeat until fatigue. Do 10 to 15 repetitions. (For extra fat-burning power, do two sets of 10 to 15 repetitions.)

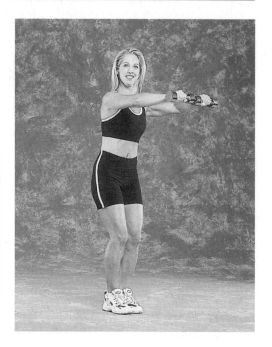

MAXIMUM RESULTS	Minimum Time
Raise your arms very slowly to shoulder level. This will prevent you from arching your back to throw momentum into the lift. If you experience lower back discomfort, do this exercise while seated.	

"Break out the **strapless dress**—you're going to have some **shapely shoulders!"**

Standing Overhead Press

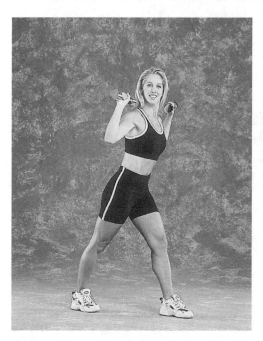

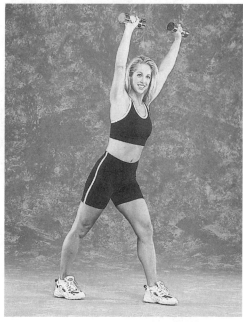

A. Stand with your feet shoulder-width apart, your abs tight, your back flat, and your knees slightly bent. Take a step forward with your left foot. Hold a pair of dumbbells at shoulder level with your arms bent, palms facing forward, and elbows open out to the sides.

B. Exhale as you press the dumbbells up, extending your arms over your head. Inhale as you lower the weights. Do 10 to 15 repetitions. (For extra fat-burning power, do two sets of 10 to 15 repetitions.)

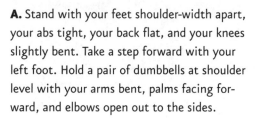

MAXIMUM RESULTS	Minimum Time

Try to keep the dumbbells directly over your shoulders, not behind them. This will isolate the top of your shoulder muscle, carving a perfectly strong shoulder line. If you experience lower back discomfort, do this exercise while seated.

THE UPPER BODY   113

STRETCH BREAK

Upper Back and Shoulder Stretch

Stand with your left foot forward and your hands at your sides. Raise your arms in front to chest level, with your arms bent and your palms facing each other.

Bring your left arm toward the right and your right arm toward the left, crossing your left arm under your right, as shown, so that your right hand points toward 10 o'clock and your left toward 2 o'clock. Inhale and exhale then lower your left hand and raise your right, bringing both hands in a semicircle until your palms meet in an intertwined prayer position. Hold for 20 seconds, breathing normally. Then switch arm positions and repeat.

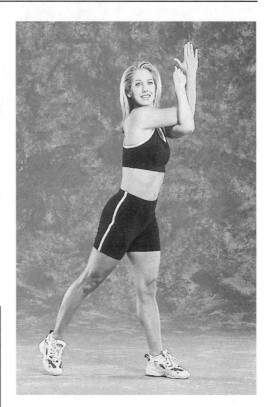

MAXIMUM RESULTS	Minimum Time

You can stretch different areas of your back and shoulders by moving your elbows up and down the centerline of your torso. You can also round your upper back slightly as you press your elbows away from your body and bring your shoulder blades farther apart to deepen the stretch.

During the next 2 weeks, you'll build upon many of the exercises you learned in weeks 1 and 2. For example, you'll be doing a slightly more challenging version of the pushup. Also, instead of isolating one side of your body and then the other, as you did in some exercises, you'll target both sides of your upper body simultaneously.

You'll also learn a series of new exercises designed to target different areas of your upper body muscles, helping you to work them from every angle. These new exercises will add variety, which will keep you mentally motivated as well as make your muscles work harder to complete each lift. You'll challenge yourself and ultimately create a more beautiful body.

➤ FIRMS YOUR OUTER CHEST MUSCLES

Chest Press

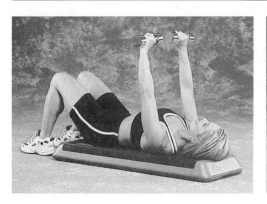 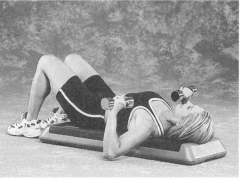

A. Lie on your back on an aerobics step, a pillow placed under your upper back, or a weight bench, with your knees bent and feet flat on the floor, holding a dumbbell in each hand.

B. Bend your arms so that your upper arms are parallel to the floor and the weights are in line with your chest. Keep your abs tight and back flat as you exhale and press the weights up, extending your arms directly above your chest but not locking your elbows. Inhale as you lower the weights. Do 15 repetitions or repeat until fatigue. (For extra fat-burning power, do two sets of 15 repetitions.)

➤ CREATES THE ILLUSION OF CLEAVAGE ➤ LIFTS YOUR BREASTS
➤ BUILDS ON THE MODIFIED PUSHUP

Pushup on Knees

A. Kneel on your mat and place your hands under your shoulders. Lift your feet and shins so that you are balanced on your hands and knees.

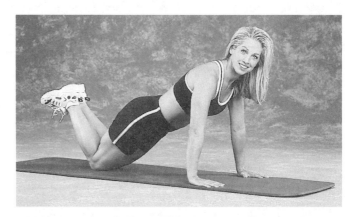

B. With a straight back and tight abs, slowly bend your elbows as you inhale and lower your chest toward the mat. Lower yourself as far as you can while still being able to press yourself up to the starting position. Exhale as you straighten your elbows and press up. Do 15 repetitions or repeat until fatigue. (For extra fat-burning power, do two sets of 15 repetitions.)

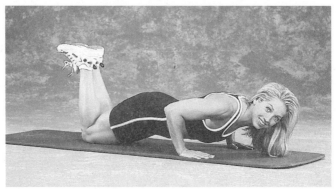

MAXIMUM RESULTS | Minimum Time

To help press yourself up, blow air out through your mouth, imagining the air pushing against your mat to raise your torso. Of course, the air won't raise you—your chest muscles and abs will. The simple visualization, however, helps to create an "I can" attitude in your brain, which in turn makes you more likely to recruit as many muscle fibers as possible to perform the pushup.

STRETCH BREAK

Chest Opener

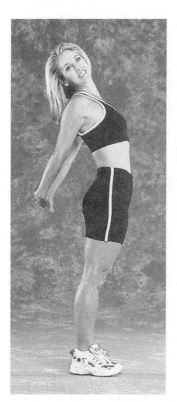

Stand with your feet aligned under your hips and your arms at your sides. Extend through your crown to lengthen your spine and straighten your back. Roll your shoulders up, back, and down, then grasp your hands behind your back, interlacing your fingers and bringing your palms close together. Inhale and then exhale and extend your arms out and up, as shown, feeling your chest open. Slightly arch your back as you lengthen back into a slight back bend. Hold for 20 seconds, breathing normally, lower, and repeat one time.

MAXIMUM RESULTS	Minimum Time

Try interlacing your fingers in a different position. Usually, when we clasp our hands behind our backs for the chest expansion, we always clasp them the same way, with the thumbs down. Holding the thumbs and index fingers on top will slightly change the stretch.

> ❝You are creating a body
> that is strong and balanced.❞

➤ TARGETS THE BACKS OF YOUR SHOULDERS
➤ SHRINKS THE FLAB THAT TENDS TO PRESS OUT OVER YOUR BRA STRAP
➤ MINIMIZES YOUR WAIST

Bilateral Row

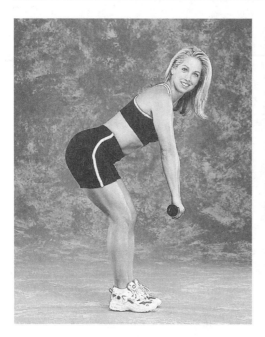 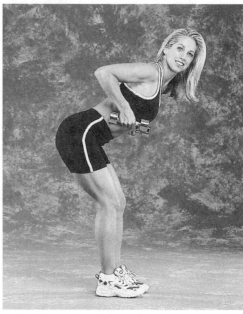

A. Standing with a slight bend in your knees, hold a dumbbell in each hand. Bend forward from the waist about 45 degrees and extend your arms toward the floor, as shown.

B. Maintain a tight tummy as you exhale and pull the weights up toward your armpits, keeping your elbows close to your torso. Inhale as you lower the weights. Do 15 repetitions or repeat until fatigue. (For extra fat-burning power, do two sets of 15 repetitions.)

MAXIMUM RESULTS	Minimum Time
Raise your elbows as high as possible, pausing for a couple seconds at the top of the contraction to really make your back muscles work to hold up the weights.	

Double-Arm Fly

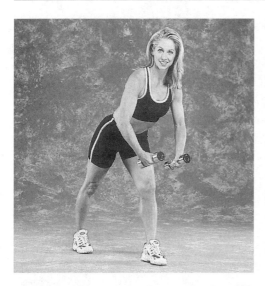 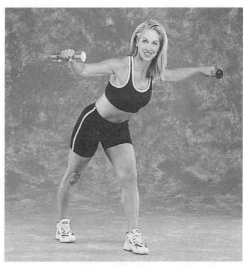

A. Stand with your feet slightly wider than shoulder-width apart and with a slight bend in your knees. Take a step forward with your left foot, bend your left knee, and lean forward from your waist about 45 degrees. Holding a dumbbell in each hand, palms facing each other, extend your arms down toward the floor, with your elbows slightly bent.

B. Exhale and bring your arms out to the sides, leading with your pinkies and squeezing your shoulder blades together. Lift until your arms are parallel to the ground. Inhale as you lower the weights. Do 15 repetitions or repeat until fatigue. (For extra fat-burning power, do two sets of 15 repetitions.)

" Remember: If the last few reps feel easy, it's time to add more weight."

MAXIMUM RESULTS	Minimum Time
Rather than focusing on lifting your hands, focus on squeezing your shoulder blades together, allowing your shoulder blades to lift the weight.	

Bear Hug

Stand with your feet aligned under your hips. Extend your arms in front of your chest with your palms facing each other. Bring your right palm past the left and your left palm past the right in a large arc, eventually reaching your right palm toward your left shoulder blade and your left palm toward your right shoulder blade, as shown, exhaling and feeling the stretch along your upper back. Hold for 20 seconds, breathing normally.

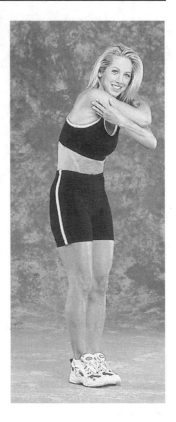

MAXIMUM RESULTS	Minimum Time

While you give yourself a big hug, try to add more space between your shoulder blades as you spread them farther apart to increase the stretch.

Standing Lateral Raise

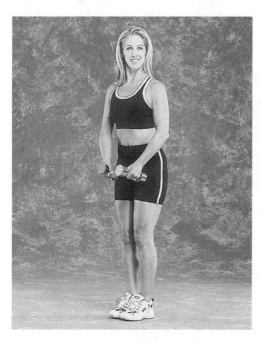

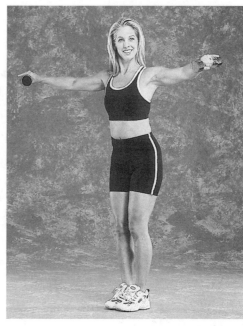

A. Stand with your abs tight, your back flat, and your knees slightly bent. Hold a pair of dumbbells at your sides.

B. Exhale as you raise your arms out to the sides with your palms down. Bring the dumbbells to shoulder level, keeping a slight bend in your elbows. Keep your neck long. Inhale as you lower your arms. Do 15 repetitions or repeat until fatigue. (For extra fat-burning power, do two sets of 15 repetitions.)

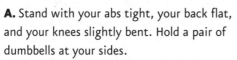

MAXIMUM RESULTS	Minimum Time

Go slowly. It's easy to use momentum, as if you were flapping a pair of wings. The more slowly and more controlled the movement, however, the more effective the exercise. Also, as you raise the weights, try to lengthen your arms by pressing outward through your knuckles.

➤ FIRMS THE BACKS OF YOUR UPPER ARMS
➤ ALLOWS YOU TO WAVE YOUR HAND WITH CONFIDENCE

Bilateral Kickback

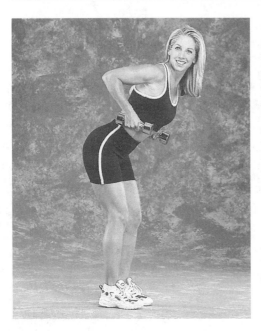
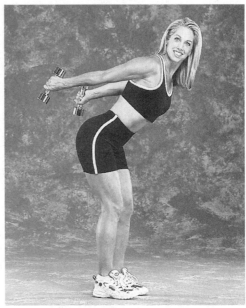

A. Stand with your feet slightly wider than shoulder-width apart and with a slight bend in your knees. Hold a pair of dumbbells at your sides. Bend forward from your waist about 45 degrees. Bend your arms, as shown, so that your upper arms rest against your sides but your knuckles point toward the floor.

B. Exhale as you slowly raise both hands behind you. Inhale as you return them to the starting position. Do 15 repetitions or repeat until fatigue. (For extra fat-burning power, do two sets of 15 repetitions.)

MAXIMUM RESULTS	Minimum Time
At the top of the contraction, hold the weights and turn your pinkies inward. This slightly changes the area of the triceps muscle that you target, helping to work all angles of the muscle.	

Low Hover

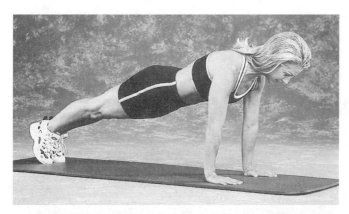

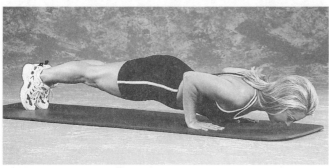

A. Kneel on your mat with your palms under your collarbones and your knees under your hips. Extend your legs and press into the balls of your feet, raising your knees off the floor into a pushup position, as shown.

B. Inhale and exhale and bend your elbows, keeping them in close to your torso, and lower your body into the hover, keeping your entire torso a few inches off your mat. Hold for 10 to 30 seconds, breathing normally, and then relax. Do 15 repetitions or repeat until fatigue. (For extra fat-burning power, do two sets of 15 repetitions.)

MAXIMUM RESULTS	Minimum Time

Resist the urge to rotate your elbows out away from your body. This will change the exercise, targeting your chest rather than your triceps. Instead, keep your upper arms as close to your torso as you can. The closer your elbows are to your body, the more effective the exercise.

LOW HOVER ON KNEES (VARIATION)

If you lack the strength to do the hover with straight legs, try it with your knees bent on the mat.

Kneel on your mat with your hands under your collarbones and knees under your hips. Walk your hands forward about 6 inches. Then inhale and lift your feet and shins off the mat, so that you are balanced on your knees and palms. Exhale and lower your torso into the hover, as shown, making sure to keep your upper arms close to your body. Hold for 10 to 30 seconds, breathing normally, and then relax. Do 15 repetitions or repeat until fatigue. (For extra fat-burning power, do two sets of 15 repetitions.)

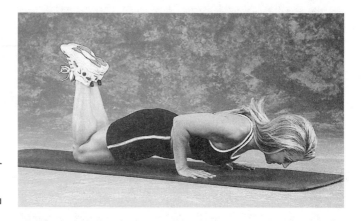

MAXIMUM RESULTS	Minimum Time

Try to keep your back long and straight as you lower yourself, pulling up through your abs to prevent your hips from sinking downward.

"This is a **challenging** exercise. Think **positive** thoughts. If you **think** you **can**, you **will**."

Lat Pulldown 1

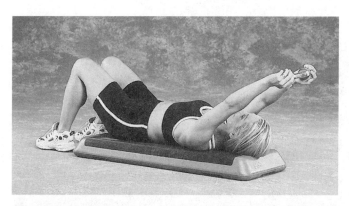

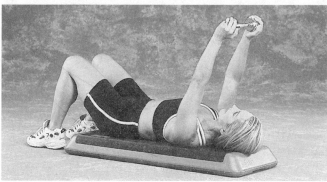

A. Lie on your back on an aerobics step, weight bench, pillow, or stability ball. Bend your knees, placing your feet flat on the ground, and hold a dumbbell with both hands, your arms extended above your eyes. Inhale as you bring your arms back, about 1 foot behind your head, as shown.

B. Imagine that someone is pressing down on the dumbbell, causing your shoulder blades to retract and press against the surface that you're lying upon. Keep your shoulders pressed down as you exhale and bring your hands forward to chest level. Don't allow your back to rise. Inhale as you bring your hands back to the starting position. Do 15 repetitions or repeat until fatigue. (For extra fat-burning power, do two sets of 15 repetitions.)

MAXIMUM RESULTS	Minimum Time

If you do this exercise correctly, you'll probably be able to complete only 5 to 10 repetitions before fatigue. If, however, you do the exercise incorrectly, you won't feel it at all. To make the move most effective, keep your shoulder blades pressed down, as if magnets were pulling them toward the center of the earth.

STRETCH BREAK

Seated Triceps Stretch

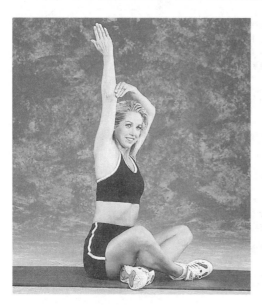 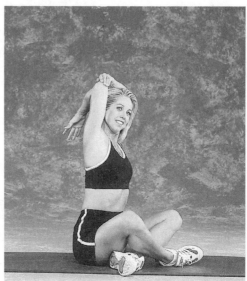

A. Sit on your mat in a comfortable, cross-legged position. Raise your right arm overhead, as shown, and then bend it, bringing your right hand toward your left shoulder blade.

B. Inhale and reach up with your left hand, then exhale and grab your right elbow, using gentle pressure with your left hand to increase the stretch. Hold for 20 seconds, breathing normally, and then repeat on the other side.

"You've worked hard, so give yourself a pat on the back."

MAXIMUM RESULTS	Minimum Time
Try not to allow your arm to press your head forward. This may hurt your neck and decrease the effectiveness of the stretch.	

During weeks 5 and 6, you'll continue to build on some of the exercises you learned during the first 4 weeks of the Upper-Body Fat Zone routines. For example, you'll now attempt a full pushup! I know you can do it. Believe in yourself!

You'll also do some of the exercises from weeks 3 and 4 while seated in a chair. This will help you to isolate your upper body muscles. Finally, you'll learn a series of new, challenging moves.

You'll need a chair, a large stability ball, an exercise mat, and dumbbells for this routine.

> ➤ FIRMS THE SIDES OF YOUR CHEST ➤ LIFTS YOUR BREASTS
> ➤ CREATES THE ILLUSION OF CLEAVAGE

Chest Press Incline

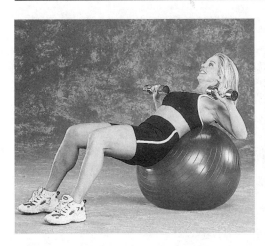 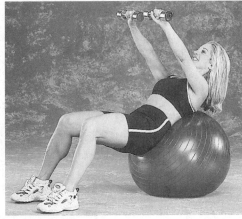

A. Sit on a large stability ball, holding a dumbbell in each hand. Slowly walk your feet forward as you slide your back down the ball until your thighs are parallel to the floor and the ball rests against your lower to middle back. Hold the dumbbells just above your collarbones with your arms bent and elbows to the sides at shoulder level, as shown.

B. Exhale and press the dumbbells up and forward, keeping them in line with your chest. Inhale as you lower them. Do 15 repetitions or repeat until fatigue. (For extra fat-burning power, do two sets of 15 repetitions.)

Pushup

A. Kneel on a mat with your palms under your collarbones and your knees under your hips. Extend one leg and then the other to balance on the balls of your feet and raise your knees off the floor into a standard pushup position, as shown.

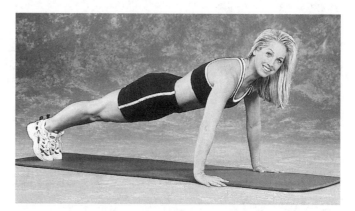

B. With a straight back, slowly bend your elbows as you inhale and lower your chest toward the mat. Lower yourself as close to the floor as you can while still being able to press up to the starting position. Exhale and straighten your elbows as you press up. Do 15 repetitions or repeat until fatigue. (For extra fat-burning power, do two sets of 15 repetitions.)

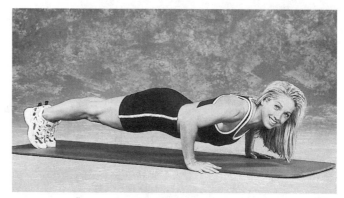

MAXIMUM RESULTS | Minimum Time

Keep your abs tight throughout the pushup, particularly if you tend to experience lower back pain. Tight abs will prevent your hips from sinking down and allow you to focus on targeting your chest.

Pushup on Ball (variation)

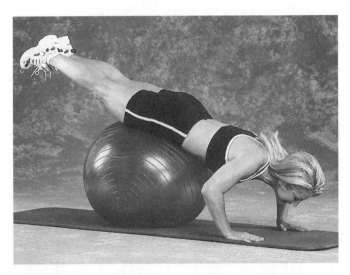

MAXIMUM RESULTS Minimum Time

Try not to allow your hips to sink down toward the floor when you do the pushup, as this will place pressure on your lower back. To keep your hips and pelvis in the proper position, pull up through your abs as you do the pushup on the ball.

To really challenge yourself, try the pushup with your legs on a stability ball. This will test your strength and balance.

Lift into a pushup position with your shins or thighs on a large stability ball and your hands under your chest. With a straight back, slowly bend your elbows as you inhale and lower your chest toward the mat. Lower as close to the floor as you can while still being able to press up to the starting position. Exhale and straighten your elbows as you press up. Do 15 repetitions or repeat until fatigue. (For extra fat-burning power, do two sets of 15 repetitions.)

> " There's no **better confidence** **builder** than the **pushup.** "

STRETCH BREAK

Seated Chest Expansion

Sit on your mat in a comfortable cross-legged position. Inhale and extend through your crown to lengthen your spine and straighten your back. Roll your shoulders up, back, and down and then exhale and place your fingertips on your mat a few inches behind your buttocks. Allow your chest to open as your sternum rises. Hold for 20 seconds, relax, and repeat one time, breathing normally.

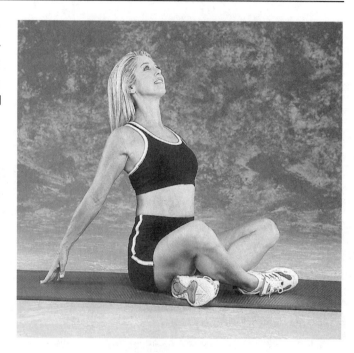

MAXIMUM RESULTS Minimum Time

Though your sternum will rise as you open your chest, don't allow your ribs to thrust forward. To keep them in position and gain an even deeper stretch, tighten your lower abdomen as you stretch.

Lat Pulldown 2

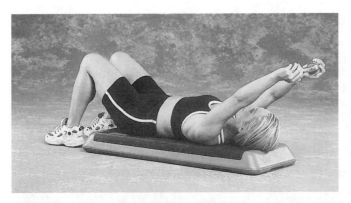

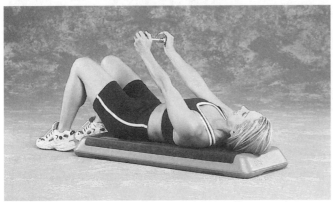

A. Lie on your back on an aerobics step, weight bench, pillow, or stability ball. Bend your knees, placing your feet flat on the ground, and hold a dumbbell with both hands, your arms extended above your eyes. Inhale as you bring your arms back, about 1 foot behind your head, as shown.

B. Imagine that someone is pressing down on your dumbbell, causing your shoulder blades to retract and press against the surface you're lying upon. Keep your shoulders pressed down as you exhale and bring your hands forward to navel level. Don't allow your back to rise. Inhale as you bring your hands back to the starting position. Do 15 repetitions or repeat until fatigue. (For extra fat-burning power, do two sets of 15 repetitions.)

MAXIMUM RESULTS | Minimum Time

If you do this exercise correctly, you'll probably be able to complete only 5 to 10 repetitions before fatigue. If, however, you do the exercise incorrectly, you won't feel it at all. To make the move most effective, keep your shoulder blades pressed down, as if magnets were pulling them toward the center of the earth.

Seated Double-Arm Row

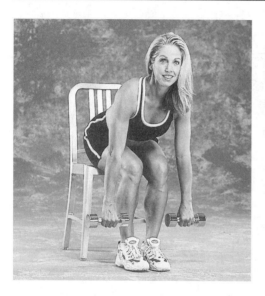

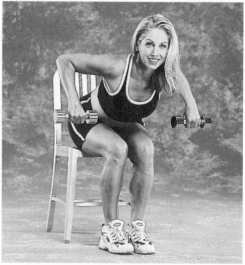

A. Sit on the edge of your chair with your knees bent and feet flat on the floor. Hold a dumbbell in each hand, with your palms facing behind you. Bend forward from the waist about 90 degrees so that your torso is nearly parallel to the floor. Extend your arms toward the floor.

B. Keep your abs tight as you exhale and pull the weights up toward your armpits. Inhale as you lower them. Do 15 repetitions or repeat until fatigue. (For extra fat-burning power, do two sets of 15 repetitions.)

MAXIMUM RESULTS	Minimum Time

Try changing your grip for every other repetition to slightly target a different area of your back. Do so simply by turning your palms forward. Do one repetition with your palms forward and another with them facing behind you, alternating back and forth.

Seated Back Fly

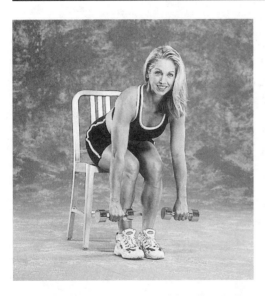 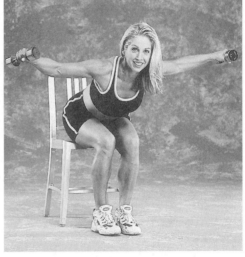

A. Sit on the edge of a chair with your knees bent and feet flat on the floor. Hold a dumbbell in each hand. Bend forward from the waist about 90 degrees so that your torso is nearly parallel with the floor. Extend your arms toward the floor.

B. Exhale and bring your arms out to the sides, leading with your pinkies and squeezing your shoulder blades together. Stop once your arms are parallel to the floor, then inhale as you lower. Do 15 repetitions or repeat until fatigue. (For extra fat-burning power, do two sets of 15 repetitions.)

> "The waif look is out. The toned look is in."

MAXIMUM RESULTS	Minimum Time
Rather than focusing on lifting your hands, focus on squeezing your shoulder blades together, allowing your shoulder blades to lift the weights.	

Seated Overhead Press

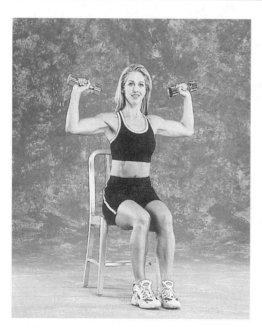 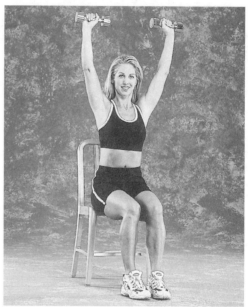

A. Sit on the edge of a chair with your knees bent and feet flat on the floor. Keep your abs tight and your back flat. Hold a pair of dumbbells, palms facing forward, at shoulder level with your arms bent and elbows open out to the sides.

B. Exhale as you press the dumbbells up, extending your arms over your head. Inhale as you lower the weights. Do 15 repetitions or repeat until fatigue. (For extra fat-burning power, do two sets of 15 repetitions.)

MAXIMUM RESULTS	Minimum Time

Keep your shoulders low and away from your ears as you do the exercise. Sometimes it helps to do a few shoulder shrugs first: With no weights in your hands, lift your shoulders as close to your ears as possible, and then exhale as you let them drop down, releasing all of the tension from your shoulders.

Seated Combined Front and Lateral Raise

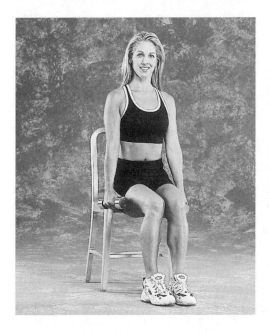 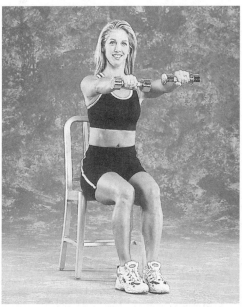

A. Sit on the edge of a chair with your knees bent and feet flat on the floor. Hold a dumbbell in each hand with your arms extended and the dumbbells on either side of your thighs.

B. Exhale as you raise your arms in front of your torso, palms down, bringing the dumbbells to shoulder level.

—continued

Seated Combined Front and Lateral Raise—*continued*

C. Inhale as you lower them, and then exhale and raise the dumbbells out to your sides to shoulder level. Continue alternating between front and lateral raises until you've completed 15 repetitions or reached fatigue. (For extra fat-burning power, do two sets of 15 repetitions.)

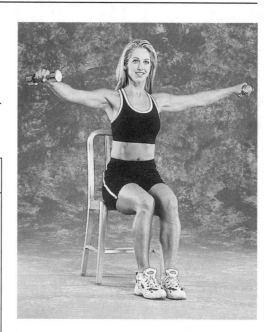

MAXIMUM RESULTS	Minimum Time

If your neck tends to feel tense when you do this exercise, put your weights down on the floor and try this simple fix: Extend your arms out to the sides. Now, focus your attention on your shoulder blades. Place all of the weight of your arms into your shoulder blades, feeling them drop down your back under the weight. This should remove tension from your neck and even your arms. Take a moment to memorize this sensation. Then pick up your weights and try the exercise again, this time concentrating on keeping your shoulder blades low on your back.

> "Use proper form. Slow down and feel the exercise."

Triceps Chair Dip

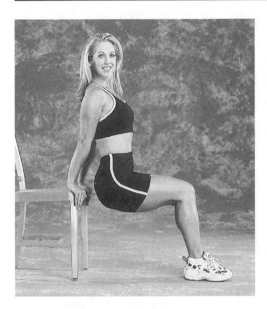

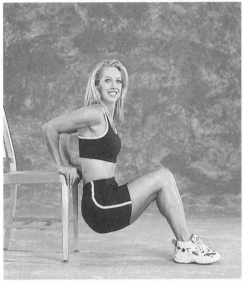

A. Sit on the edge of a chair. Place your palms on the front edge of the chair on either side of your buttocks. Press into your hands to lift your buttocks and move them forward off the chair. Once in the starting position, you should have a 90-degree angle bend in your knees, as shown.

B. Inhale and slowly bend your elbows as you lower your buttocks toward the floor. Once your arms bend 90 degrees, exhale and press back up. Do 15 repetitions or repeat until fatigue. (For extra fat-burning power, do two sets of 15 repetitions.)

MAXIMUM RESULTS	Minimum Time
Bend your arms straight back, not to the sides. Also, try not to press into your feet to rise to the starting position. You can also try this with your legs extended in front for more of a challenge.	

➤ FIRMS THE BACKS OF YOUR UPPER ARMS

Triceps Chair Dip on One Leg

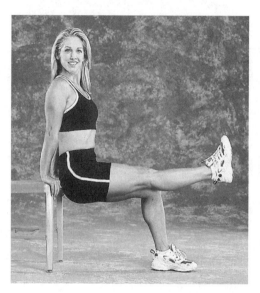 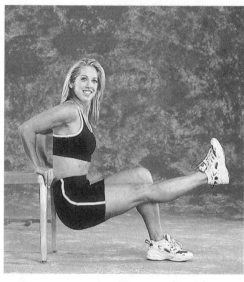

A. Sit on the edge of your chair. Place your palms on the front edge of the chair on either side of your buttocks. Press into your hands to lift your buttocks and move them forward off the chair. You should have a 90-degree angle bend in your knees. Lift and extend your right leg so that your right thigh and calf are parallel to the floor, as shown.

B. Inhale and slowly bend your elbows as you lower your buttocks toward the floor. Once your arms bend 90 degrees, exhale and press back up. Repeat five times with your right leg extended. Then lower your right foot to the floor and extend your left leg. Repeat five more times.

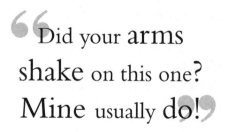

"Did your **arms** **shake** on this one? **Mine** usually do!"

MAXIMUM RESULTS	Minimum Time
This is a tough move, particularly after just doing standard chair dips. Try your best. I know you can do it!	

STRETCH BREAK

Seated Arm Stretch

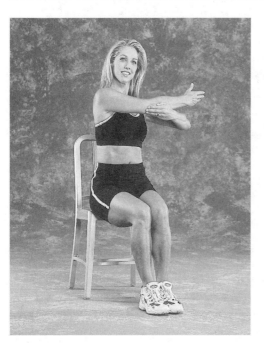

Sit on your chair with your knees bent and feet flat on the floor. Inhale and raise your right arm across your chest, pressing your right elbow with your left hand. Exhale as you use your left hand to gently press your right arm to the left. Hold for 20 seconds and then repeat on the other side.

MAXIMUM RESULTS	Minimum Time
Try to keep your right shoulder low instead of hunched up toward your ear. If you allow your right shoulder to rise toward your right ear, you won't feel as much of a stretch.	

"Congratulations. You did it.
You're doing a **great job."**

CHAPTER 6

The Midsection

I'm known for my tummy. I'll admit this image wasn't accidental. During my twenties, I often showed off my tight abs, asking anyone and everyone to "feel my tummy." Back then, people used to snicker, "You just wait until you have a baby. Then we'll see how flat it is!"

Well, I had a baby at age 33 and then another at age 37. Guess what? I still have a flat tummy!

I'm living proof that any woman can whip her abdominal area into shape. With each of my pregnancies I gained a total of 35 pounds, and by the time I left the hospital I'd lost only 10 of those extra pounds. I still looked as if I were pregnant!

But I worked the extra pounds off, and slowly but surely flattened my midsection. I went from a 44-inch waistline at 9 months pregnant to a 24-inch waistline within 3 months.

Now that I'm 46, I still ask people to feel my tummy. It seems that no matter where I go, people tell me how much my ab workouts have really helped them. Husbands love to tell me how much I've helped their wives get back into shape after a baby. Their comments always make me feel good.

I can tell you, keeping my abs flat and firm after age 40 isn't as simple as it was during my twenties. Twenty years ago, I could occasionally slack off on my abdominal routine, sometimes for as long as 2 weeks and not notice a difference. Today, I have to stick with it. If I go as little as 4 days without working my abs, I notice them starting to soften.

So you see, I'm not a genetic anomaly. I do work at keeping my abs firm, and you can achieve the very same results by doing my favorite tummy-tightening exercises. Before I get to those midsection-shrinking routines, however, let's take a look at the physiology behind tummy flab.

The Anatomy of a Tight Tummy

Your abdominal area can stretch out, lose strength, and begin to bulge for numerous reasons. Simple lack of use allows your internal organs to press against your abdominal wall, creating a rounded appearance, even if you carry no extra fat in your abdomen. Few of us use our abs enough during everyday life—which usually finds us sitting most of the day!—to keep our abs strong enough to hold our internal organs in place.

Big life events such as pregnancy and menopause weaken your midsection further. As your baby grows, it stretches out your abs. If you don't tighten up those muscles after delivery, your abs remain loose and weak. Also, any surgery you may have had during delivery sometimes could have cut through abdominal muscle, overstretching it and weakening it even more.

As I mentioned in chapter 1, changing hormone levels at menopause cause women to store more fat in their midsections than in their butts, hips, and thighs. My friends who are over age 50 and who used to have naturally flat tummies in their youth now tell me that they are noticing them getting poochy. They also notice extra flab at the lower end of their backs, like two unwanted fatty packages. Each one of these friends, however, firmed up those tummies and shrunk those love handles after just 6 weeks on this midsection routine, along with my healthy eating plan.

My Midsection Fat Zone routine will help you sculpt a toned, tight, sexy midsection, just as it has for me, my sisters, my girlfriends, and the countless

I Shrunk My Female Fat Zones!

Robyn Smyles gained anywhere from 45 to 60 pounds during each of her five pregnancies. Home-based exercise provided her postpregnancy formula for success.

I have five children, and with each additional child I have found it harder to find time to exercise. I simply can't get five kids out the door to a gym! That's why I was so excited to learn about Denise's workouts, routines that I could do at home with my children in the room.

I gave birth to my fifth child less than a year ago, and over the past year I've still managed to lose 47 pounds!

Because I'm breastfeeding, I can't restrict my caloric intake. I've found, however, that healthy eating combined with exercise has reshaped all of my trouble spots and kept me strong and energetic.

Some days I can work in only 10 minutes of exercise at a time. I try to amass 30 to 40 minutes most days, even if that means I complete three or four mini workouts. I work exercise around my life, doing bits and parts of routines whenever I find a few spare minutes.

I've never had a weight problem, and I'm confident that Denise's workouts are one of the main reasons.

They are so fast and effective! They are not terribly strenuous, but they've helped my body to gradually take a better shape, especially my stomach. Plus I feel great!

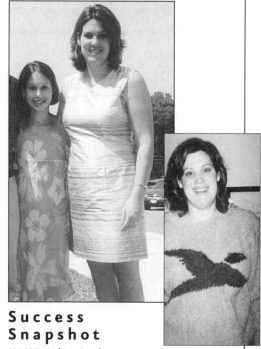

Success Snapshot

NAME: Robyn Smyles

AGE: 35

TOWN: Annapolis, Maryland

OCCUPATION: Mother of five

WEIGHT LOST: 47 pounds

OTHER ACCOMPLISHMENTS: Boosted her energy and emotional health

Robyn's Secret to Success

"You have to take the time to get your body healthy. I don't go by the scale. I go by the way I feel and the way my clothes fit. My body is different now than before I had children. Different, but better."

numbers of women who exercise to my show and videos. It will help you stand taller, slimming your overall appearance.

Besides your abdomen, these Midsection Fat Zone routines will also work your lower back muscles, helping to cinch your natural midsection "corset" a little tighter and shrink those love handles.

Here are the specific muscles that these workouts target and why.

■ **Your upper and lower rectus abdominis.** When most of us picture rock-hard abs, we picture this muscle. Fibrous bands of tissue break up this large muscle that runs from your pubic bone to your ribs along the front center of your abdomen, creating the "six-pack" appearance.

Though the rectus abdominis really is one large muscle, I like to think of it as two distinct ones: one below the navel and one above it. Many women are much weaker in the lower end of this muscle, the part below the navel. Weakness here allows our internal organs to press out, creating a rounded appearance even if we have little body fat. You use this section of the abdomen the least during daily life.

Because the lower end of the muscle is weaker than the upper end, all of these fat zone workouts target the lower rectus abdominis first, allowing you to fully work that area so that you won't feel too fatigued. Oftentimes, if you work the upper abs first, you might feel too tired by the time you get to the lower abs.

■ **Your transverse abdominis.** This deepest layer of the abdomen lies underneath your rectus abdominis. This muscle helps you contract your abdomen and draw your belly inward. Strengthening it creates a natural girdle for the front of your midsection. It also adds power and stability to everyday movements such as walking.

■ **Your obliques.** Internal and external obliques form your sides and waist. Your external obliques sit closest to the surface toward the front of your waist, with the internal obliques sitting deeper and closer to your back. These muscles help you bend from side to side as well as rotate your trunk to look behind you. Toning them will help shrink your waist as well as any love handles.

▪ **Your lower back.** Your lower back contains numerous muscles. One group of muscles, called the erector spinae, contains a trio of muscles called the iliocostalis, longissimus, and spinalis. These muscles attach to your spinal column at different points along your back, allowing you to bend it forward and backward and from side to side.

Toning these muscles helps prevent back pain as well as tightens and firms your entire lower back, shrinking love handles as well as any other back flab that may stick out when you wear a bikini.

Denise's Midsection Do's and Don'ts

The exercises in my Midsection Fat Zone routines contain a blend of Pilates, traditional crunches, and my own signature moves. Taken together, they provide you with the most effective exercises from every fitness discipline to help you carve a fit and firm midsection.

If your midsection is your personal fat zone, do these routines three times a week or more. I personally work my abs a little every day. Unlike other muscles in your body, your abdominal muscles recover quickly from exercise. You don't need to skip a day between abdominal workouts.

I've also incorporated numerous stretches throughout each routine, allowing you to rest and recover between exercises, make your workout more effective, and elongate your midsection, helping you to stand taller.

Here are some do's and don'ts to help you get the most out of these workouts.

" Eventually, keeping your tummy pulled in and up will become as second nature as breathing. Just zip it up! "

DO . . .

- **Zip up your abs all day long.** Whenever you get a free moment, look down. Are you allowing your abs to pooch outward? Pull them in! Imagine that you're zipping up a corset, starting at your pelvic bone. As you zip it up, your tummy pulls in and up. The more often you zip up your abs, the less often you'll need to remind yourself to do so.

- **Protect your back.** Do this by keeping your lower back pressed down to the floor and bringing your navel toward your spine during any type of abdominal crunch.

- **Keep your head in a neutral position.** Do this for every exercise. To know what that feels like, stand against a wall, aligning your buttocks, shoulder blades, and head against the wall. Now walk forward. Take a moment to memorize that feeling.

- **Stay smooth.** Resist the urge to use your arms to jerk your head forward during abdominal-crunching exercises that require you to place your hands behind your head. Imagine that you are holding a peeled orange under your chin. Look too far up, and you'll lose the orange. Look too far down, and you'll squeeze the juice out of it.

- **Exhale at the proper time.** You need to exhale whenever you contract your abdomen during an exercise. If you inhale on a contraction, you'll press your tummy out. Exhale on the way up, scoop and hollow and feel as though you're deflating a balloon.

- **Stay consistent.** Fortunately, your abdominal muscles respond quickly to toning—no matter what your age. I spend only 3 to 4 minutes a day on my abs, and look at my tummy! My secret is consistency. You must work your abs and back at least three times a week, particularly after age 40, to keep them fit and firm.

Repeat As Needed

THE THREE MIDSECTION Fat Zone routines include the most effective exercises for trimming and strengthening your abs, waist, and lower back. Every 2 weeks, you'll take on a new set of exercises, helping you to fully strengthen and tone your entire midsection.

Your current fitness level will determine how many repetitions you can perform for each exercise. Tune in to your body. Whether you are working your abs, waist, or back, pay attention to how those muscles feel as you move. When they start to burn and feel fatigued, do two more repetitions and then move on to the next exercise.

Here's a rule of thumb for the right number of repetitions as you progress on the program.

WEEKS 1 AND 2: 8 to 12

WEEKS 3 AND 4: 12 to 15

WEEKS 5 AND 6: 15 to 20

DON'T . . .

■ **Focus only on your abdomen.** As I mentioned in chapter 2, you need a total-body conditioning program to shed fat effectively. Do your midsection routine according to your body type prescription, found on pages 20 to 21.

■ **Get discouraged.** Ab work can feel tough, especially in the beginning. Short of getting out of bed, few movements in life mimic the abdominal crunch, so your abs get little work throughout your natural day. They may well rank as the weakest muscles in your body. Just do your best. As a general rule, go until you start to feel the burn, and then do two more.

■ **Rush.** The more slowly you do each exercise, the more effective the movement.

■ **Ignore stretching.** These routines all take 20 minutes or less. Don't try to shorten them even more by skipping the suggested stretches. These stretches help you to make the most of your abdominal work by allowing you to recover between exercises, helping you to work each movement to your fullest potential.

During the first 2 weeks, you'll focus on the best traditional abdominal moves as well as exercises from the Pilates method, a series of moves developed by European gymnast Joseph Pilates that place intense concentration on your abs, particularly the deepest layer of muscle in your abdomen. Pilates exercises lengthen as they strengthen, helping you to appear leaner and stand taller.

You will first learn the beginner version of many different Pilates exercises. In the coming weeks, you'll build on those same exercises to challenge your abdominal muscles even more.

> ➤ TARGETS THE BELT AREA OF YOUR WAIST ➤ PULLS IN YOUR TUMMY
> ➤ CREATES AN AMAZING BIKINI BELLY

Roll-Down 1

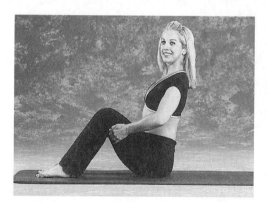 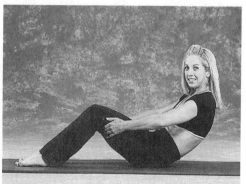

A. Sit on your mat with your legs bent and feet flat on the mat. Sit tall, extending the crown of your head toward the ceiling to create a nice, long, flat back. Gently grasp your thighs with your hands, as shown.

B. Starting from your tailbone, slowly roll back toward the floor one vertebra at a time as you exhale and bring your tummy in and up, forming a C shape with your spine and creating length between each vertebra. Once your head reaches the mat, reverse the direction by curling upward one vertebra at a time as you inhale, starting with your neck, and then your upper back, then middle back, then lower back, until you return to the starting position. Do 8 to 12 repetitions.

➤ TARGETS THE FRONT OF YOUR ABDOMEN ABOVE YOUR NAVEL
➤ HELPS YOU TO ZIP UP THOSE TIGHT JEANS

Pulsing Crunch 1

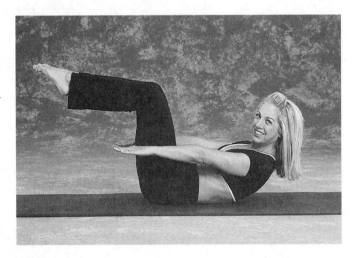

Lie on your back with your knees bent and feet flat on your mat. Raise your feet as you keep your knees bent, forming a 90-degree angle between your thighs and your torso. Extend your arms at your sides so that they are parallel to, but a few inches above, the floor.

Press your lower back into the mat, tighten and contract your abs, and exhale as you slowly raise your shoulders off the mat, as shown, bringing your fingertips past either side of your buttocks. Keep your head in a neutral position. Inhale as you lower slightly, then exhale as you reach forward with your fingers again, pulsing up and down without lowering your shoulder blades onto the mat. Do 8 to 12 repetitions. (For extra fat-burning power, do two sets of 8 to 12 repetitions.)

MAXIMUM RESULTS | Minimum Time

As you raise your torso, lengthen your abdomen by reaching out and up with the crown of your head. This length will help target a larger area of your abdomen.

Note: For a greater challenge, you can also do this crunch while seated on a large stability ball.

➤ FLATTENS THE ENTIRE FRONT OF YOUR TUMMY ➤ BORROWED FROM
THE PILATES METHOD ➤ AN EXTREMELY EFFICIENT TUMMY TIGHTENER

Single-Leg Stretch

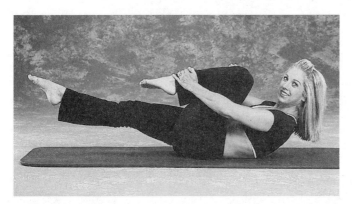

A. Lie on your back with your knees bent and feet flat on your mat. Bring your left knee in toward your chest. Tighten your abs, exhale, and extend and raise your right leg off the floor only as far as you can while keeping your back flat against the mat. Place your right hand on your left knee and your left hand on your left ankle, as shown. Inhale as you flatten and tighten your tummy and raise your shoulders.

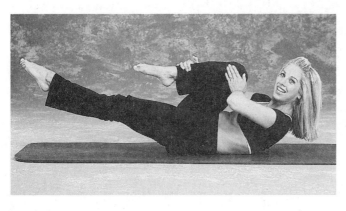

B. Switch legs, as shown, without lowering your head to the floor as you exhale. Press outward through your toes and make the movement as smooth and controlled as possible. Continue to alternate your legs and hands, moving with your breath, until you've completed 8 to 12 repetitions. (For extra fat-burning power, do two sets of 8 to 12 repetitions.)

MAXIMUM RESULTS	Minimum Time

Focus your gaze on your navel to help maintain your lift during this exercise.

Twisting Crunch

Lie on your back with your knees bent and the soles of your feet on the mat. Place your fingers behind your head with your elbows open to the sides. Exhale and lift your right shoulder toward your left knee, as shown. Inhale as you lower your shoulder. Then exhale and lift your left shoulder toward your right knee. Continue to alternate from right to left, repeating until you've done 8 to 12 repetitions. (For extra fat-burning power, do two sets of 8 to 12 repetitions.) Throughout, keep your elbows open out to the sides, not closed around your head. Relax your head back into your fingers, trying not to use your hands and arms to yank your upper body toward your knees.

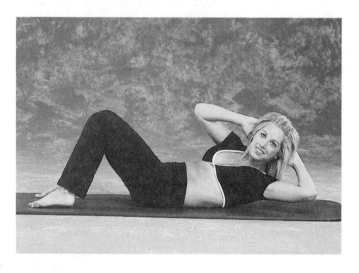

MAXIMUM RESULTS | Minimum Time

When you lower between twists, keep your upper back from completely resting on the floor. This will create constant work in your abs, making the exercise more effective.

"**Ab muscles** act like a **girdle.** They'll keep your **tummy flat.**"

Twisting Crunch on Ball (variation)

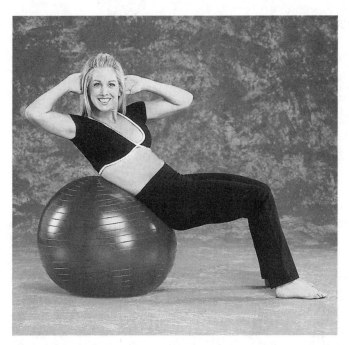

You can do the same exercise on a stability ball, increasing the challenge and benefit of the exercise.

Sit on a large stability ball. Walk your feet away from the ball as you slide your back down the ball, stopping once your lower and middle back press against the ball. Place your fingers behind your head with your elbows open to the sides. Exhale as you lift your left shoulder to the right. Inhale as you lower to center and then exhale as you lift your right shoulder to the left. Continue to alternate from left to right, repeating until you've done 8 to 12 repetitions. (For extra fat-burning power, do two sets of 8 to 12 repetitions.)

"Because the **ball makes** you **work harder,** you may not be **able** to **do** as **many** repetitions on the **ball** as you can on your **mat.**"

STRETCH BREAK

Full-Body Reach

A. Lie on your back with your legs extended. Extend your arms overhead.

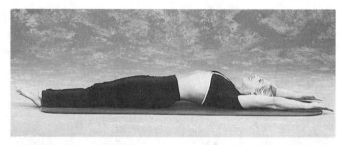

B. Bend your left knee and place your left foot on the mat. Exhale as you reach through your right arm and right leg. Inhale. Then exhale and switch, bending your right knee and reaching through your left arm and leg. Continue alternating for 20 seconds, adding more and more length to your body.

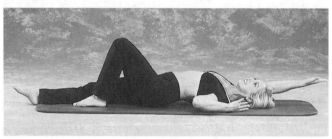

MAXIMUM RESULTS Minimum Time

As you exhale, visualize breathing into any tight spots. This will help them to lengthen and release.

➤ CARVES A WAIST FASTER THAN YOU CAN SAY, "LOVE HANDLE"

Modified T-Stand

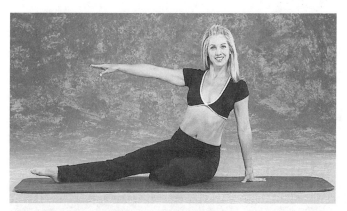

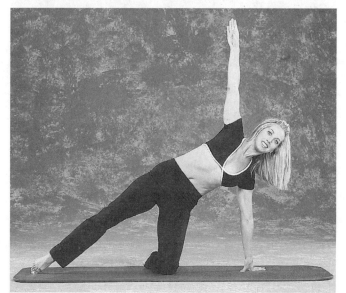

A. Sit with both knees bent, your legs toward the right side of your torso, with your right thigh and shin on top of your left, and your left shin and thigh against your mat. Place your left palm against the mat, directly under your left shoulder. Extend your right leg, as shown.

B. Press into your left palm as you exhale, lift your right hip, and sweep your right hand up and to the left in an arc until it reaches overhead, with your upper arm near your right ear. Inhale as you lower. Do 8 to 12 repetitions or repeat until fatigue. Then switch sides.

MAXIMUM RESULTS Minimum Time

When in the "up" position, try to lift your hips as much as possible, as if an imaginary belt were wrapped around your hips and pulling them toward the ceiling.

➤ TARGETS THE DEEPEST OF ABDOMINAL MUSCLES,
THE TRANSVERSE ABDOMINIS ➤ HELPS YOU STAND TALLER AUTOMATICALLY
➤ CREATES A NATURAL CORSET TO HOLD IN YOUR TUMMY

Plank

Get on all fours, with your hands flat on the mat directly under your shoulders and your knees under your hips. Extend one leg behind and balance on the ball of that foot. Extend the other leg, bringing yourself into the plank position, as shown. Pull up through your abs to form a straight line from your shoulders to your feet. Breathing normally, tighten your abs—zip it up—and hold for up to 1 minute.

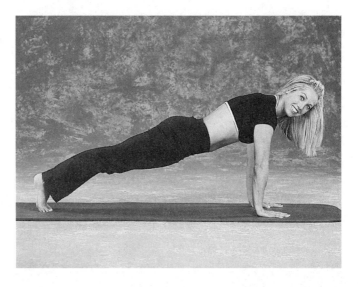

MAXIMUM RESULTS Minimum Time

Do this in front of a mirror or ask someone to watch as you do it. Many women allow their hips to sink down, forming a slight arch in their lower backs. This can strain the back. Others jut their rear ends toward the ceiling, forming a slight triangle with their bodies. This makes the move less effective.

> "You want a straight line from your feet to your shoulders. To create that line, you must zip your abs in and up."

Lower Back Strengthener

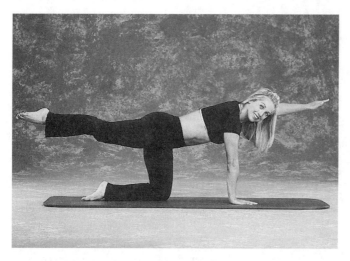

Get on all fours, with your hands flat on the mat under your shoulders and your knees under your hips. Pulling your abs in, exhale and extend your left arm as you simultaneously extend your right leg until both are parallel to the floor, as shown. Return your left arm and right leg to the starting position as you inhale. Then exhale and extend your right arm and left leg. Continue alternating until you've completed 8 10 12 repetitions. (For extra fat-burning power, do two sets of 8 to 12 repetitions.)

MAXIMUM RESULTS | Minimum Time

As you alternate extending your arms and legs, keep your tummy tight and pulled in and up. This will help you to continue to use your abs as you work your back, giving you a two-for-one workout.

STRETCH BREAK
Child's Pose

Get on all fours, with your knees under your hips and your hands flat on the mat under your shoulders. Pull your tummy toward your spine as you bring your buttocks back toward your heels, as shown. Once your buttocks rest against your heels, bend forward with a long spine, lowering your forehead to the floor and your torso to your thighs. Then slide your arms along the floor and bring them behind your body, palms facing the ceiling. Take three deep breaths as you relax.

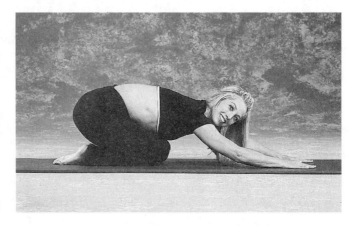

MAXIMUM RESULTS | Minimum Time

Before sliding your arms behind your buttocks, reach forward with your fingers as far as you can and then press your palms into the mat to help you further lengthen your spine and bring your buttocks even closer to your heels.

❝I love this one. I do it whenever I need a break!❞

Now you're ready to step up the difficulty of your abdominal routine. You'll encounter many exercises that you did during weeks 1 and 2. Only now I've changed them slightly to make them a bit more challenging. If you're not quite ready to increase the level of difficulty, however, feel free to stick with the less-challenging versions. Just do your best.

> ➤ TARGETS THE DEEP TRANSVERSE MUSCLE ➤ HELPS TO CINCH IN YOUR TUMMY AND WAIST ➤ BUILDS ON THE ROLL-DOWN FROM WEEKS 1 AND 2

Roll-Down 2

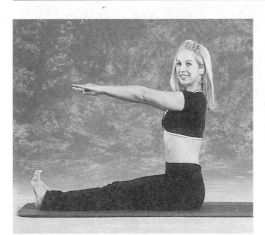 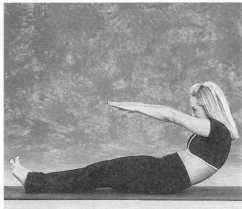

A. Sit on your mat with your legs extended. Sit tall, extending the crown of your head toward the ceiling and creating a nice, long, flat back. Extend your arms in front of your chest, as shown. Squeeze the backs of your thighs together. This will help keep your legs and lower back against the mat as you roll up and down.

B. Starting from your tailbone, exhale and slowly roll back one vertebra at a time as you bring your belly in and up, forming a C shape with your spine and creating length between each vertebra. Once your head reaches the mat, reverse the direction by rolling back up, one vertebra at a time, as you inhale. Do 12 to 15 times or repeat until fatigue. (For extra fat-burning power, do two sets of 12 to 15 repetitions.)

➤ THIS IS A GREAT OVERALL TUMMY FLATTENER
➤ SIMILAR TO THE PULSING CRUNCH IN WEEKS 1 AND 2

Pulsing Crunch 2

Lie on your back with your knees bent and feet flat on your mat. Press your lower back down into the mat, extend your arms from your chest, tighten your abs, and exhale as you raise your shoulders off the mat, as shown, crossing the right hand over the left and reaching between your knees. Lower slightly as you inhale and then reach forward with your fingers again, pulsing up and down without lowering your shoulder blades onto the mat. Do 12 to 15 repetitions or repeat until fatigue. (For extra fat-burning power, do two sets of 12 to 15 repetitions.)

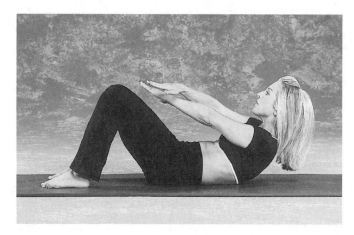

MAXIMUM RESULTS Minimum Time

Lift your shoulders off the mat the entire time, keeping constant tension in your abdominals—really feeling them work.

PULSING CRUNCH 2 ON BALL (VARIATION)

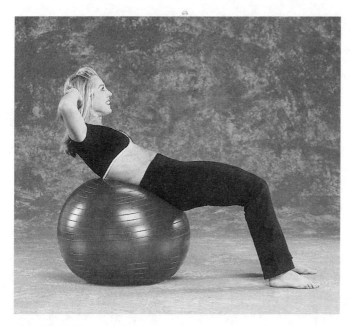

You can also try the pulsing crunch while seated on a stability ball.

Sit on a large stability ball. Walk your feet away from the ball as you slide down it, stopping once your lower and middle back press against the ball. Place your palms behind your head, with your elbows open to the sides. Tighten your abs and exhale as you lift your shoulders. Inhale as you lower just an inch or two and then pulse back up, keeping constant tension in your abdominals. Do 12 to 15 repetitions or repeat until fatigue. (For extra fat-burning power, do two sets of 12 to 15 repetitions.)

"**Imagine** a heavy **brick** resting on your **lower belly,** keeping it **pressed down** as you **crunch.**"

> ➤ BORROWED FROM THE PILATES METHOD ➤ STRETCHES THE BACKS
> OF YOUR LEGS ➤ TIGHTENS THE ENTIRE FRONT OF YOUR TUMMY
> ➤ TARGETS YOUR TRANSVERSE ABDOMINIS

Single Straight-Leg Stretch

A. Lie on your back with your knees bent and feet flat on your mat. With your abs tight, exhale as you extend and raise your right leg toward the ceiling. Then inhale as you lift and extend your left leg a few inches above the mat. Grasp your right leg with both hands. Contract your abs, navel in toward your spine, and raise your shoulders, as shown.

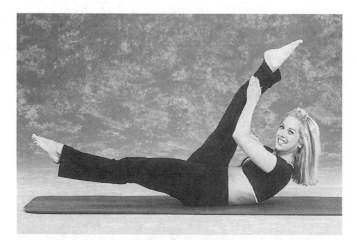

B. Exhale and switch legs without lowering your head to the floor. Alternate your legs and hands in a smooth, controlled motion, moving with your breath, until you've completed 12 to 15 repetitions or until fatigue. (For extra fat-burning power, do two sets of 12 to 15 repetitions.)

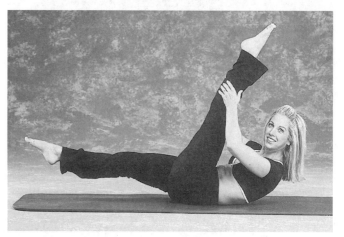

MAXIMUM RESULTS | Minimum Time

Try to keep your hips square and motionless throughout the exercise. To do so, you must use your lower abs and transverse abdominis, making the exercise more effective.

WEEKS 3 & 4

➤ FIRMS YOUR OBLIQUES, THE SIDES OF YOUR ABDOMEN
➤ SHRINKS YOUR WAISTLINE ➤ BUILDS ON THE TWISTING CRUNCH
IN WEEKS 1 AND 2

Twisting Crunch with Straight Legs

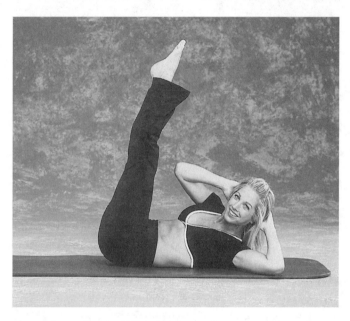

MAXIMUM RESULTS | Minimum Time

When you lower between twists, keep your upper back from completely resting on the floor. This will create constant tone in your abs, making the exercise more effective.

Lie on your back with your knees bent and feet flat on your mat. Lift your feet toward the ceiling as you extend your legs, forming a 90-degree angle between your legs and your torso. Place your fingers behind your head with your elbows open to the sides.

Exhale as you lift your right shoulder toward your left leg, as shown. Inhale as you lower your shoulder. Then exhale and lift your left shoulder toward your right leg, alternating until you've completed 12 to 15 repetitions on each side or until fatigue. (For extra fat-burning power, do two sets of 12 to 15 repetitions.) Throughout, keep your elbows open out to the sides, not closed around your head. Relax your head back into your fingers, but try not to use your hands and arms to yank your upper body toward your knees.

➤ STRETCHES THE FRONT AND SIDES OF YOUR ABDOMEN
➤ GIVES YOU A NICE MINI REST

STRETCH BREAK

Full-Body Reach

A. Lie on your back with your legs extended. Extend your arms overhead.

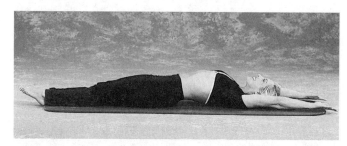

B. Bend your left knee and place your left foot on the mat. Exhale as you reach through your right arm and right leg. Inhale. Then exhale as you switch, bending your right knee and reaching through your left arm and leg. Continue alternating for 20 seconds, adding more and more length to your body.

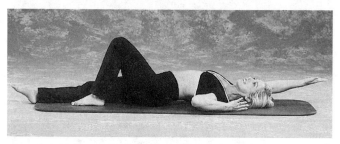

MAXIMUM RESULTS	Minimum Time

As you exhale, visualize breathing into any tight spots. This will help them to lengthen and release.

Ultimate Tummy Trimmer

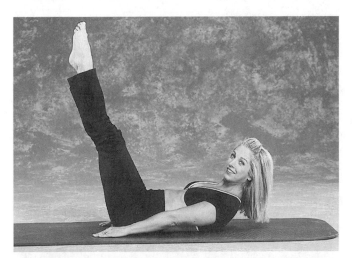

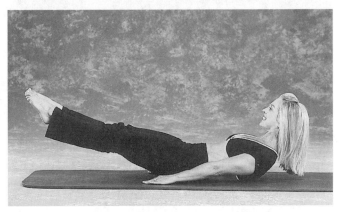

A. Lie on your back, with your knees bent and feet on the mat. Rest your arms at your sides, palms down. Lift your feet toward the ceiling as you extend your legs, forming a 90-degree angle between your legs and torso. Lift your upper torso off the mat until your shoulder blades hover just above the surface of the mat, as shown.

B. Exhale as you slowly lower your legs, tightening your abs. To keep your back in a neutral position, imagine your abs lengthening as you lower your legs. Stop once you can no longer keep your spine neutral. Inhale as you lift your legs back to the previous position. Do 12 to 15 repetitions or repeat until fatigue. (For extra fat-burning power, do two sets of 12 to 15 repetitions.)

MAXIMUM RESULTS	Minimum Time

Squeeze your buttocks as you lift and lower your legs to boost the effectiveness of the exercise.

T-Stand

A. From the modified T-stand position, as shown, extend both legs to the right as you bring your body weight onto your left hip and side of your left leg. Place your left palm on the mat directly under your left shoulder. Your right leg should be directly on top of your left.

B. Press into the outer edge of your left foot and your left palm as you exhale, tighten your abs, and lift into the T-stand. Extend your right arm toward the ceiling, as shown, forming a T shape with your arms and body. Hold for 10 to 30 seconds, lifting hips up as you inhale and exhale, then release. Repeat on the other side.

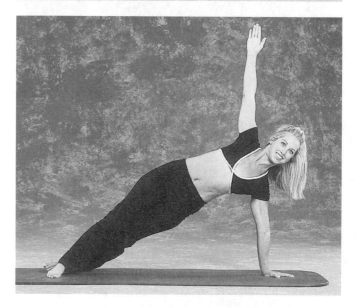

"Believe in yourself. Your inner confidence will help you remain balanced and hold the exercise for a longer period of time."

> CHALLENGING, BUT WELL WORTH THE EFFORT ➤ TARGETS THE DEEPEST ABDOMINAL MUSCLES ➤ IMPROVES POSTURE ➤ BUILDS ON THE PLANK LEARNED IN WEEKS 1 AND 2

Plank with Leg Tuck

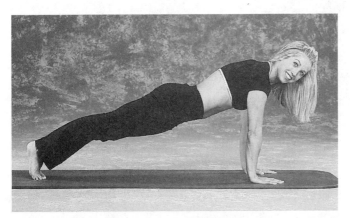

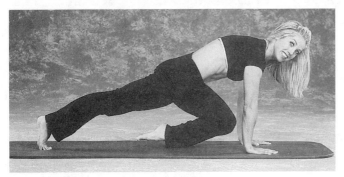

A. Get on all fours, with your hands directly under your shoulders and your knees under your hips. Extend one leg behind and balance on the ball of that foot. Extend the other leg, bringing yourself into the plank position, as shown. Pull up through your abs to form a straight line from your shoulders to your feet.

B. Adjust your body weight onto your left foot. Lift your right foot and bend your right knee, bringing your right thigh toward your tummy. Then press back through your left foot as you extend your right leg back to the floor. Repeat with the left leg, alternating legs until you've completed 12 to 15 repetitions or until fatigue. (For extra fat-burning power, do two sets of 12 to 15 repetitions.) Exhale as you bring a knee toward your chest, inhale as you extend it back, and alternate legs with your breath.

MAXIMUM RESULTS	Minimum Time

You want a straight line from your feet to your head throughout the entire exercise. Don't allow your hips to sink down or your buttocks to press up toward the ceiling. Also, as you balance on one leg, keep your hips square to the floor. Don't allow one hip to rise up or sink down.

❝This is a **tough move,** but it's also **very effective!**❞

Superwoman

Lie with your tummy on your mat and your arms and legs extended. Tighten your abs and buttocks as you exhale and lift your legs and arms, as shown. Create length in your spine as you do so by pressing out with your fingers and toes. Hold for five breaths and then lower your arms and legs. Repeat two times.

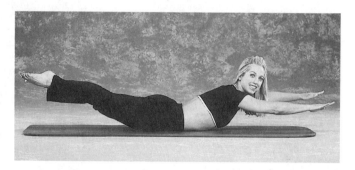

MAXIMUM RESULTS | Minimum Time

The more length you create in your spine, the lower you'll fly, but the more effective—and safe—the exercise.

STRETCH BREAK
Spinal Twist

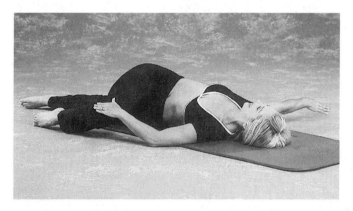

MAXIMUM RESULTS | Minimum Time

Try to keep both shoulders against the floor as you stretch. To do so, reach through the fingers on the hand that's on the side of the raised leg.

Lie on your back with your legs extended and arms out to your sides. Inhale as you raise your right knee and place your right foot on the mat near your left knee. Exhale as you rotate your torso to bring your right knee toward the left and onto or near the floor, as shown. Hold for 20 seconds, breathing normally, and then release. Repeat on the other side.

During the next 2 weeks, you'll again see many exercises that you learned during the previous 4 weeks. I've added some extremely challenging tweaks to them, however. I also show even more challenging moves as variations, for those of you who really want to feel your tummies burn. Plus, you'll encounter some brand-new exercises, some of the most effective abdominal exercises around.

If you're not quite ready to increase the level of difficulty of your routine, that's fine. Just stick with the less-challenging versions—but keep pushing yourself. As soon as you find yourself completing a routine and not feeling fatigued, it's time to increase the difficulty.

> ➤ STRENGTHENS YOUR DEEPEST ABDOMINAL MUSCLE
> ➤ CARVES OUT YOUR LOWER TUMMY

Roll-Down with Arms Overhead

A. Sit on your mat with your legs extended. Press your inner thighs together as you turn out your feet, heels touching. Sit tall, extending the crown of your head toward the ceiling and creating a nice, long, flat back. Extend your arms overhead, as shown.

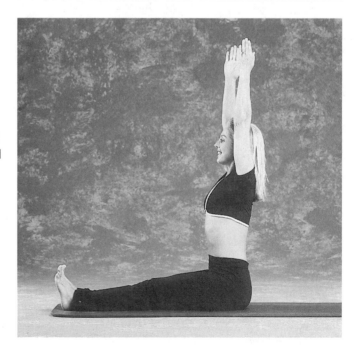

"Let's get rid of that paunch once and for all."

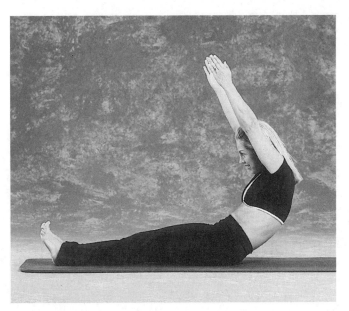

B. Starting from your tailbone, exhale and slowly roll back one vertebra at a time as you bring your belly in and up, forming a C shape with your spine and creating length between each vertebra. Once your head reaches your mat, reverse the direction by rolling back up, one vertebra at a time, as you inhale. Do 15 to 20 repetitions or repeat until fatigue. (For extra fat-burning power, do two sets of 15 to 20 repetitions.)

MAXIMUM RESULTS	Minimum Time

Squeeze the backs of your thighs together as you roll up and down. This will help you to keep your legs and lower back against your mat.

> ➤ FLATTENS YOUR UPPER AND LOWER TUMMY IN ONE MOVEMENT

Double Crunch

Lie on your back with your knees bent and feet flat on your mat. Place your fingers behind your head with your elbows open to the sides. Lift your feet as you keep your knees bent, forming a 90-degree angle between your thighs and torso. Simultaneously curl your pelvic bone toward your ribs and exhale as you lift your shoulders, as shown, bringing your knees toward your chest and your shoulder blades slightly off the mat. Inhale as you lower. Do 15 to 20 repetitions or repeat until fatigue. (For extra fat-burning power, do two sets of 15 to 20 repetitions.)

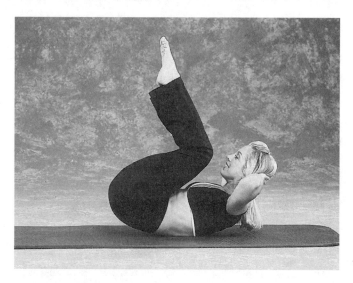

MAXIMUM RESULTS Minimum Time

As you crunch, exhale using your tummy muscles to press out all of the air. This will help keep your tummy flat as you crunch, sculpting muscles that hold it in rather than muscles that push it outward.

“You don't have to lift your tailbone much— just 3 to 5 inches from the floor—to really work your lower tummy during this exercise.”

Bicycle

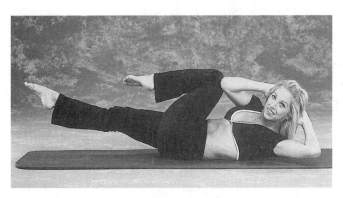

MAXIMUM RESULTS Minimum Time

It's easy to lose control and move too quickly. Try to slow down your movement as you concentrate on keeping your navel tight and your lower back pressed to the mat. Try to create a flat, hollow tummy throughout the exercise.

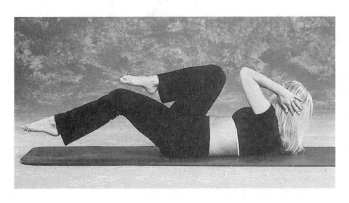

A. Lie on your back with your knees bent and feet flat on the mat. Lift your feet and thighs, keeping your knees bent, until you form a 90-degree angle between your torso and thighs. Place your fingers behind your head with your elbows open to the sides. Firmly press your lower back into the mat. Tighten your abs and lift your upper torso so that your shoulder blades hover just above the mat surface. Rest your head back into your hands, keeping your neck and shoulders relaxed. Exhale as you bring your right shoulder and left knee toward one another, as shown, and simultaneously extend your right leg.

B. Lower your right shoulder, inhale, and extend your left leg as you bring your left shoulder and right knee toward one another. Continue alternating you've completed 15 to 20 repetitions or until fatigue. (For extra fat-burning power, do two sets of 15 to 20 repetitions.)

Ultimate Tummy Trimmer 2

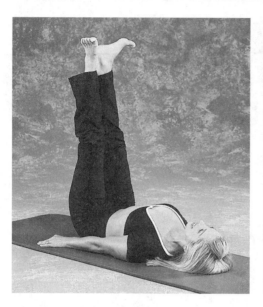
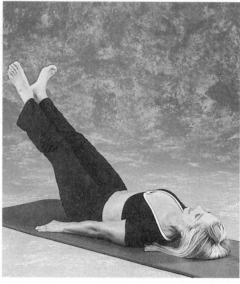

A. Lie on your back with your knees bent and feet on the mat. Rest your arms at your sides. Lift your feet toward the ceiling as you extend your legs, forming a 90-degree angle between your legs and torso. Press your inner thighs and heels together as you rotate your toes outward, as shown, to isolate the middle and lowest areas of your lower abs.

B. Lift your upper torso off the mat until your shoulder blades hover just above the surface of the mat. Slowly lower your legs as you tighten your abs and exhale. To keep your back in a neutral position, imagine your abs lengthening as you lower your legs. Stop once you can no longer keep your spine neutral. Inhale as you rise to the starting position. Do 15 to 20 repetitions or repeat until fatigue. (For extra fat-burning power, do two sets of 15 to 20 repetitions.)

Ultimate Tummy Trimmer 2 (variation)

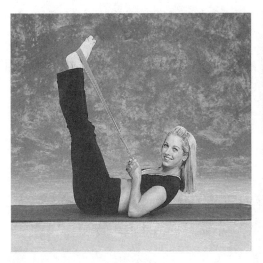 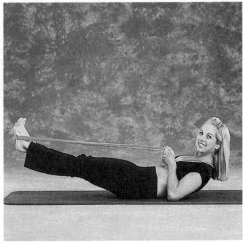

A. For a greater challenge and additional resistance, try this move with a resistance band.

Lie on your back with your knees bent and feet flat on the floor. Lift your feet toward the ceiling and place the middle of the resistance band across your arches, holding the ends of the band with your hands. Form a 90-degree angle between your legs and torso. Lift your upper torso off the mat until your shoulder blades hover just above the surface of the mat, as shown.

B. Slowly lower your legs as you exhale. Keep your hands stationary, stretching the band. Stop once you can no longer keep your spine neutral. Inhale and rise to the starting position. Do 15 to 20 repetitions or repeat until fatigue. (For extra fat-burning power, do two sets of 15 to 20 repetitions.)

MAXIMUM RESULTS	Minimum Time
Continue to press your inner thighs together as you lower and raise your legs. This will allow you to work them, too.	

WEEKS 5 & 6

➤ TRIMS YOUR WAIST ➤ IMPROVES YOUR BALANCE
➤ STRENGTHENS YOUR BACK AND DEEP ABDOMINAL MUSCLES
➤ BUILDS ON THE T-STAND FROM WEEKS 3 AND 4

T-Stand with Twist

A. From the modified T-stand position, as shown, extend both legs to the right as you bring your body weight onto your left hip and side of your left leg. Place your left palm on the mat directly under your left shoulder. Your right leg should be directly on top of your left.

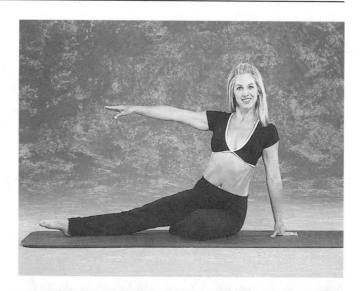

B. Press into the outer edge of your left foot and your left palm as you exhale and lift into the T-stand. Inhale and extend your right arm toward the ceiling, forming a T shape with your arms and body.

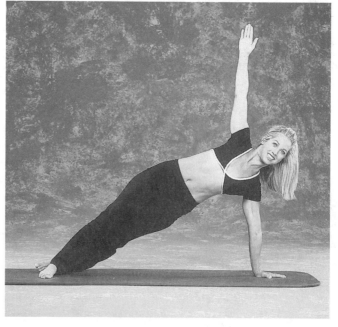

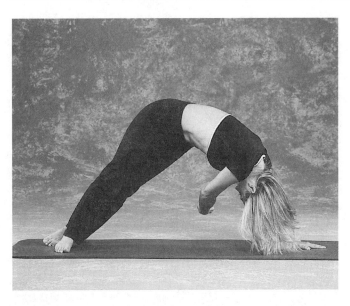

C. Exhale as you slowly sweep your extended right arm forward, extending through your waist and back. Then reach your right hand under your body as you inhale. Feel your upper back open up, fanning open your upper rib cage. Your obliques and rectus abdominis are working together to keep you up. Then exhale and use your abs to unfold and raise your torso to the previous position. Do as many repetitions as you can—shooting for 15 to 20—before switching to the other side.

MAXIMUM RESULTS	Minimum Time

To help keep your balance as you fold forward and under, focus on your navel, your center of gravity. Keep this area tight, and you won't wobble.

"You may only be able to do a few repetitions of this exercise before feeling fatigued. Good work!"

STRETCH BREAK

Spinal Twist

Lie on your back with your legs extended and arms out to your sides. Inhale as you raise your right knee and place your right foot on the mat near your left knee. Exhale as you rotate your torso to bring your right knee toward the left and onto or near the floor, as shown. Hold for 20 seconds, breathing normally, and then release. Repeat on the other side.

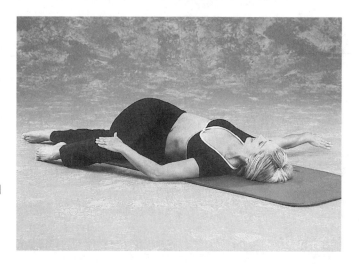

MAXIMUM RESULTS	Minimum Time

Try to keep both shoulders against the floor as you stretch. To do so, reach through the fingers on the hand that's on the side of the raised leg.

66 Be aware of your posture all day long. Good posture helps retrain your abdominal muscles, helping to tone them around the clock. 99

Bent-Arm Plank with Knee Kiss

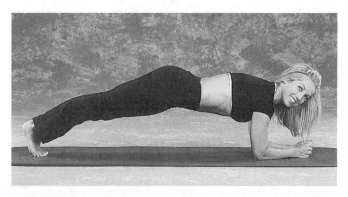

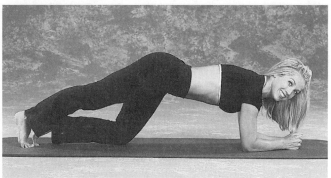

A. Get on all fours, with your hands directly under your shoulders and your knees under your hips. Bend your elbows, lowering yourself onto your forearms. Clasp your hands together. Extend one leg behind and balance on the ball of that foot. Extend the other leg, bringing yourself into the plank position, as shown. Pull up through your abs to form a straight line from your shoulders to your feet.

B. Adjust your body weight onto your right foot. Exhale and lift your left foot and bend your left knee, bringing your left thigh toward your tummy. Inhale and press back through your left foot as you extend your leg back to the floor. Repeat with the right leg, alternating legs until you've done 15 to 20 repetitions. (For extra fat-burning power, do two sets of 15 to 20 repetitions.)

MAXIMUM RESULTS Minimum Time

Imagine that you have a yardstick attached to your spine. If you allow your hips to sink down or press upward, you'll push the yardstick off your back.

Swimming

Lie on your tummy with your arms extended in front of you and your legs extended behind. Press through your fingertips and toes to create length in your spine. Raise both arms and legs a few inches off the mat. Then exhale and raise your right arm and left leg a few inches higher than your left arm and right leg.

Inhale and switch positions, lowering your right arm and left leg slightly and raising your left arm and right leg. Alternate your arms and legs repeatedly, as if you were swimming, until until you've done 15 to 20 repetitions or until fatigue. (For extra fat-burning power, do two sets of 15 to 20 repetitions.)

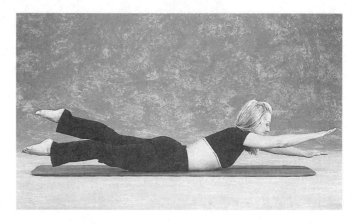

MAXIMUM RESULTS	Minimum Time

Lengthen through your spine as you keep your arms and legs elevated off the mat throughout the entire exercise, keeping a constant contraction in your back muscles.

STRETCH BREAK
Child's Pose

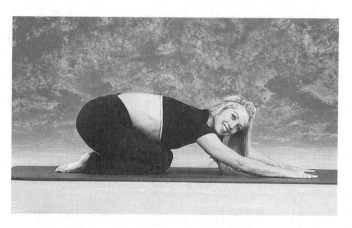

Get on all fours, with your knees under your hips and your hands flat on the mat under your shoulders. Pull your tummy toward your spine as you bring your buttocks back toward your heels, as shown. Once your buttocks rest against your heels, bend forward with a long spine, lowering your forehead to the floor and your torso to your thighs. Then slide your arms along the floor and bring them behind your body, palms facing the ceiling. Take three deep breaths as you relax.

MAXIMUM RESULTS Minimum Time

Before sliding your arms behind your buttocks, reach forward with your fingers as far as you can and then press your palms into the mat to help you further lengthen your spine and bring your buttocks even closer to your heels.

CHAPTER 7

THE FAT ZONE WORKOUTS

The Lower Body

All women point to a trouble spot or fat zone on their bodies, the place where every single excess calorie seems to quickly migrate. My fat zone? My thighs.

Whenever I overindulge—usually by eating too much dessert—I see the results in my thighs. The backs of my thighs start to lose their smoothness as the hints of cellulite threaten to turn them into "cottage cheese." When my jeans feel too tight, I know I need to cut back on the desserts and step up my Lower-Body Fat Zone workouts. In just 2 weeks, the backs of my thighs resume their smooth, toned appearance, and my jeans feel roomy again. These workouts really do the trick!

The Anatomy of Long, Lean, Sexy Legs and Buns

We all want legs that look great in shorts and pretty dresses. So why are they so hard to get?

Before menopause, most of us store a disproportionate amount of fat in our lower bodies, particularly in our hips and thighs. Thousands of years ago, excess hip, butt, and thigh fat served an important purpose for early humans.

During drought and long winters, women burned this fat to fuel both pregnancy and lactation. Women with more lower body fat tended to survive harsh conditions and consequently pass on their genes to their children, whereas women with more slender proportions did not.

In modern times, we no longer need this fat reserve because we have plenty of food to support pregnancy and lactation. Unfortunately, as we discussed, it takes thousands of years for genetics to change, and our bodies simply haven't caught up with the times.

As we age, many of us also notice a type of fat called cellulite beginning to appear on the backs of our thighs—even if we've had slender thighs most of our lives. This cottage-cheese-looking fat lies just under your skin between your muscles and the connective tissue fibers that attach your muscle to your skin. These connective tissue fibers form a web. If weakened, the tissue allows the fat to push through the tiny holes between its web, just as a mattress bulges between the stitching.

My Lower-Body Fat Zone routines will help you blast away both types of fat. You'll firm your inner thighs, lift your buns, and shape and slim your legs by doing specific exercises that target the following areas.

- **Inner thighs.** Numerous muscles along your inner thighs work together to stabilize your knees and hips as you walk. These muscles are known collectively as your adductors and include the adductor magnus, minimus, longus, and brevis. My fat zone routines will help you tone and firm your adductors, stopping any inner thigh jiggling or rubbing when you walk. Working these muscles will also help to strengthen your knees, protecting them from injury.

- **Outer thighs and hips.** The muscles that help you do the standard leg lift are called your abductors and include the gluteus medius and minimus along your hips. Toning these muscles helps you smooth away saddlebags. It also helps to draw them inward, creating sexy indentations in your outer hips.

- **Front thighs.** The muscles that form the fronts of your thighs include your quadriceps, a series of four muscles that help you to extend your knee

I Shrunk My Female Fat Zones!

For Betsy Gammons, a consistent fitness plan helped fend off age-related weight gain.

I have maintained a healthy weight throughout life, and Denise's workouts are part of my successful formula. At 5 feet 6 inches and age 50, I still wear a size 10, the same size I wore in my twenties!

I had four children by the age of 28, yet I always managed to get back into shape pretty quickly after each pregnancy. (Part of my rigorous exercise routine was raising children!)

I've been exercising most of my life, doing Denise's unique program for more than 10 years. I particularly like how Denise targets every body area within each week, rather than focusing on just one trouble spot. Her kickboxing moves are my favorites. The punching and kicking create a fun, yet powerful workout. I really feel as if I've accomplished a lot when I'm done!

The most important thing I have learned from Denise is that consistency is key. Since I have been using her workouts, I've never worked out more than ½ hour a day, but I've also never taken a break from my routine.

I'm proud to say that my fitness routine rubbed off on my children. One of my daughters who gave birth last spring is now regularly doing Denise's program, too!

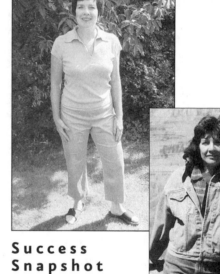

Success Snapshot

NAME: Betsy Gammons
AGE: 50
TOWN: Essex, Massachusetts
OCCUPATION: Photo editor
FITNESS GAINED: Has maintained a clothing size 10 throughout life
OTHER ACCOMPLISHMENTS: Overall feeling of strength and health

Betsy's Secret to Success

"Age is only a number. Feeling strong and healthy can improve your outlook on just about everything in life!"

and lift your leg. Near the top of the front of your thighs is another series of small muscles collectively called your hip flexors (the psoas major, psoas minor, and iliacus), which also help you lift your leg as well as propel your leg forward when you walk or climb stairs.

Many women don't think about their hip flexors when toning their legs, as these smaller muscles pale in size when compared to the larger quadriceps group. These muscles are extremely important to your appearance, however, because they help you to stand with proper posture. Overly tight hip flexors tend to tilt your pelvis forward, arching your lower back and causing your tummy to press out. Each of my fat zone routines contains not only exercises to shape the fronts of your thighs but also stretches to elongate your hip flexors, helping you to stand taller automatically.

Rear thighs. Your hamstrings form the backs of your thighs, from your knees to your buttocks. These muscles help to bend your knees, and toning them provides a great rear view and helps prevent cellulite. Besides helping to shape beautiful thighs, toning and stretching your hamstrings helps to pull your pelvis into optimal alignment, flattening your tummy and reducing pressure on your lower back.

Buttocks. Sometimes it may not seem as if you have any muscle in there, but you do! Collectively called your gluteals, your buttocks are formed by your gluteus minimus, medius, and maximus, which work together to help you lift your leg behind your torso, walk uphill, or climb steps. Since few of us perform these tasks often enough throughout the day, our buttocks muscles tend to weaken, allowing fat to jiggle. My fat zone routines will firm these muscles, helping to shrink, shape, and lift your buns.

Calves. Though your calves rarely serve as a fat depot, these important muscles, called the soleus and gastrocnemius, help flex your knees, stabilize your ankles, and flex your feet. Toning them gives you more push off during your walking workouts, helping you to boost your calorie burn.

Denise's Lower Body Do's and Don'ts

The exercises in my Lower-Body Fat Zone routines contain a blend of ballet, Power Yoga, Pilates, and traditional calisthenic exercises. Taken together, they provide you with the most effective exercises from every fitness discipline to help you make your lower half your better half! If your lower body is your personal fat zone, do these routines three times a week or more.

I've also incorporated numerous stretches throughout each routine, allowing you to rest and recover between exercises, make your workouts more effective, and elongate your leg muscles.

Here are some do's and don'ts to help you get the most out of these workouts.

DO . . .

- **Use proper form.** Just the smallest variation can make a great difference between simply going through the motions and getting the most out of each exercise. For most leg exercises, I've given you careful tips on using proper form. Keep them in mind when doing the routines.

- **Breathe correctly.** Exhale when contracting your leg and butt muscles and inhale when relaxing them. This will help you perform each exercise to your best potential. In each exercise description, I've prompted you on when to breathe in and out.

- **Squeeze the muscle group you're targeting.** Whether you're working the backs of your thighs or your butt or your hips, squeeze the area, particularly at the top of the contraction. Pretend the muscle that you are targeting is a sponge and that you're trying to squeeze every last drop of effort out of it.

- **Hold that last repetition.** During just about every exercise I do, and particularly for leg exercises, I hold my last contraction as long as I can. For example, if I'm doing leg lifts, on my last lift I hold my leg in the up position, completely fatiguing my outer thigh.

DON'T . . .

- **Focus only on your lower body.** As I mentioned in chapter 2, you need a total-body conditioning program to shed fat effectively. Do your lower body routine according to your body type prescription, found on pages 20 to 21.

- **Rush.** The more slowly you do each exercise, the more effective the movement will be.

- **Ignore stretching.** These routines all take 20 minutes or less. Don't try to shorten them even more by skipping the suggested stretches. These stretches help you to make the most of your lower body work by allowing you to recover between exercises and helping you to work each movement to your fullest potential.

- **Lock your joints.** Even when your legs are extended during an exercise, always keep your knees soft and slightly bent to prevent any pressure on your knee joint.

Repeat As Needed

THE THREE LOWER-BODY Fat Zone routines include the most effective exercises for toning and firming your buns, hips, thighs, and calves. Every 2 weeks, you'll take on a new set of exercises, helping you to fully strengthen, firm, and tone your entire lower body.

During week 1, try the exercises without extra weight. This will help you concentrate on doing the exercise correctly. After week 1, if you can easily do 10 to 15 repetitions of each exercise, consider using 3- to 5-pound ankle weights when indicated.

Your current fitness level will determine how many repetitions you can perform for each exercise. Tune in to your body. Whether you are working your buns, hips, or thighs, pay attention to how those muscles feel as you move. When they start to burn and feel fatigued, do two more repetitions and then move on to the next exercise.

Here's a rule of thumb for the right number of repetitions as you progress on the program.

WEEKS 1 AND 2: 8 to 12

WEEKS 3 AND 4: two sets of 8 to 12 reps, running through the routine twice

WEEKS 5 AND 6: 16 to 24

Your Lower-Body Fat Zone routine for weeks 1 and 2 includes numerous exercises from the Pilates method, an exercise system developed by European gymnast Joseph Pilates many years ago. These are the same exercises in my book and video, *Pilates for Every Body*.

In addition to the Pilates moves, I've also added in my favorite tried-and-true butt, hip, and thigh shapers. These are the leg exercises that I do to blast away cellulite and tone and shape my legs. They *really* work.

You'll do most of the exercises during weeks 1 and 2 while lying or sitting, so pull out your exercise mat, concentrate on using proper form, and really fatigue those leg muscles. Go slowly. I know you can do it!

> ➤ SHRINKS YOUR SADDLEBAGS ➤ TONES YOUR OUTER THIGHS
> ➤ FIRMS YOUR HIPS

Outer Thigh and Hip Lift

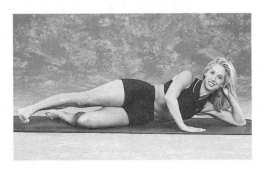

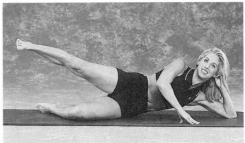

A. Start without weight, but gradually add ankle weights. Lie on your left side with your left leg bent for support and your right leg extended. Prop up your head with your left hand just behind your ear. Place your right palm on the mat in front of your torso for support. Your head, shoulders, and hips should all align, as shown.

B. With your foot flexed, exhale as you lift your right leg slowly and then inhale as you lower. You don't have to raise your leg very high to achieve results. The key here is slow, controlled movement, leading with your heel. Extend out through your top foot as you raise it, creating length in your outer thigh. Do 8 to 12 repetitions or repeat until fatigue. Then switch sides. (For extra fat-burning power, do two sets of 8 to 12 repetitions.)

➤ STRENGTHENS YOUR LOWER BACK ➤ FIRMS YOUR HIPS
➤ TIGHTENS YOUR BUTTOCKS ➤ BORROWED FROM PILATES

Front/Back

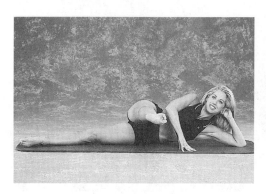
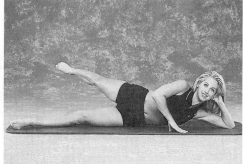

A. Lie on your left side with both legs extended. Align your left side with the edge of your mat so that your shoulders, back, and buttocks are parallel with the mat's edge.

Prop your head with your left hand just behind your left ear. Place your right palm on the mat in front of your abdomen for support. (For a greater challenge, you can place your right hand on your head.)

Then bring your legs forward 45 degrees in front of your body, keeping your buttocks, hips, back, and shoulders aligned with the mat's edge.

Lift your right leg about an inch above your left. As you inhale, slowly sweep your right leg forward, as shown. Only sweep your leg as far forward as you can without losing the alignment in your hips. Your right hipbone should remain stacked above your left, not tilting forward or back.

B. Once you've swept your leg as far forward as you can, exhale as you sweep it back behind your body and slightly up. Keep your abs strong throughout and squeeze your buttocks. Do 8 to 12 repetitions or repeat until fatigue. Then switch legs. (For extra fat-burning power, do two sets of 8 to 12 repetitions.)

MAXIMUM RESULTS	Minimum Time
Start with just a small motion on this exercise, taking care to keep your shoulders, torso, and hips from rocking back and forth as you move your leg. Eventually, as your abdominal muscles and thigh muscles stretch and strengthen, you'll be able to sweep your leg farther forward and back while keeping your hips and shoulders stacked.	

Inner Thigh Firmer

Lie on your left side with both legs extended. Align your left side with the edge of your mat so that your shoulders, back, and buttocks are parallel with the mat's edge. Then bring your legs forward 45 degrees in front of your body, keeping your buttocks, hips, back, and shoulders aligned with the mat's edge.

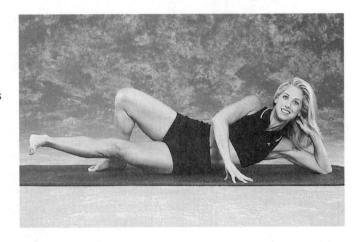

Prop your head with your left hand just behind your left ear. Place your right palm on the mat in front of your abdomen for support.

Bend your right leg and place your right foot on the mat just behind your left knee. Exhale and lift your left leg with your left foot flexed, as shown, feeling the movement in your left inner thigh. Inhale and lower, repeating 10 times. Then point your toes outward and repeat 8 to 12 times or until fatigue. Then switch sides. (For extra fat-burning power, do two sets of 8 to 12 repetitions.)

MAXIMUM RESULTS	Minimum Time

Hold your last repetition, squeezing your inner thighs until you can't hold your leg up any longer.

STRETCH BREAK

Outer Thigh and Hip Stretch

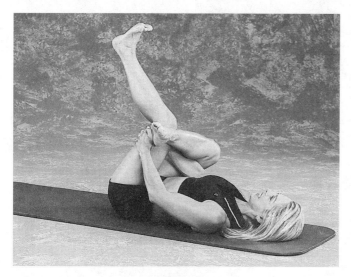

Lie on your back with your knees bent and feet flat on your mat. Inhale and lift your right foot, placing your right ankle just above your left knee on your left thigh, allowing your right knee to open to the side.

Exhale and raise your left foot, bringing your left knee in toward your chest. Hold for 20 seconds, breathing normally, then release. Switch legs and repeat.

MAXIMUM RESULTS	Minimum Time

To deepen the stretch, grasp the back of the thigh that's on the bottom with both hands, as shown, gently pulling it closer to your chest. Simultaneously, use your elbow to gently nudge the thigh that's on top outward, opening your top knee farther to the side. Ah-h-h . . . doesn't that feel wonderful?

Butt Lift

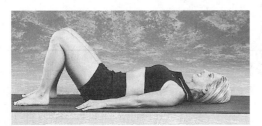

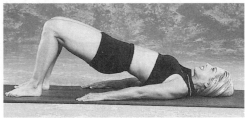

A. Lie on your back with both legs bent and feet flat on your mat. Rest your arms by your sides.

B. Exhale and press your hips toward the ceiling as you contract your buttocks, abs, and the backs of your thighs, lifting your buttocks 3 to 6 inches from your mat.

MAXIMUM RESULTS	Minimum Time

When you're in the lifted position, squeeze your buttocks for a few seconds, as if you were trying to squeeze every last drop out of a sponge.

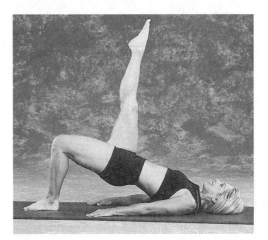

C. Inhale. Then exhale and lift and extend your right leg toward the ceiling. Lower your hips slightly as you inhale and then press back up, continuing to pulse up and down for 8 to 12 repetitions or until fatigue. Then lower to the starting position and repeat with your left leg extended. (For extra fat-burning power, do two sets of 8 to 12 repetitions.)

Leg Circles

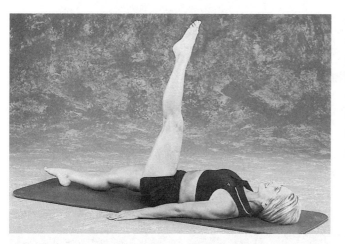

A. Lie on your back on your mat with your hands at your sides and your legs extended. Raise and extend your left leg until your left big toe points directly toward the ceiling, as shown.

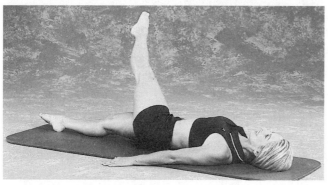

B. Engage your abs and circle your left leg counterclockwise, making sure to keep your hips level and motionless. As you circle, exhale as you lower your leg to the left and inhale as you raise it to the right. Once you've made three complete revolutions, switch direction, circling clockwise three times. Then switch legs and repeat the sequence.

MAXIMUM RESULTS | Minimum Time

Imagine that you're drawing circles on the ceiling with a crayon that's attached to your big toe. Start with small circles, and as your strength improves, draw larger ones. Only advance to larger circles if you can keep your upper body and hips motionless and your lower back pressed into your mat throughout the exercise. To work your inner thighs even more, turn your leg out slightly, bringing your heel in and toes out.

LEG CIRCLES WITH BAND (VARIATION)

For more of a challenge, try the leg circles with a resistance band.

Lie on your back with your left leg extended on the mat and your right leg extended toward the ceiling, with the exercise band wrapped around the arch of your right foot. Hold both ends of the band in your right hand at chest level with your elbow bent. Extend your left arm out to the side for balance.

Engage your abs and slowly circle your right foot counterclockwise, dipping down to the floor as you move your foot around the circle. Make three large circles—exhaling as you lower your leg and inhaling as you raise your leg—and then switch direction, circling clockwise. Then switch legs and repeat.

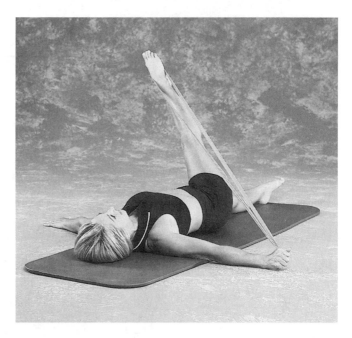

"You'll **look great** from **behind.** You'll get the **lean** legs you've always **wanted.**"

Butt Toner

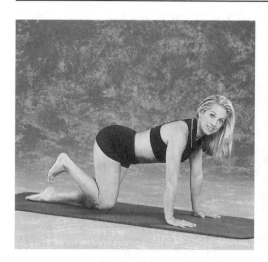 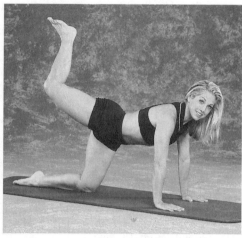

A. Get on your hands and knees, as shown, with your hands under your shoulders and your knees under your hips. Bend and lift your right leg so that your right thigh is parallel with your mat and your right calf and thigh form a right angle.

B. Exhale and lift your right foot toward the ceiling as far as you can, as shown, squeezing your buttocks as you do so. Inhale and lower, repeating 8 to 12 times or until fatigue. Switch legs and repeat. (For extra fat-burning power, do two sets of 8 to 12 repetitions.)

MAXIMUM RESULTS	Minimum Time
Keep your back flat, abs tight, and hips square to the floor throughout the exercise.	

STRETCH BREAK

Down Dog

Get on your hands and knees. Press back through your palms and bring your buttocks close to your heels. Lower both heels toward the floor and extend through both legs, raising your tailbone toward the ceiling, as shown. Allow your shoulder blades to widen apart and your chest to open. Gaze at your navel to keep your neck in a neutral position. Hold for 20 seconds, breathing deeply, and release.

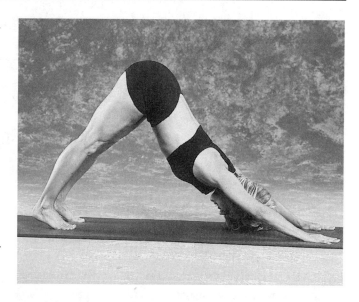

MAXIMUM RESULTS | Minimum Time

To intensify the stretch, try lifting and extending one leg. This will place your body weight onto your other heel, pressing it toward the floor. Try this only if your heels are nearly touching the floor when in the regular down dog position.

"You've really worked your thighs, so take a break and try one of my favorite stretches."

Thigh Toner

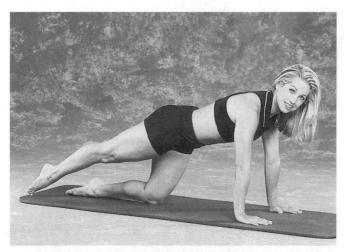

A. Get on all fours, with your hands under your shoulders and your knees under your hips. Extend your right leg and lift your right foot with your toes pointed out and held just above the mat, as shown. Make sure that your back is flat, your abs are tight, and your hips are square to the floor.

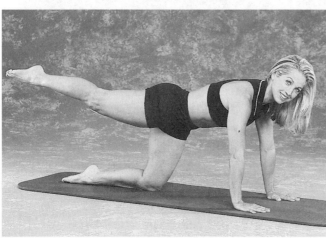

B. Exhale and lift your right leg as far as you can. Inhale and lower, repeating 8 to 12 times or until fatigue. Switch sides and repeat. (For extra fat-burning power, do two sets of 8 to 12 repetitions.)

MAXIMUM RESULTS Minimum Time

Squeeze your buttocks as you lift your leg to increase the effectiveness of the exercise.

WEEKS 1 & 2

➤ FIRMS, TONES, AND TIGHTENS THE FRONTS OF YOUR THIGHS
➤ HELPS YOU LOOK GREAT IN SHORTS ➤ STRENGTHENS MUSCLES THAT HELP PROTECT YOUR KNEES FROM INJURY

Thigh Blaster

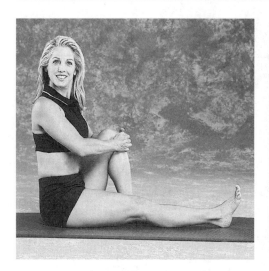 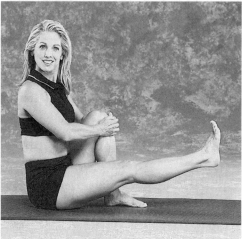

A. Sit with your right leg extended and left leg bent, left knee pulled in toward your chest and left foot flat on your mat. Try to bring your left foot as close to your body as you can. Grasp your left knee with your hands, as shown.

B. Exhale as you lift your right leg and inhale as you lower it, repeating 8 to 12 times or until fatigue. Then switch legs. (For extra fat-burning power, do two sets of 8 to 12 repetitions.)

MAXIMUM RESULTS	Minimum Time

The farther forward you position your torso to the foot that's flat on the floor, the harder the exercise. If you can't do the exercise while holding on to your bent knee, place your hands on your mat and lean back slightly, making sure to keep your back straight. Eventually, work your way forward, hugging your knee to your torso as you do the exercise.

STRETCH BREAK

Pigeon

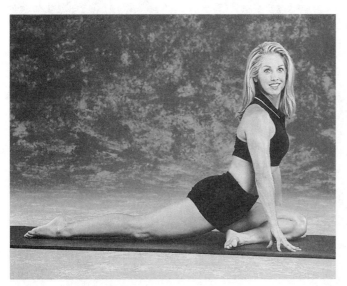

Get on your hands and knees. Bring your left knee forward between your hands, just to the inside of your left wrist, placing your left foot closer to your right hand. Exhale and extend back through your right leg, sinking deeper into the stretch. Hold for 20 seconds, breathing normally, then release and repeat with the other leg.

MAXIMUM RESULTS   Minimum Time

If your buttocks and hips are extremely tight, place a pillow or cushion under the buttock of your bent leg. This will reduce the angle of the stretch, making it less intense. Breathe into any tight spots as you exhale, imagining your breath opening and loosening your muscles.

My Lower-Body Fat Zone routine for weeks 3 and 4 contains numerous moves I learned during my childhood ballet classes. These moves—typically done at a ballet bar—will help you to develop the long, lean legs of a ballerina. You'll do all of these moves while standing, which will increase your calorie burn during your workout, as your standing leg also has to work hard to keep you balanced.

Since you probably don't have a ballet bar in your home, you'll need a sturdy chair for these exercises. Place one hand on the back of the chair as you do the moves, as if it were a bar. Over time, rely on the chair less and less, making your standing leg and abs work harder.

> ➤ TARGETS THE FRONTS OF YOUR THIGHS
> ➤ STRENGTHENS THE MUSCLES THAT PROTECT YOUR KNEES

Ballet Lift

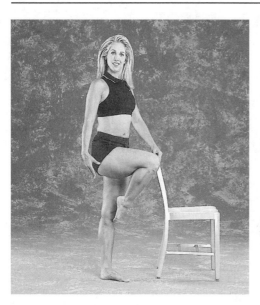
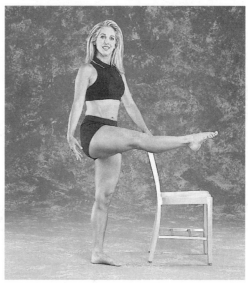

A. Stand next to a chair, with your left hand on the chair back for balance. Bend and lift your right knee until your right thigh is parallel to the floor, as shown.

B. With your abs tight, exhale and extend your right leg by lifting your right shin. Inhale and lower your shin, without lowering your thigh, repeating 8 to 12 times. Switch sides and repeat, then do another set on both sides.

Ronde de Jambe

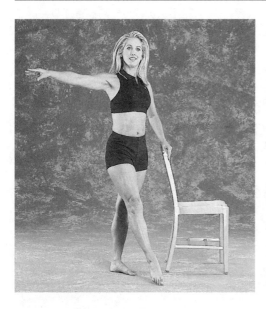

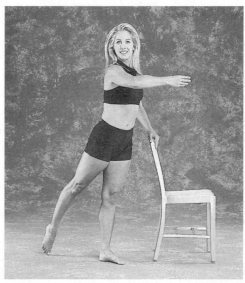

A. Stand with one foot in front of the other and your toes turned out. Place your left hand on a chair back for balance.

MAXIMUM RESULTS	Minimum Time

Keep your hips pointed forward and level throughout the exercise. Also, try the ronde de jambe at different levels, with your leg extended about 2 feet above the floor, for example, or at hip level. This will slightly change the area of the inner and outer thighs that you target, shaping the entire muscle.

B. Inhale and then slowly sweep your extended right leg out to the right, then behind your torso and to the left in a large arc, as if you were drawing a semicircle on the floor with your big toe. Then exhale and reverse the motion. Touch in front and touch behind. Repeat 8 to 12 times before switching sides. Do two sets total.

Standing Front/Back

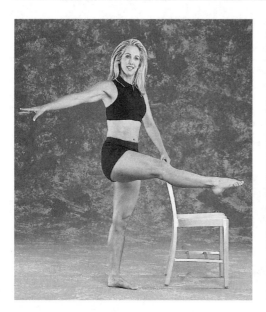

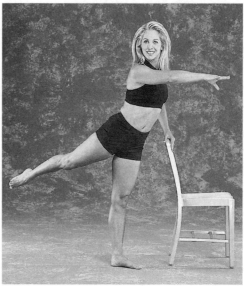

A. Stand with your feet in ballet's second position, with your feet aligned under your hips and your toes turned out. Place your left hand on a chair back for balance. Lift and extend your right leg in front of your torso, as shown. Bend your left leg slightly.

B. Exhale and sweep your extended right leg behind your torso. Inhale and bring it forward, repeating 8 to 12 times before switching legs. As your leg goes back, your free arm should lift forward, and vice versa. Repeat for another set of 8 to 12 repetitions.

MAXIMUM RESULTS	Minimum Time
Squeeze your buttocks as you sweep your leg behind your torso. Also try to keep your hips level and pointing forward throughout the move.	

Thigh Stretch

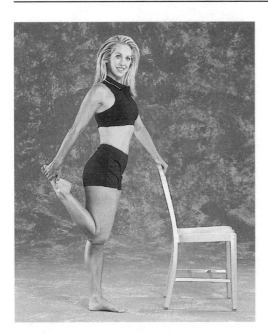

Stand with your left hand on a chair back for balance. Shift your body weight to your left foot and then lift and bend your right leg behind you, bringing your right calf toward your right thigh. Reach back with your right hand and grab your right foot, as shown, gently pulling your right foot even closer to your buttock as you exhale. Hold for 20 seconds then release. Repeat with your left leg.

MAXIMUM RESULTS	Minimum Time
To increase the stretch, you don't need to pull your knee behind the plane of your torso. Rather, drop your body weight through your bent knee, lowering that knee toward the floor. Then tighten your lower abs to tuck your pelvis.	

Inner Thigh Beats

Stand with your feet in ballet's first position, in which your heels are together and your toes are turned out. Place your left hand on a chair back for balance. Bring your body weight onto your left foot and lift your right foot a few inches off the ground and about a foot in front of your body. Exhale and bring your right heel toward the left heel and pulse back and forth toward the left for 8 to 12 repetitions. Relax and then repeat on your left side. Finish with another set of 8 to 12 repetitions on both sides.

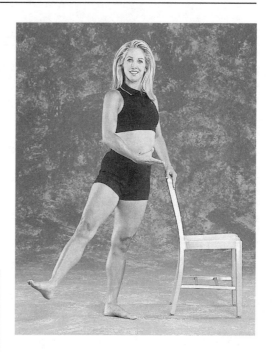

MAXIMUM RESULTS	Minimum Time

On the last repetition, hold your leg in the up position as long as you can as you squeeze that inner thigh muscle, getting the most out of the exercise.

➤ ONE OF THE MOST EFFECTIVE LEG EXERCISES
➤ WORKS YOUR HIPS, BUTT, THIGHS, AND CALVES

Lunge with Chair

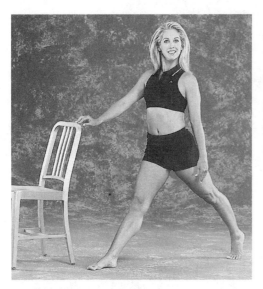 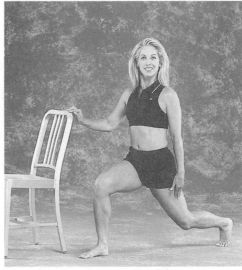

A. Stand with your right hand on a chair back for balance. Take a large step back with your left foot, forming the shape of open scissors with your legs. Evenly adjust your body weight between the ball of your left foot and the bottom of your right foot.

B. With your back straight and tummy tight, inhale as you lower your torso by bending both knees and sinking into a lunge. Bring your left knee close to the floor, but not touching, and bend your right leg to a 90-degree angle.

> "If lunges were the only exercise you did for your legs, your legs would still look terrific."

—continued

THE LOWER BODY   203

Lunge with Chair—continued

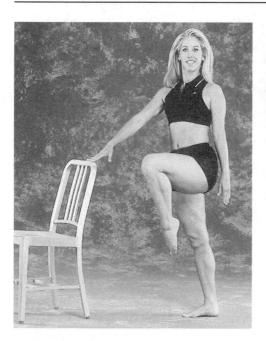

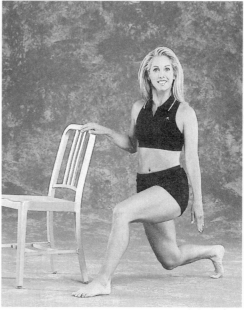

C. Exhale as you press into your feet and straighten your legs. Then lift your left foot, as shown, bringing your left knee in toward your chest.

D. Bring your left foot forward, planting your legs again in the scissors position with your left leg in front, and then sink into a lunge. Repeat 8 to 12 times, switch legs, and repeat. Then do another set of 8 to 12 on both sides.

MAXIMUM RESULTS	Minimum Time
Don't allow your front knee to jut forward beyond your ankle. If it does, slide your front foot forward a few inches. If you have weak knees, don't bend your knees fully to 90 degrees. Only bend them as far as you can without discomfort and then rise back to the starting position.	

STRETCH BREAK

Standing Hip Opener

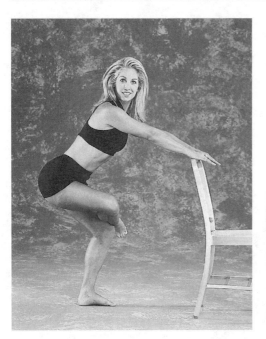

Stand with your hands on a chair back for balance. Inhale as you bend your right leg and place your right ankle on top of your lower left thigh. Exhale as you bend your left leg and lightly press into your right knee with your right hand, feeling the stretch in your right hip. Hold for 20 seconds, rise to the starting position, and repeat on the other side.

MAXIMUM RESULTS	Minimum Time
To achieve a deeper stretch, you don't need to bend the knee of the leg you're standing on all the way to 90 degrees. Rather, just simply lean forward from your hips and press your buttocks back.	

"Breathe into tight spots. Imagine your breath opening and soothing any tension in the muscle, helping you to increase the stretch."

Plié

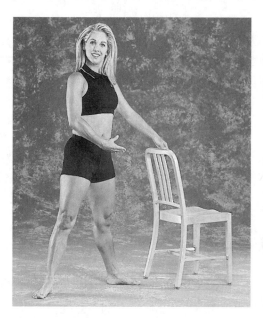 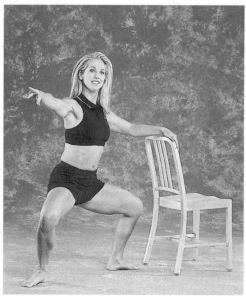

A. Begin in ballet's second position, with your feet wider than hip-width apart, your toes turned out and abs pulled toward your spine. Place your left hand on a chair for balance.

B. Inhale as you plié down, bringing your knees out to the sides. Exhale as you press through your inner thighs to rise. Repeat 8 to 12 times, holding your last repetition in the down position for as long as you can, trying to open your knees outward as you do so. Then do an additional set of 8 to 12 repetitions.

> "This exercise will prevent jiggle and keep your thighs from rubbing together."

MAXIMUM RESULTS	Minimum Time
To get the most from this exercise, concentrate on your inner thighs and groin, being sure that you contract and squeeze those muscles as you rise.	

> ➤ TONES YOUR QUADRICEPS, ALONG THE FRONTS OF YOUR THIGHS
> ➤ FIRMS YOUR HAMSTRINGS, ALONG THE BACKS OF YOUR THIGHS
> ➤ LIFTS YOUR BUNS

Butt-Tap Squat

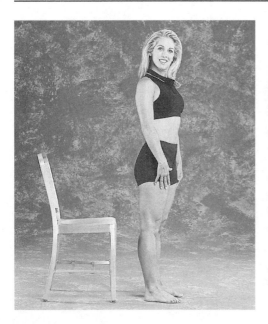

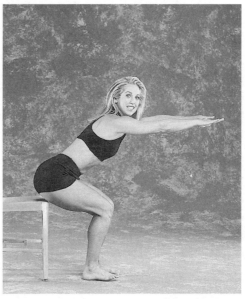

A. Stand in front of a chair with your feet slightly wider than hip-width apart. Extend through your crown to lengthen and straighten your spine. Tighten your abs.

B. Extend your arms in front of your chest for balance. Inhale and slowly bend your knees as you sit back, as if you were going to sit in the chair. As you do so, keep your body weight over your heels. As soon as you feel your buttocks touch the seat, exhale and press up through your inner thighs and buttocks. Repeat 8 to 12 times, then rest briefly. Finish with one last set of 8 to 12 repetitions.

MAXIMUM RESULTS	Minimum Time
You can also do this exercise from a wide-leg stance with your toes pointed out to tighten your inner thighs and buttocks at the same time.	

Standing Hamstring Curl

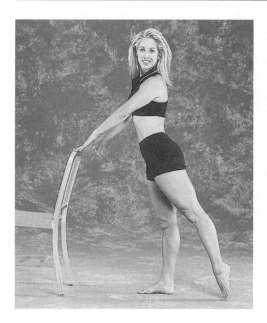 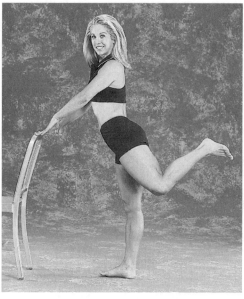

A. Stand with your hands on a chair back for balance. Extend your left leg about 2 feet behind your body, as shown. Lean forward slightly from your waist.

B. Exhale and bend your left leg, curling your left heel toward the back of your left thigh. Inhale as you lower. Repeat 8 to 12 times before switching legs. Rest briefly, then do a final set of 8 to 12 with each leg.

MAXIMUM RESULTS	Minimum Time
Tighten your abs, pressing them in and up toward your spine. This will tilt your pelvis slightly, lengthening the backs of your thighs and making the exercise more effective.	

STRETCH BREAK

Half-Forward Bend

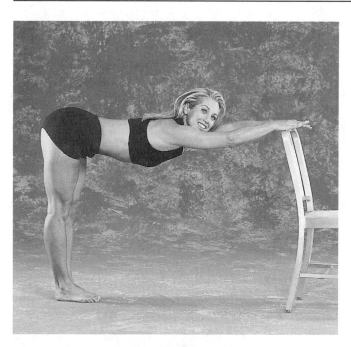

Stand with your feet aligned under your hips several feet behind a chair. Inhale as you lengthen your spine and tighten your abs. Then exhale as you bend forward from the waist, reaching your hands out and resting them on the chair back. Press back through your hips as you lengthen your spine and the backs of your thighs. Hold for 20 seconds and then release.

MAXIMUM RESULTS Minimum Time

To stretch your thighs and back even more, raise your tailbone up toward the ceiling.

For this Lower-Body Fat Zone routine, I've incorporated numerous moves from yoga, helping you to shape lean yet pliable and balanced yoga legs. These moves will help you to improve your balance as well as help you properly align your hips, preventing age-related injuries.

Other moves come from kickboxing. I love these exercises. I've found that my legs and backside look their best when I focus on doing this series of kicks. For some of these exercises, you'll place your body weight against a wall or use a wall for balance, so find a wall in your house that's clear of pictures, shelves, or other hindrances.

➤ FIRMS YOUR BUTTOCKS ➤ TONES YOUR THIGHS

Wall Sit

Stand with your back against a wall, your legs extended, and your feet about 2 feet in front of the wall. Inhale and then exhale and slide your back down the wall as you bend your legs to a 90-degree angle. Make sure that your knees do not go past your toes. If they do, slide your feet out farther. Hold for 10 to 30 seconds.

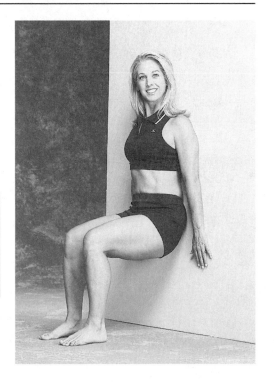

MAXIMUM RESULTS	Minimum Time
When in the sitting position, press your lower back into the wall and firm your abs, bringing them in and up.	

WALL SIT WITH BALL (VARIATION)

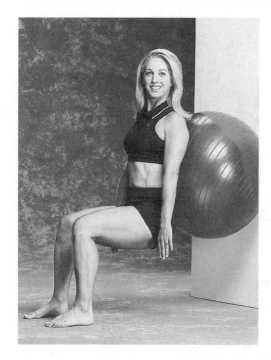

Doing the wall sit with a large stability ball between your back and the wall works your core muscles as they attempt to stabilize your upper body.

Stand with a stability ball held between your back and a wall. Lean your back into the ball and then exhale and sit as you bend your knees, rolling the ball down the wall as you do so.

MAXIMUM RESULTS	Minimum Time
From the sitting position, try pulsing up just an inch or two and then lowering your buttocks back to the sitting position with your legs bent at a 90-degree angle. This will help you hold the position longer by keeping your mind off your thighs as well as helping you more fully target your butt and thigh muscles.	

"This move helps carve that sexy separation between your buns and thighs, creating a beautiful line that defines your buttocks."

STRETCH BREAK

Standing Quad Stretch

Stand with your feet aligned under your hips. Place your left hand against a wall for balance. Inhale and bend your right leg behind you, bringing your right foot toward your right thigh. Exhale and grasp your right foot with your right hand, as shown, bringing the foot closer to your buttocks and feeling the stretch in the front of your right thigh. Hold for 20 seconds, release, and repeat with your left leg.

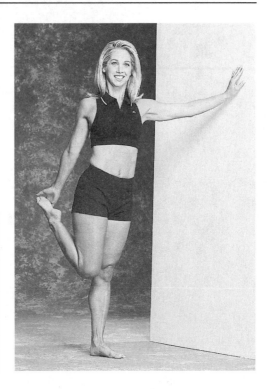

MAXIMUM RESULTS	Minimum Time

To increase the stretch, you don't need to pull your knee behind the plane of your torso. Rather, drop your body weight through your bent knee, lowering that knee toward the floor. Then tighten your lower abs to tuck your pelvis.

Diagonal Lunge

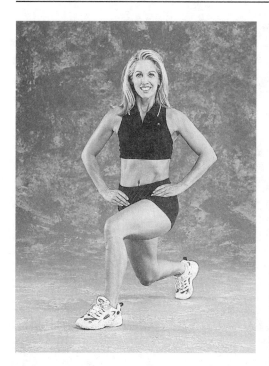

Stand with your feet aligned under your hips. Exhale and take a large step diagonally forward with your left foot, aiming to plant it at 2 o'clock. Square your hips as you inhale and sink into the lunge, bending your left leg at a 90-degree angle. Exhale and press through your left foot to rise to the starting position and then repeat on your right, stepping out toward 10 o'clock. Continue alternating until you've completed 16 to 24 repetitions on each side. (For extra fat-burning power, do two sets of 16 to 24 repetitions.)

MAXIMUM RESULTS	Minimum Time
As you sink into the lunge, try to drop your hips directly down, not forward. This will help you protect your front knee by preventing it from jutting in front of your ankle.	

"Don't let those buns go south!"

➤ STRETCHES YOUR INNER THIGHS, BUTTOCKS, AND HIPS
➤ GREAT FOR LEAN LEGS

STRETCH BREAK

Wide-Angle Forward Bend

Stand with your feet 3 to 3½ feet apart. Place your palms against your thighs. Inhale and lengthen your spine and tighten your tummy. Then exhale and bend forward from your hips, as shown, as you slide your hands down your thighs to your shins then ankles and possibly even to the floor. Hold for 20 seconds and then release.

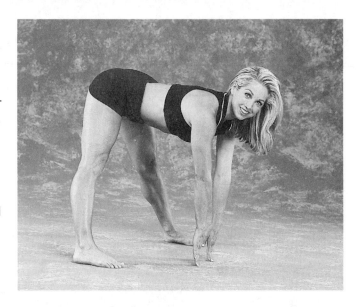

MAXIMUM RESULTS	Minimum Time

Try not to round your back as you bend forward. You'll get a better stretch by bending forward only slightly with a straight spine than by rounding your back and reaching your head close to the floor.

Warrior

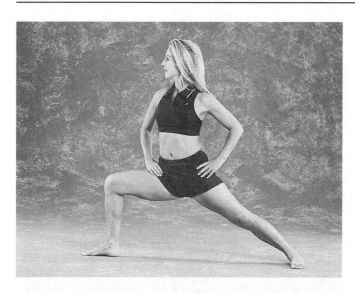

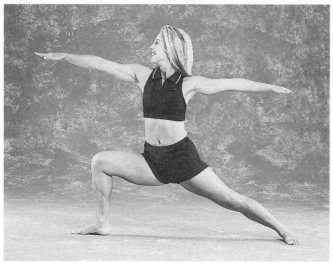

A. Start with your feet aligned under your hips. Inhale as you slightly bend your knees and take a large step to the left with your left foot, spreading your feet about 3½ to 4 feet apart. Turn out your right toes 90 degrees and allow your left heel to move back slightly. Exhale and sink into a deep lunge, with your right knee bent at a 90-degree angle and your left leg extended. You'll be looking out over your right knee. Your right foot should be pointed to the right, and your left foot will be pointed to the front, at a 90-degree angle from your right foot.

B. Extend your arms laterally from your shoulders. You should resemble a warrioress ready to throw a spear with her left arm. Stretch through your fingertips, creating length in your arms and upper back.

—continued

Warrior—*continued*

C. Lift your right heel, bringing part of your body weight onto the ball of your right foot, intensifying the work done by your inner thigh. Hold for 10 to 30 seconds and then relax. Repeat on the other side. (For extra fat-burning power, repeat exercise.)

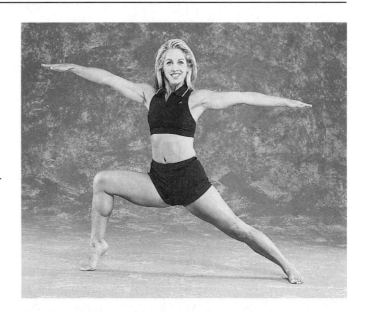

MAXIMUM RESULTS | Minimum Time

To help encourage yourself to hold the pose longer, try breathing percussively as you throw your imaginary spear. To do so, bend your rear arm as if you were holding a spear. Then press your lower tummy in quickly to force out a breath of air as you simultaneously launch your spear forward at an imaginary target. If you feel yourself lose your balance as you do so, your body weight is too far forward over your bent leg. Continue to throw numerous spears with each percussive breath.

Front Kick

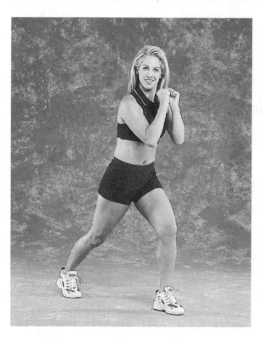 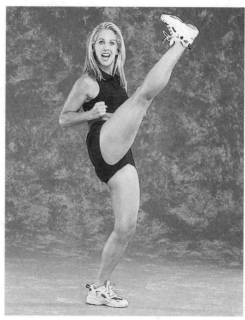

A. Stand in a fighter stance with your arms bent and hands in loose fists in front of your chin, palms facing each other. Your feet will be hip-width apart, with your left foot about a foot in front of the right.

B. Tighten your abs, lift your right knee to waist height, and exhale as you kick out your right foot, as if you were trying to whack your opponent in the chin. Inhale as you lower. Repeat 16 to 24 times and then switch legs. (For extra fat-burning power, do two sets of 16 to 24 repetitions.)

MAXIMUM RESULTS	Minimum Time
Try not to hyperextend your leg as you kick. This will help protect your knee joint.	

Back Kick

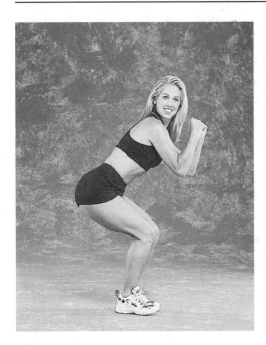

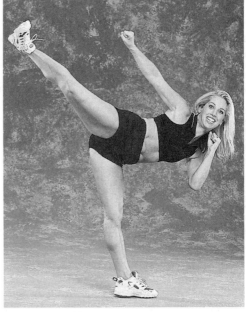

A. Stand in a fighter stance with your arms bent and hands in loose fists in front of your chin, palms facing each other. Place your feet under your hips, and tighten your abs as you sit back into a squat, as shown.

MAXIMUM RESULTS	Minimum Time
If you feel wobbly at first, know that your balance will improve quickly. One tip: Gaze at a point on the wall at eye level or higher. Looking up will help you keep your balance.	

B. Lift your right knee toward your chest and then gaze to your right side at your imaginary opponent. As you move your gaze, allow your arms and torso to rotate to the right. Exhale and extend your right leg to the right, as shown, pressing through your right heel as if you were kicking your opponent in the stomach or chest. Your right foot should be parallel to the floor, with your heel slightly higher than your toes. Inhale as you recoil. Repeat 16 to 24 times and then switch legs. (For extra fat-burning power, do two sets of 16 to 24 repetitions.)

> STRETCHES THE BACKS OF YOUR THIGHS AND BUTTOCKS > RELEASES ANY LOWER BACK
> TENSION THAT MAY HAVE RESULTED DURING THE WARRIOR

STRETCH BREAK

Forward Bend

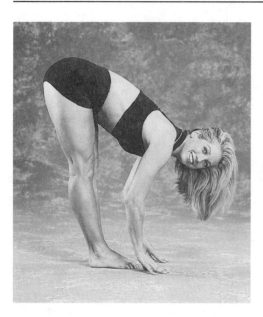

Stand with your feet together. Lengthen your spine, tighten your abs, and then exhale as you bend forward from the waist. Gently place your hands against your thighs to slowly lower your torso. Hold for 20 seconds and then release.

MAXIMUM RESULTS	Minimum Time
Many women round their backs as they attempt a forward bend. This places more of the emphasis on your back muscles and much less on your leg muscles. Also, if you are prone to spinal problems such as a herniated disk, doing a forward bend with a curved spine can create discomfort. As you lean forward, keep your spine long. To encourage yourself to lengthen, gently press your hands against your thighs or shins.	

> ➤ STRETCHES YOUR BUTTOCKS, HIPS, AND OUTER THIGHS
> ➤ FEELS WONDERFUL ➤ THIS IS ANOTHER OF MY FAVORITES

STRETCH BREAK

Standing Hip Opener

Stand with your feet aligned under your hips. Place your left hand against a wall for balance. Inhale as you bend your right leg and place your right ankle on top of your lower left thigh. Bend your left leg as you exhale, lightly pressing into your right knee with your right hand, as shown, and feeling the stretch in your right hip. Hold for 20 seconds and then rise to the starting position. Repeat on the other side.

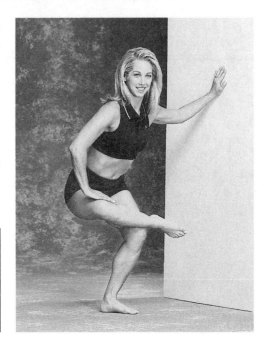

MAXIMUM RESULTS	Minimum Time
Lean forward from your hips and press your buttocks back to increase the stretch.	

CHAPTER 8

Total-Body Shape-Ups

We all have those days when we can't possibly add one more thing to our "to do" list, let alone fit in a workout.

Perhaps your child wakes up with a fever, your boss calls you into the office early for an emergency meeting, your best friend calls with a personal crisis, or one of your pipes bursts. Whatever the reason, you suddenly find yourself with five new tasks to do that you hadn't originally on your "to do" list—and not enough time or energy to get it all done.

That's when this 10-minute fat-burning blast comes in handy.

My Upper-Body, Midsection, and Lower-Body Fat Zone routines all take 20 minutes to complete. But I know some days you simply won't have 20 minutes. That's why I've included this fallback plan that combines cardio with toning, helping you to rev up your metabolism and tone your trouble spots from head to toe, even on those frenzied days.

This 10-Minute Total-Body Blast presents you with the best way to start a jam-packed day on the right foot—literally. I suggest doing it in the morning because research shows that's when you're most likely to fit in exercise. When women wait until later in the day—particularly on a busy day—other tasks take precedence, and exercise often falls to the bottom of the "to do" list.

I know. It happens to me, too. If I haven't exercised in the morning, I know that by the time evening rolls around, I have the best excuse not to workout: I have to make my family dinner. And, of course, I feel justified.

Getting your total-body blast out of the way in the morning allows you to face the rest of your day with the peace of mind of knowing that you've already worked out. You won't have to muddle up your already busy brain with thoughts of how you'll fit in your workout—or with the guilt associated with not fitting it in.

Think of this routine as an emergency backup plan. On a busy day, set your alarm clock 10 minutes earlier and get right out of bed. Splash some water on your face, put on your exercise clothes, lace up those shoes, and just do it.

That said, do keep this as your *backup* plan. To truly shrink your fat zones, you need your longer, more targeted toning workouts coupled with daily stretching and regular walking. If you find yourself opting for this 10-minute routine every day, reexamine your priorities. Whenever you're thinking of cutting a longer workout short, ask yourself the following:

Do I really need to do all of these errands today? I ask myself this question a lot. It seems as the day goes on, I find myself adding more and more to my mental "to do" list. Sometimes I have to step back and take a good, hard look at what I'm trying to accomplish. Oftentimes, I realize that many of those tasks can wait.

Am I really busy—or am I procrastinating? Sometimes we come up with things to keep us from working out. What is filling your day? Are you talking on the phone a lot? Watching television? Get off the phone, turn off the TV, and move your body.

Denise's Fast Workout Do's and Don'ts

No matter your personal fat zone, my 10-Minute Total-Body Blast will target and tone your entire body. Here are some do's and don'ts for making the best of this workout.

DO . . .

- **Fidget.** On days when you cut your workout short to just 10 minutes, try to fit in as much exercise as you can throughout the day. Walk whenever you get the chance. Climb every flight of stairs that you see. Do butt or abdominal squeezes when standing in line. Blow-dry your hair from a squatting position. You get the idea.

- **Stretch.** No matter how busy your day, try not to eliminate your three stretching routines. They will clear your mind, boost your performance at work, and allow you to feel better all day long. This in turn prevents the stress of your busy day from destroying your energy levels. That way, when you arrive home with an unexpected 5 to 10 minutes to spare, you'll have the energy to go for a quick walk.

- **Make it social.** Involving family or friends in your exercise routine helps you to multitask. Invite your girlfriends over for a total-body blast (or even your 20-minute fat zone workout). Or meet them for a walk. Do some fun cardio with your kids. I love playing tag with my daughters. It really gets my heart rate up. We also take our Portuguese water dog, Madonna, for a walk after dinner every day together as a family.

DON'T . . .

- **Make excuses.** Everyone has 10 minutes. No matter how busy your day, don't let yourself get in the habit of skipping your workouts altogether. This will start a bad precedent of putting exercise last on your priorities list.

- **Rush.** This routine takes only 10 minutes, so there's no need to rush through it. Take your time during each exercise, making sure to work until muscle fatigue and to perform each repetition with proper form.

Your 10-Minute Total-Body Blast

I've included the best exercises for toning and working your muscles from head to toe, particularly your trouble spots. This workout includes numerous combination moves that work at least two muscle groups in one exercise. This allows you to fit more moves into your allotted time.

This workout also includes several lunges and squats, some of them off the back of an aerobics step. These will not only tone your buns and legs but also rev up your heart rate and boost your calorie burning.

Use a step that's 6 to 8 inches high. If you don't have an aerobics step, do these exercises on a stair step or without any step at all. You'll also need your dumbbells and exercise mat.

➤ SHAPES YOUR ARMS ➤ LIFTS YOUR BUNS ➤ FIRMS YOUR THIGHS

Biceps Curl
with Off-the-Back Lunge

A. Stand on the middle of your step with a dumbbell in each hand, palms up, and your feet aligned under your hips.

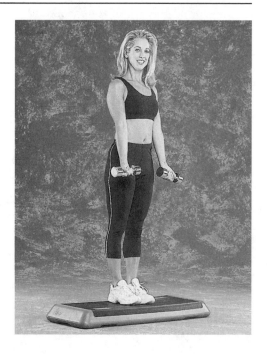

"You are creating beautiful, sexy curves."

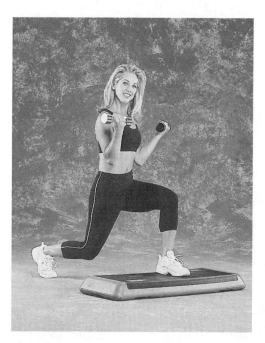

B. Tighten your abs, exhale, and take a large step back with your right leg as you simultaneously curl the dumbbells toward your shoulders. While continuing to curl the dumbbells, plant the ball of your right foot on the floor and sink into the lunge, bending your right leg as much as 90 degrees, as shown.

Inhale and press up through your left foot as you lift back to the starting position, lowering the dumbbells back to your sides as you do so. Then repeat by stepping back with your left leg as you curl the dumbbells. Continue alternating right and left for 15 repetitions on each leg.

MAXIMUM RESULTS	Minimum Time
Do your lunges with energy, really pressing through your feet to lift your torso back onto the bench, as if your body were an elevator heading straight up. This will help speed up your heart rate—burning more calories—and more quickly fatigue your leg muscles.	

Triceps Kickback with Rear Leg Lift

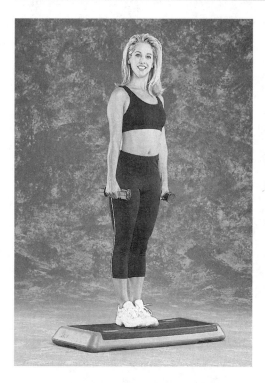

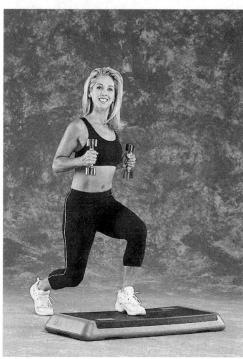

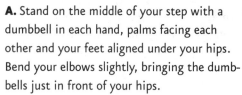

A. Stand on the middle of your step with a dumbbell in each hand, palms facing each other and your feet aligned under your hips. Bend your elbows slightly, bringing the dumbbells just in front of your hips.

B. Inhale and take a large step back with your right leg and plant the ball of your right foot firmly on the floor. Simultaneously, bend your elbows, raising the dumbbells to chest level.

"Your body is an **investment** that **pays off** numerous **dividends** over time. **Two** of those dividends are **more energy** and **better health.** Those **errands** can **wait. Your body can't."**

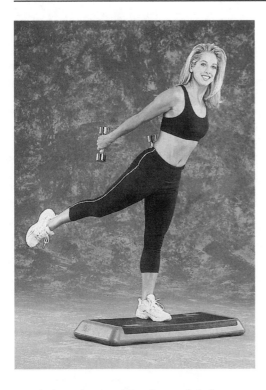

MAXIMUM RESULTS	Minimum Time
Lift your leg as high as you can behind your torso, squeezing your buttocks as you do so. Remember, if you don't squeeze them, no one else will!	

C. Exhale and press through your left foot as you straighten your left leg and lift your extended right leg behind your torso. As you do so, kick back the dumbbells by extending your arms, bringing the dumbbells up past your thighs and behind your torso, as shown.

Inhale as you lower your arms and right leg and return to the starting position. Repeat with your left leg, then continue to alternate right and left for 15 repetitions on each leg.

Overhead Raise
with Side Lift

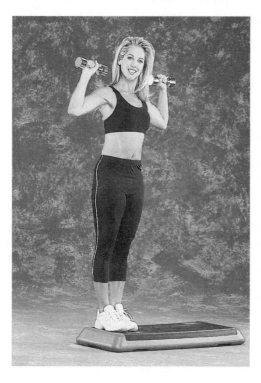

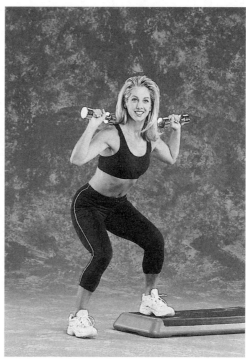

A. Stand near the right end of your step with a dumbbell in each hand. Bend your arms and raise the dumbbells to shoulder level, with your palms facing forward.

B. Inhale and take a step to the right with your right foot.

"Slow it down. Use proper form. Get a quality workout."

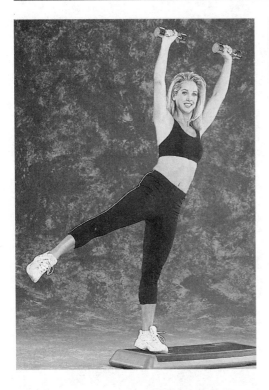

MAXIMUM RESULTS	Minimum Time
Pay attention to your form on this one. You want to raise the weights directly above your shoulders. Try not to let the momentum of your side kick allow your upper torso to lean forward, causing you to raise the weights on a forward diagonal.	

C. Exhale and press through your left foot to lift your torso as you simultaneously lift and extend your right leg to the side, feeling the movement in your right outer thigh. At the same time, lift the dumbbells overhead by extending your arms.

Inhale and bring your right leg back to the step as you lower the dumbbells to your shoulders. Repeat with your left foot, stepping out toward the left. Alternate right and then left for 15 repetitions on each leg.

Lunge with Upper Back Fly

A. Stand on the end of your step with a dumb-bell in each hand, palms facing each other, by your sides. Bend your arms and bring the dumbbells slightly in front of your torso. Exhale and take a large step back with your right foot. Plant the ball of your right foot and sink into the lunge, bending your left leg as much as 90 degrees.

B. Inhale and lean forward from your waist about 45 degrees as you hold the lunge, holding your hands at arm's length below your chest. Exhale as you slowly raise your hands out to your sides in a large arcing motion, as shown, bringing your shoulder blades closer together. Inhale as you lower. Repeat six times while continuing to hold the lunge.

Then lower your arms and press through your left foot to return to the starting position. Repeat by stepping back with your left foot and performing six upper back flies.

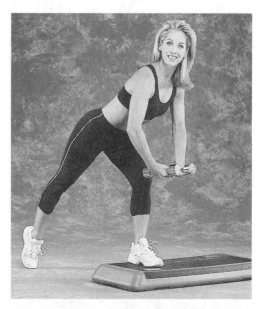

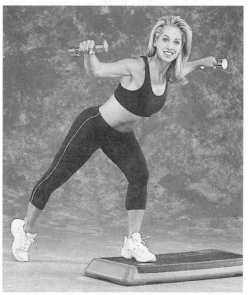

MAXIMUM RESULTS	Minimum Time
Keep your back long and straight. Try not to allow your spine to slump forward.	

STRETCH BREAK

Forward Bend

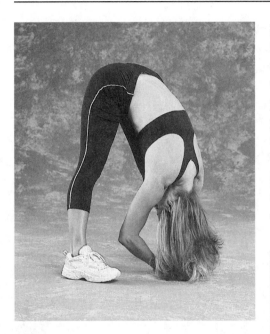

Stand with your feet aligned under your hips. Inhale and lengthen your spine, tighten your abs, and then exhale and bend forward from the waist. Gently place your hands against your thighs to slowly lower your torso. Once you've lowered as far as you can with a straight back, allow your hands to drop toward the floor, as shown, and hang effortlessly, releasing any tension that you may have built up during the previous exercises. Hold for 20 seconds, breathing normally, and then release.

MAXIMUM RESULTS	Minimum Time

Many women round their backs as they attempt a forward bend. This places more of the emphasis on your back muscles and much less on your leg muscles. Also, if you are prone to spinal problems such as a herniated disk, doing a forward bend with a curved spine can create discomfort. As you lean forward, keep your spine long. To encourage yourself to lengthen, gently press your hands against your thighs or shins.

> "You just **blasted** your **legs.** Give them a **nice, relaxing rest** before moving **on to** your abs."

Bicycle

A. Lie on your back on your mat. Bend your knees and lift your feet and thighs until you form a 90-degree angle between your torso and your thighs. Place your fingers behind your head with your elbows open to the sides. Lift your upper torso off the mat so that your shoulder blades hover just above the mat's surface. Exhale and bring your left shoulder and right knee toward one another and simultaneously extend your left leg.

B. In quick succession, inhale and lower your left shoulder and right knee as you exhale and bring your right shoulder and left knee toward one another while extending your right leg. Continue alternating for 10 to 15 repetitions on each side.

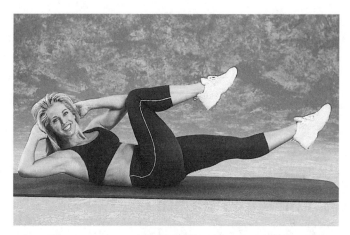

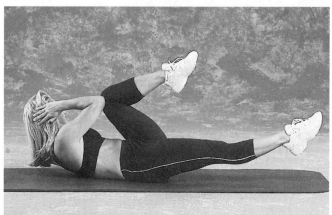

MAXIMUM RESULTS	Minimum Time

It's easy to lose control and move too quickly. Try to slow down your movement as you concentrate on keeping your navel tight and your lower back pressed to the mat. Try to create a flat, hollow tummy throughout the exercise.

Double-Leg Stretch

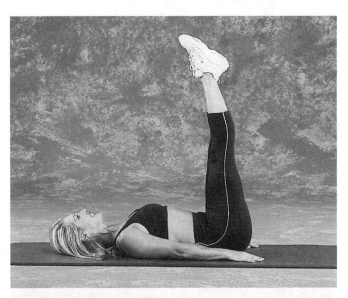

A. Lie on your back on your mat, with your knees bent and feet flat on the floor and your arms at your sides. Lift your feet toward the ceiling as you extend your legs, forming a 90-degree angle between your legs and torso, as shown. Press your inner thighs and heels together as you turn out your toes. Lift your upper torso off the mat until your shoulder blades hover just above the surface of the mat.

B. Exhale and slowly lower your legs as you tighten your abs. To keep your back in a neutral position, imagine your abs lengthening as you lower your legs. Stop once you can no longer keep your spine neutral. Inhale and raise your legs to the starting position. Repeat 10 times.

MAXIMUM RESULTS   Minimum Time

Continue to press your inner thighs together as you lower and raise your legs. This will allow you to work them, too!

➤ FLATTENS YOUR ABS BELOW THE NAVEL

Rollover

A. Lie on your back on your mat, with your knees bent and feet flat on the floor and your arms at your sides. Lift your feet toward the ceiling as you extend your legs, forming a 90-degree angle between your legs and torso, as shown. Press your inner thighs and heels together as you rotate out your toes.

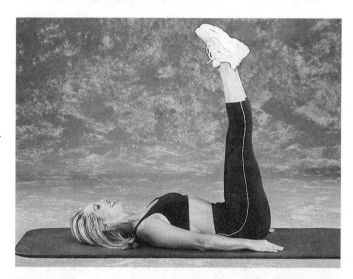

B. With flat, tight abs, exhale and curl your hips toward your ribs, curling up slowly just one vertebra at a time. Once you cannot curl your lower body any farther, inhale and slowly uncurl your torso, lowering just one vertebra at a time. Once you finish uncurling, repeat 10 times.

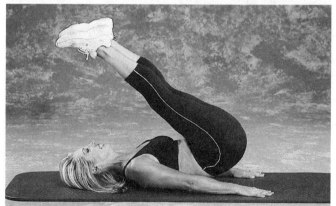

MAXIMUM RESULTS Minimum Time

As you roll over, concentrate on lifting from your hips. Try not to let the weight of your legs pull you into the rollover. You want to work those lower abs, not let gravity do the work for you!

Plank with Leg Lift

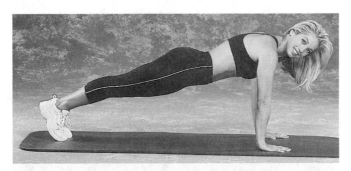

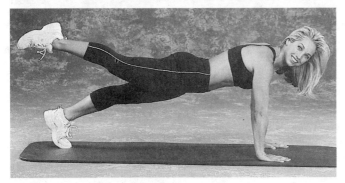

A. Get on all fours, with your hands under your shoulders and your knees under your hips. Extend one leg behind and balance on the ball of that foot. Extend the other leg, bringing yourself into a pushup position. Pull up through your abs to form a straight line from your shoulders to your feet, as shown.

B. While keeping your torso firmly in the plank position, exhale and lift your extended right leg as high as you can without losing your balance or shifting or dropping your hips. Lower as you inhale. Repeat with your left leg. Continue alternating back and forth for 15 repetitions.

MAXIMUM RESULTS Minimum Time

When you lift your leg, you should feel your lower abdominal area tighten to hold your hips in place. Try not to swivel your hips or let them drop as you lift and lower your legs.

"Pretend that you're balancing a yardstick sideways along your lower back. Don't let it slide off!"

STRETCH BREAK

Cobra Stretch

A. Lie with your tummy on your mat and your legs extended behind you. Place your palms on the floor under your shoulders.

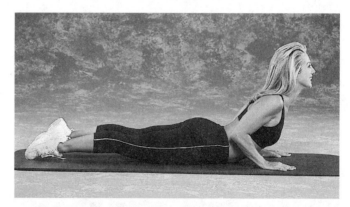

B. Exhale as you push your nose forward slightly and then press into your palms to pull your chest forward and up, arching your back. Feel your chest open and your ribs lengthen away from your hips as you lift your head and shoulders, creating a long arch in your back. You should feel no pinching in your spine. If you do, you haven't created enough length by pulling forward as you lift. Hold for four breaths, lower, and repeat one time.

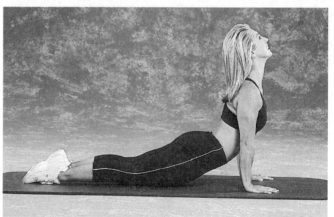

MAXIMUM RESULTS	Minimum Time

Imagine yourself lengthening between each vertebra in your back as you lift, creating a long, arched spine.

Pushup

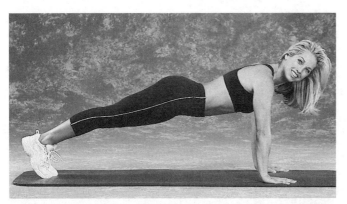

A. Get on all fours, with your palms under your collarbones and your knees under your hips. Extend one leg behind and balance on the ball of that foot. Extend the other leg, bringing yourself into a pushup position.

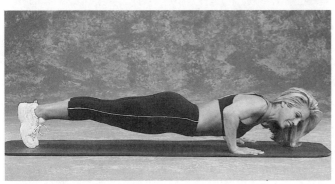

B. With a straight back, slowly bend your elbows as you inhale and lower your chest toward the mat. Lower your chest as far as you can while still being able to press up to the starting position. Straighten your elbows as you press up and exhale. Repeat as many times as you can, up to 10 to 15 repetitions.

MAXIMUM RESULTS	Minimum Time

If you are just starting out, try it with your knees on the floor and with your hands elevated on a step. Once that becomes too easy, continue to do it with your knees bent but with your hands on the floor, not on the step. Then, once you can do that, try the full pushup shown here.

STRETCH BREAK

Child's Pose

A. Get on all fours, with your knees under your hips and your hands on the mat under your shoulders.

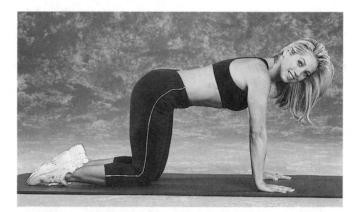

B. Pull your tummy toward your spine as you bring your buttocks back toward your heels. Once your buttocks rest against your heels, bend forward with a long spine, lowering your forehead to the floor and your torso to your thighs. Then slide your arms along the floor and bring them behind your body, palms facing the ceiling. Take three deep breaths as you relax.

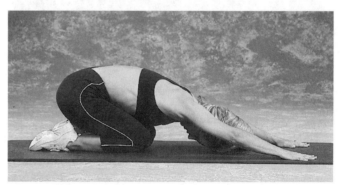

MAXIMUM RESULTS | Minimum Time

Before sliding your arms behind your buttocks, reach forward with your fingers as far as you can and then press your palms into the mat to help you further lengthen your spine and bring your buttocks even closer to your heels.

Back Extension

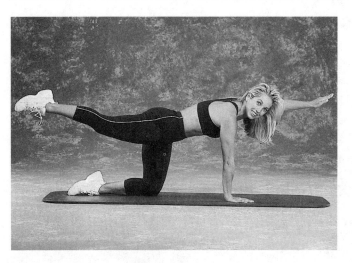

Get on all fours, with your hands on the mat under your shoulders and knees under your hips. Exhale and extend your left arm as you simultaneously extend your right leg. Inhale and return your left arm and right leg to the starting position. Then extend your right arm and left leg. Continue alternating until fatigue.

MAXIMUM RESULTS Minimum Time

As you extend your arm and leg, make sure that your tummy is tight and back is long and flat. Don't let those hips drop! Also, press through your fingers and toes as you extend your arm and leg to lengthen your back muscles as you strengthen them.

STRETCH BREAK

Circular Hip Opener

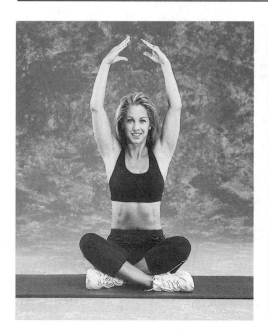

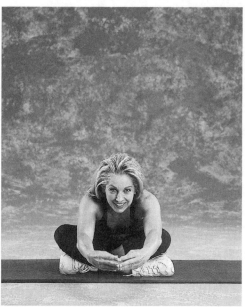

A. Sit on your mat in a comfortable cross-legged position with your right leg in front of or on top of your left. Extend through your crown and lift your arms overhead, as shown, with your palms facing each other.

B. With firm abs, slowly lean forward from your waist, keeping both butt cheeks against the mat.

MAXIMUM RESULTS	Minimum Time
Try not to round your back as you circle. Keeping your back long and extended may mean that your chest remains farther away from the floor. It also means, however, that you'll achieve a better stretch in your hips, thighs, and buttocks.	

"I love this stretch. I do it whenever I've been sitting for a long time and need a quick break."

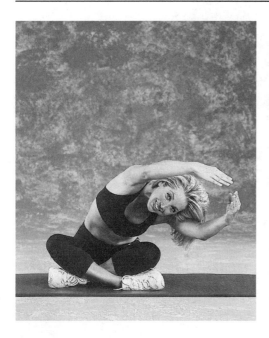 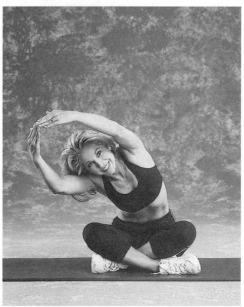

C. Circle your torso and extend arms to the left, breathing normally.

D. Continue circling, bringing your torso back to the previous position and then over to the right, to the middle, and then to the left. Make three large semicircles and then switch directions for three circles. Then rearrange your legs so that your left leg is in front and repeat the entire sequence.

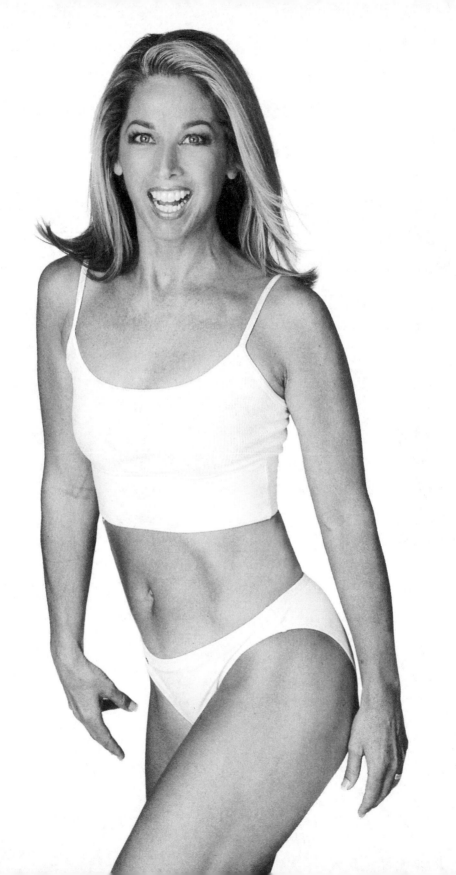

PART 4

The Shrink Your Female Fat Zones Diet

CHAPTER 9

THE SHRINK YOUR FEMALE FAT ZONES DIET

The Shrink-Fat Eating Plan

I love to eat, and I love to cook—only when it's quick and easy and I have the time to do it! But even when I'm rushing from a photo shoot to pick up my kids at school, I try to have yogurt or something else healthy.

I've learned that you *can* have a busy life and still have a nutritious—and slimming—diet. That's what this plan is all about: easy, nutritious meals and snacks, along with the right exercises, that will help you drop the pounds.

I'm a big believer in balance. I've never found that cutting out a whole universe of food—like desserts or foods containing carbs or fat—has worked for me. I always wind up craving what I can't have and feeling like a failure when I "cave in." Instead, I've learned that moderation is the key. With that in mind, I've devised a delicious eating plan that allows you to eat your favorite foods—even treats!—and still shed pounds quickly and safely.

I do not want you to feel as though you're on a diet over the next 6 weeks. You're not; you're on a healthy eating plan to lose weight. I want you to promise me right now that you won't get upset at yourself or feel like a failure because you slip. Don't worry, it won't happen much on my 6-week plan anyway because I give you treats and real-life foods like chili and cornbread or a brownie sundae as part of your overall eating plan. No negative thinking with me around, okay? Think positively—you can do it!

Let's begin!

How This Plan Works

When it comes to female fat zones, scientists still haven't discovered foods that melt away stomach fat or whittle down thighs or other areas. (They have discovered, however, that being stressed-out can give you a bigger belly; more on this in week 6.) But the great news is that you'll shed fat all over your body on this plan.

Over the next 6 weeks, I'll teach you a way of eating to keep your weight down for life. Unlike fad diets that work for a few weeks before you can't stand all the meat or all the cabbage soup (or whatever), this is one you'll want to stick with.

One of the biggest reasons why fad diets don't work is that they expect you to change overnight. But think about this: It took you a lifetime to accumulate all of your fattening habits—how could you change all of them in one day?

That's why the Shrink-Fat Eating Plan is smart but simple—you have a week to unlearn one of six fattening habits and exchange each of them for a new slimming strategy that's worked for me.

By the time the 6 weeks are up, you'll be armed with all the tools you need to keep losing weight—or to maintain what you've lost. As a huge bonus, you'll automatically be helping to protect yourself from osteoporosis, cancer, diabetes, heart disease, and dozens of other health conditions. You'll instinctively make better food choices—and love the way they taste!—without even trying.

Here are your six healthy slimming strategies.

■ **Week 1: Eat the right portions.** You'll find out what a reasonable portion looks like and stop being misled by the oversize portions in restaurants and on the snack aisles of the grocery store. But I'm not one to constantly measure out my food, so I'm going to teach you how to eyeball a serving and get a sense for what a *real* portion looks like.

Healthy Bites for Kids

I TRY TO SET A GOOD EXAMPLE for my two girls by eating healthy foods and offering them nutritious snacks and meals. The following go over big with my kids.

BREAKFASTS

- Less sugary, higher fiber (3 grams or more per serving) kids' cereals, such as Cheerios
- Go Lean toaster waffles with a little butter and syrup and whatever fruit they'll eat
- Flavored yogurt and some trail mix
- Whole grain toast with jam

LUNCHES

- Chicken noodle soup (with corn and peas slipped in) and a slice of wheat bread
- Chicken or bean tortilla with salsa
- Grilled cheese sandwich with reduced-fat cheese (about 5 grams of fat per ounce)—not fat-free—and fruit
- Hummus in pita bread and a vegetable or fruit
- Peanut butter and jelly sandwich with a glass of milk and baby carrots
- Turkey sandwich and a fruit or vegetable

SNACKS

- Frozen banana on a stick
- Baby carrots
- Cereal and milk (try a mix of unsweetened and sweetened cereals)
- Crackers and a cheese stick
- Fresh fruit
- Fruit yogurt
- Nuts
- Reduced-fat popcorn
- Smoothies (make the ones from this book; add an extra teaspoon of honey, if necessary)
- Yogurt pops (combine chopped fruit with vanilla yogurt and freeze in paper cups with pop sticks)

DINNERS

- Chicken with baked beans and a vegetable
- Morningstar Farm Chik Nuggets (made from soy) and a vegetable
- Pizza topped with lots of vegetables
- Spaghetti with tomato-based meat sauce
- Turkey burger on a soft whole wheat bun and a vegetable
- Whole wheat macaroni and cheese and a vegetable

▪ **Week 2: Eat more fiber.** Sounds too simple to be true, but lots of studies show that just increasing the fiber in your diet speeds up weight loss—and fat loss, too.

▪ **Week 3: Eat more good fat and less bad fat.** Turns out that fat—in moderation—can actually help you stick with a weight-loss plan. Hooray!

- **Week 4: Eat more fruits and vegetables.** These beauties fill you up on fewer calories and help ward off cancer and other diseases. As you'll see on this plan, eating more fruits and vegetables is so much easier than you ever thought.

- **Week 5: Eat in response to hunger.** This strategy is about reconnecting to your hunger signals and trusting your body to tell you when you need food and when you don't.

- **Week 6: Stop overeating.** If cravings and bouts of overeating sabotaged your past diet attempts, then you are going to love this part of the plan. I'll help you conquer that problem (and you still get to enjoy ice cream, chips, and other treats!).

You will not go hungry on this plan. Here's why: I've teamed up with registered dietitian Janis Jibrin to create nutritionally balanced meals designed to keep you satisfied and energized so that you don't have to think about food all day. It's no magic: We simply loaded your diet with fruits, vegetables, and whole grains—nature's appetite suppressors.

Don't worry. This isn't rabbit food! You get pizza, beer, ice cream, even the occasional burger on this plan. You'll also discover some amazingly effortless new dishes, like easy homemade chili (the fastest chili ever!) and Mexican lasagna (a crowd pleaser with leftovers to freeze!). You'll find a wide variety and range of foods that you will love. The recipes are easy and delicious. It's truly a way of living healthfully for life.

Pick Your Calorie Level

Your other insurance against hunger is that I give you three different calorie levels to choose from: 1,400, 1,600, and 1,800. Figuring out your target calorie level involves a little trial and error. You will know you've hit it right when you're losing ½ to 2 pounds a week without feeling hungry. You may find that you'll lose more for the first 2 weeks; the body often sheds both fat and water weight at first. But by week 3, dropping more than 2 pounds a week could be unhealthy. If this is happening to you, you're probably starving—literally! Your body may not be getting enough nutrition, and your metabolism could slow down. In this case, move up a calorie level.

Here are guidelines on where to begin.

- **1,400 calories:** If you tend to gain weight very easily and you suspect that you have a slow metabolism, try this calorie level first. If you're losing more than 2 pounds a week, you can always move up to 1,600 calories. Also, on those rare days when you don't exercise at all, definitely stick to 1,400.

- **1,600 calories:** If past experience shows that you lose weight pretty easily without having to cut calories too low, then try the 1,600 level. If you're not losing at least ½ pound a week, drop back to 1,400 calories or alternate between 1,400- and 1,600-calorie days. If you're losing weight too quickly (more than 2 pounds a week), shift up to 1,800 calories or alternate 1,600- and 1,800-calorie days.

- **1,800 calories:** If past experience shows that you lose weight easily without having to cut calories too low, try 1,800 calories a day. And if you're getting extra exercise outside this plan, you may need 1,800 calories. If you're not losing at least ½ pound a week, move down to 1,600. If you're losing more than 2 pounds a week, then add 100 to 200 calories a day. Each of these foods comes to 100 calories: ½ cup (4 ounces) 2% cottage cheese, 1¼ cups fat-free milk, ½ cup brown rice, 1 banana, 16 almonds.

"Food is not the enemy— sitting still is!"

I Shrunk My Female Fat Zones!

Daily exercise and a no-dieting mentality helped transform Lori J. Delgado's body—and her life.

Denise has helped me to completely change my outlook on fitness and nutrition. Before my first pregnancy, I weighed about 30 pounds more than I wanted, and I gained an additional 26 pounds during my pregnancy. After giving birth, I wanted the excess weight off—fast. I first tried Slim-Fast and other drastic diets. None of them kept the weight off long term—until I turned to Denise and her exercise and eating program.

I began exercising nearly every day during the week and reading everything I could about nutrition. As a result, my diet changed dramatically—and I lost all of my excess weight within a year!

I no longer consider myself to be "on a diet." As Denise often says, this is a lifestyle change that I will continue forever! Rather than dieting, I am fueling my body with healthy and nutritious foods—and I also eat a portion of organic dark chocolate chips every day!

The last time I had my body fat measured, it was 21 percent, down from 24. My cholesterol has gone from 183 to 170. I feel so great and am so proud of my success.

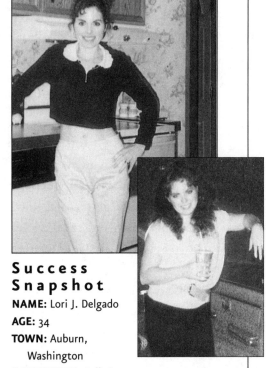

Success Snapshot

NAME: Lori J. Delgado
AGE: 34
TOWN: Auburn, Washington
OCCUPATION: Full-time mom
WEIGHT LOST: More than 52 pounds
OTHER ACCOMPLISHMENTS: Lowered her blood cholesterol and body fat

Lori's Secret to Success

"Love who you are! Know that taking time for yourself doesn't mean that you're selfish. You have to love yourself and be happy with yourself to be your best for you and your family. I know that I am a better person, wife, mom, and friend because I am happy with me."

Meals Designed for Women's Needs

Besides keeping calories in check, Janis and I also made sure that this plan is loaded with all the vitamins, minerals, and other healthy nutrients you need to help ward off diseases facing women: heart disease, osteoporosis, cancer, and other conditions. While we also recommend taking a multivitamin/mineral supplement each day as great insurance, nutrition is best derived from food. Here's how we've got you covered.

■ **Dairy.** Milk, yogurt, and cheese (or calcium-fortified soy milk) are mainstays of this plan because they are such concentrated sources of calcium. You need 1,000 milligrams of calcium daily up until age 50 and 1,200 milligrams after that. This diet averages about 1,050 milligrams calcium daily. So if you're over 50 years old, take a daily calcium supplement or check your multivitamin/mineral supplement. All you need is an extra 200 milligrams a day, the amount in many multis.

Sadly, the average American woman gets only 570 milligrams of calcium daily, about half of what's needed. And that's a setup for the bone-thinning disease osteoporosis. As we age, our bones tend to lose calcium, but with enough calcium—and vitamin D—we can minimize or prevent bone loss. Because dairy is the richest calcium source, I make sure to get at least two servings of milk or yogurt—or calcium-fortified soy milk—every day. That's just what you'll get on this plan: dairy or soy milk every morning for breakfast and a calcium-rich snack later in the day.

■ **Fruits and vegetables of every color.** Strawberries, blueberries, oranges, cantaloupe, watermelon, plums, broccoli, sweet potatoes . . . You get these and more on this plan. The more colors you eat, the more vitamins and phytonutrients you get. Phyto-what? These are beneficial compounds in plant-based foods that fight aging and age-related conditions such as cancer and heart disease. You've probably heard of beta-carotene; that's what gives carrots their orange color. But there are hundreds of other phytonutrients, and I'll teach you about them in the little "Nutrient Booster!" boxes scattered throughout the 6-week plan.

The best way to ensure that you're getting a wide range of phytonutrients is to keep your diet colorful. Those plant pigments are actually disease fighters! Tomatoes and watermelon get their red color from the antioxidant lycopene (more on this in week 1). Spinach and other dark, leafy greens have compounds that protect your eyes, and they're loaded with folate (also known as folic acid), a vitamin that's absolutely crucial for us women (more in week 6). Blueberries and other berries have a host of health-promoting compounds (check it out in week 2). Each week introduces you to the benefits of delicious, colorful foods!

• **Whole grains.** Whole wheat, brown rice, whole rye, and other whole grains are particularly important for women. It's not just for the fiber; these foods give us important phytonutrients that fight breast cancer, other cancers, and heart disease.

For instance, flax and whole rye flour contain phytoestrogens, plant compounds that look very much like human estrogen. (I'm such a believer in flax that I add a few tablespoons of ground flax to my cereal or smoothies every day. Try to grind your own, a week's worth at a time, and make sure to keep ground flax in the fridge, because its oils can spoil when left out in the heat.) These phytoestrogens may protect us from estrogen-triggered breast and colon cancers by lowering the potentially harmful impact of real estrogen on sensitive tissues.

You'll be eating plenty of whole grain foods on this plan. You'll notice, however, the occasional "bread (preferably whole wheat)" or "rice (preferably brown)" in the menu plans. That's in case you wind up at a restaurant that doesn't serve whole grain foods. In that case, it's okay to have the white flour version.

"Don't think of this plan as a diet—think of it as a choice for energy and strength!"

• **Fish.** Eat fish twice a week. That's the recommendation from the American Heart Association, because there's so much amazing research showing that fish helps prevent heart disease and heart attacks. Remember: Heart disease isn't just a man's problem. It's the biggest killer of women in this country. Fish's famous omega-3 fats protect your heart by helping prevent blood clots, normalizing heart rhythms, and lowering cholesterol and other blood fats. They can alleviate stiff arthritic joints as well, and exciting new research shows that they can help prevent depression.

Breakfast: Don't Even Think of Skipping It!

Breakfast eaters are thinner. Cereal eaters are thinner. Breakfast eaters are more alert. People who skip breakfast get fewer vitamins. Those are the results of dozens of scientific studies that all point to the amazing benefits of breakfast. If you're serious about losing weight, you have to eat breakfast. I've given you 6 weeks of super-healthy breakfasts, so promise me that you'll eat them!

If you need more convincing, look at all you get from eating breakfast.

• **For starters, it revs up your metabolism.** Skip it, and your body may start slowing down, afraid it's not going to get fed. That means you may be burning fewer calories at the beginning of the day.

• **Breakfast prevents late-night bingeing.** So many people tell me, "Denise, I've been good all day, but then at night I polish off cookies or ice cream or other snack foods." Well, that's your body's way of telling you that you didn't give it enough calories that day, because you skipped breakfast!

• **Eating good carbs at breakfast gives you energy.** Fiber-rich foods such as oatmeal, high-fiber cereals, and fresh fruit help keep blood sugar on an even keel, giving you steady energy. Danishes and doughnuts, on the other hand, send blood sugar—and energy levels—soaring, then crashing.

(continued on page 257)

THE SHRINK-FAT EATING PLAN 253

Treat Yourself

ONE OF THE REALLY GREAT THINGS about this eating plan is that each day you get a treat. Knowing that you can still include fun foods like cookies, chips, and ice cream makes a weight-loss plan so much easier to stick to. Sometimes, I suggest a treat (like the brownie sundae!). But often, I just specify a calorie count and leave the choice up to you. The treat calories vary from day to day depending on how many calories were left after your three meals and a snack were accounted for.

Some of these treats—particularly the baked foods—do contain a little hydrogenated oil. Such oils contain trans fats, which raise cholesterol. But since the rest of the meal plan is very low in trans fat, the little bits you get from these treats shouldn't hurt you.

For easy reference, I've drawn up this list of treats, according to calorie count. As always, check labels to verify serving sizes and calories.

70 TO 75 CALORIES

- 1 Creamsicle frozen bar (1.75 ounces)
- 1 Frozfruit frozen fruit bar, such as cantaloupe, watermelon, or cherry
- 1 tube Yoplait Exprèsse
- 2 wedges Light Laughing Cow cheese
- 2 Pepperidge Farm Bordeaux cookies
- 3 Hershey's Kisses

80 TO 90 CALORIES

- ¾ ounce fat-free pretzels
- 1 Dole Fruit-n-Gel Bowl
- 1 Edy's or Dreyer's whole-fruit frozen fruit bar (except coconut)
- 1 Fudgsicle (2.7 ounces)
- 1 giant Tootsie Pop
- 3 gingersnaps
- 4 cups Orville Redenbacher's Butter Light popcorn or General Mills' Pop Secret Light
- 4 ounces applesauce
- 4 ounces wine
- 7 Milk Duds
- 8 Junior Mints

100 TO 110 CALORIES

- ¾ cup Jell-O
- 1 frosty lemon cookie
- 1 Good Humor Creamsicle (2.5 ounces)
- 1 M&M fun-size pack (20.9 grams), plain or peanut
- 1 tablespoon peanut butter
- 1 ounce pretzels
- 1¼ cups Baked Bugles
- 2 Fig Newtons
- 2 Nestlé Crunch fun-size bars (10 grams each)
- 2 Oreo cookies
- 12 ounces light beer
- 25 small jelly beans or 10 large jelly beans

120 TO 130 CALORIES

⅔ cup Fiddle Faddle

1 Starbucks frozen coffee bar, such as Mocha Frappuccino or Java Fudge Frappuccino

2 low-fat Fig Newmans

2 Newman-O's sandwich cookies

4 Twizzlers

6 cups Orville Redenbacher's Butter Light popcorn or General Mills' Pop Secret Light

6 ounces wine

8 Barnum's Animals crackers

140 TO 150 CALORIES

⅔ cup light ice cream or frozen yogurt (with no more than 110 calories per ½ cup)

1 ounce reduced-fat potato chips

1 ounce tortilla chips

5 Twizzlers

7 graham crackers (amaranth or oat bran)

10 or 11 Sunchips

15 Junior Mints

30 Goobers

35 small jelly beans

160 TO 170 CALORIES

1 Milky Way Lite (44.5 grams)

2 Keebler Sandies cookies

3 Oreo cookies

4 mini Reese's peanut butter cups

200 CALORIES

1 Chunky bar (1.4 ounces)

1 Dove chocolate bar (1.3 ounces)

1 cup light ice cream or frozen yogurt (with no more than 110 calories per ½ cup)

2 frosty lemon cookies

2 sugar cookies

5 Keebler Fudge Shoppe Grasshopper Fudge Mint cookies

15 Sunchips

210 TO 220 CALORIES

1 Edy's Creamy Banana Chocolate fruit bar

2 ounces pretzels

5 Chips Ahoy! cookies

27 reduced-fat potato chips

I Shrunk My Female Fat Zones!

Consistent exercise and healthful eating helped Janice Cammon maintain a healthy weight for life.

I love Denise and have followed her exercise programs for the past 25 years. Now that I'm 51, I need all the advice she can give—and her advice has always been top notch! Her Shrink Your Female Fat Zones program is no exception.

Consistent exercise has truly helped me to shrink my female fat zones. I have found that exercise and diet are the answers. Cellulite may not completely go away, but it will improve tremendously.

I also love Denise's recipes. I was one of those women many years ago that people made fun of for eating a healthy breakfast instead of doughnuts. I've always been mindful of drinking a lot of water throughout the day, especially after Denise taught me about keeping a spare water bottle in the car, at work, and around the house to encourage drinking. I now have water bottles everywhere!

I'm proud to say that, at age 51, I do not take hormones or medications, and I exercise 6 days a week, strive for a healthy diet, and feel better now than when I was in my twenties and thirties. I have more energy and an overall sense of well-being!

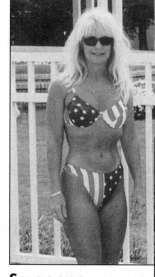

Success Snapshot

NAME: Janice Cammon

AGE: 51

TOWN: Panama City, Florida

OCCUPATION: Merchandiser

FITNESS GAINED: Has maintained the same weight of 110 pounds throughout life

OTHER ACCOMPLISHMENTS: Boosted her energy and mental outlook

Janice's Secret to Success

"You have to control your health—and doing so is simple. Educate yourself about exercise and nutrition and your body. Reading this book is a great start! Exercise and nutrition have to become a way of life, part of your normal everyday routine. I'm proud to say that it's a way of life for me!"

- **Breakfast sharpens your brain.** British studies show that breakfast eaters do better on memory tests and feel calmer and more positive than breakfast skippers.

- **Cereal eaters are healthier.** Two British studies looking at 262 people, ages 21 to 85, found that morning-cereal eaters are in better shape, both mentally and physically. An ongoing study tracking 31,000 women in Iowa found that those who ate whole grain, fiber-filled cereal at least three times a week cut their risk of getting heart disease by one-third and had one-quarter less diabetes risk than people eating low-fiber breakfasts. As you'll see, this plan is loaded with high-fiber breakfasts.

My Eating Philosophy

There are no magic bullets or "cures" for a person's appetite. There is no miracle diet or drug that leads to permanent weight loss. But here's the truth: It's all about calories in . . . and calories out. Take in fewer calories than you burn, and you'll lose weight. Do the opposite, and you'll gain weight.

It's also about choices: our *personal* choices about what goes into our mouths. Just as it's *we* who determine how much we move each day. It's all up to us—we have the power and the control to change our own lives. What I'm going to do is show you the easiest and best way to lose weight and get healthy. I know this works. Remember: It's in our hands—and in our mouths.

As you go through these weeks, you'll start to be more comfortable with

> "I'm here for you. I want you to lose weight and keep it off for a lifetime. This is a long-term plan. You'll keep it up for your lifetime."

choosing healthier foods instead of high-calorie ones. I'll show you how. Food is not your enemy. Sitting still is!

Food is a pleasure. It fuels us and gives us energy and the nutrients our bodies need to be replenished and rejuvenated. We're going to think that way from now on. I'll teach you why you should believe in food.

Fasting or starving will be counterproductive because it slows the metabolism. If you eat consistently throughout the day, just like I'll teach you, you will keep your metabolism steady and revved up throughout the day.

As we age, our metabolism slows down, so we need to increase our moving time and slightly decrease our calorie intake. And if you do eat an extra ½ cup of ice cream, for example, you need to walk about an extra mile. It's 100 calories in and 100 calories out.

Finally, I want to encourage you to get your family together for dinner as often as you can. Try to rearrange your plans, wherever you are, to have a wonderful time together at the dinner table. This is very helpful to your weight-loss success, and here's why: Gathering around the dinner table is a very comforting feeling for all of us—doubly so if you're a mom. There's no better "family feeling" of gratification for me as a mom. There I am, sitting down for dinner where everyone is talking about their day and eating wholesome foods and being together. It's a great stress reliever, and as you'll find out in week 6 of the eating plan, lowering stress can shrink one of your toughest female fat zones—your belly.

Also, talking with your family and taking your time when you eat help you slow down so that you don't mindlessly stuff your face. You are able to see your portions, and you will register that you are full and that you don't really want those seconds. (More on hunger and fullness in week 5.)

"Take time to enjoy your food— it's one of life's greatest pleasures."

So, as often as you can, have a *real* dinnertime with your family. If your schedules absolutely won't allow it at the traditional dinner hour, then make another special time to sit down together and eat. (Maybe it could be breakfast, but I know in my family, I'm always rushing to get the kids off to school on time.) The more you eat together, the more calmly you will eat, and the more your digestive system will thank you!

Let's Make a Deal

You will lose weight and keep it off if you follow this 6-week plan—both the eating and exercise parts—and make it your lifestyle. If you do your part on this plan, it will pay you back with pure success.

I never want you to feel unhappy about yourself. You are a wonderful person with great qualities. Just keep forging ahead. You are worth it! Your health is worth it. Your family loves you and wants you around a long time. So do it now!

CHAPTER 10

Go on Portion Patrol

"I'm so full."

"I ate way too much!"

"Why did I eat so much?"

How often do you say these things to yourself? I say them, but less than I used to. Now I know to eat smaller portions and then wait. It takes about 15 minutes for the brain to register "I'm full."

One reason we stuff ourselves is because portions have ballooned out of control. Does that big bagel have 100 calories or 400? What *is* a normal portion? Knowing the answers to these questions may make or break your weight-loss success. No matter how you dress it up, weight loss is about calories, and calories are about portions. In this "Land of Expanding Portions," pretty much everything you buy—and everything served to you in a restaurant—is too much.

To get around this problem, my husband, Jeff, and I sometimes share an entrée at a restaurant, and we each get our own salad or soup as an appetizer. Not only does this help us maintain our weight, we're also trying to set a good example for our girls. We want them to learn to define their own healthy portions and not let any restaurant do it for them.

Whether you're eating out or in your own home, help your kids figure out what's a reasonable portion. Children need positive influences about food, and your attitude is contagious. If you practice balance and moderation, so will they.

How Much Is That?

This week you'll find out what a reasonable portion looks like. As you follow the week 1 menu plan, measure any foods you're not sure about. A cup of soup, 2 tablespoons of granola, 1 cup of pasta—you might be surprised at what these portions really look like! Here's what I do.

▪ **Measure.** Just get out your measuring cups and spoons and keep them handy. The only way to really, truly know whether you're eating 1 cup of cooked pasta (200 calories) or 3 cups (600 calories) is by measuring. Don't worry; you won't have to keep measuring forever! Here's the trick: Measure foods into the bowls you usually use and keep using those exact same bowls. For instance, measure the bran flakes into a cereal bowl, looking carefully at the level in the bowl. Next time, measure again, using that same bowl. By the third time, you probably won't need to measure; you can simply eyeball it.

Salad dressing and spreads—as well as peanut butter—are a little trickier. After measuring and tasting a few times, you get a feel for a lightly dressed salad, and you'll know when you've drenched it. And after measuring out 2 tablespoons of peanut butter, cream cheese, or other spreads, you'll recognize a light-to-medium layer on your bread or cracker.

▪ **Read labels.** The Nutrition Facts panel on food labels is a powerful portion-control tool. Always check both the calories and the servings per package. For instance, on Wednesday you'll choose a 200-calorie treat. You might pick up a snack cake with "200 calories" on the label. Sounds great! But now look at the serving size: "Servings per package: 2." Oops, that's 400 calories for the little cake.

ESTIMATING PORTIONS

These examples will help you make quick-and-dirty portion assessments.

	WEIGHT/DIMENSIONS	ABOUT THE . . .	CALORIES
BAGEL			
OLD STANDARD SIZE	2 oz; 3" diameter; 1" high	Diameter of a credit card (remember the old Lender's bagels?)	157
BIGGER SIZE	4 oz; 4½" diameter; 1¼" high	Size of a CD	302
EVEN BIGGER SIZE	6–7 oz; 5" diameter; 2" high	Size of a teacup saucer	470–550
PASTA (COOKED, WITHOUT SAUCE)			
WEIGHT-CONTROL SIZE	1–1¼ cups	Size of your fist (for 1 cup)	200–250
RESTAURANT PORTION (THINK OLIVE GARDEN)	3½ cups	Size of the whole dinner plate and a thumb-length deep	700
COOKIE			
OLD STANDARD	⅓ oz; 2¼" diameter	Size of a little roll of transparent tape	48
SUPER-SIZE COOKIE	4 oz	Size of a CD, even a little bigger sometimes	550
MUFFIN			
OLD STANDARD	2 oz; 2¾" diameter; 2" high	Size of a tennis ball, just a little smaller	170
BIGGER MUFFIN	6 oz; 3½" diameter; 3½" high	Size of a softball	500
EVEN BIGGER MUFFIN	10–12 oz; 4½" diameter, 4" high	Size of both hands cupped, fingers spread	850–1,020

1,400 CALORIES: 24% calories from fat, 20% protein, 56% carbohydrates
1,600 CALORIES: 24% calories from fat, 20% protein, 56% carbohydrates
1,800 CALORIES: 25% calories from fat, 19% protein, 56% carbohydrates

▪ **Divvy up your plate.** Let's be real—we're not about to take our measuring cups into a restaurant. Instead, use this handy rule of thumb: Draw an imaginary line through your plate. Fill the top half of your plate with vegetables or salad. (No fries or other fried foods. C'mon, you can do it!)

Now look at the bottom half of the plate and divide it in two. In one section, check out your piece of fish, chicken, or meat. If it's too big for that space, then the portion is too large. Just don't eat the excess—ask for a doggie bag later. In the other section, place your starch: a roll, rice, potato, or pasta. Again, if the starch doesn't fit on that quarter of your plate, they served you too much. Into the doggie bag!

Lasagna, eggplant Parmesan, and other mixed dishes shouldn't fill more than a third of your dinner plate. There should always be enough room to fill half the plate with vegetables or a salad.

These tips should help you get a portion reality check, a key to weight loss. If you can master portion control, you've mastered weight control for a lifetime.

Chart Your Weight-Loss Progress

Today, before you begin this eating and exercise plan, get a sense of where you stand now. As we talked about in chapter 1, in addition to stepping on the scale, try on a pair of very tight pants or measure your waist (at the smallest point), your hips (at the biggest point), and any other fat zone. (If you're burned out by weight-loss attempts and feel anxious about measuring, then don't! It's okay; you'll know how much better your body feels.)

Each week, I'll remind you to chart your progress.

SHOPPING LIST

THIS LOOKS LIKE A LOT OF FOOD, but much of it will carry over to the upcoming weeks. Portions will vary depending on how many people are in your family and which calorie level you are following. So just go through the menu plan and note how much of everything you'll need.

If you don't like something, substitute with a close equivalent. For instance, have strawberries instead of blueberries or mozzarella instead of Cheddar. But don't substitute white flour products (like white bread) for whole grain products (like whole wheat bread). Whole grains are important weight-loss tools.

FRESH FRUIT

Apples or berries (such as blueberries or raspberries)

Bananas

Grapes (for 1,800-calorie plan only)

Lemons (Don't buy if you're eating dinner out on Monday.)

Mangoes (for 1,600- and 1,800-calorie plans)

Oranges

Pears

Strawberries

FRESH VEGETABLES AND HERBS

Avocado, Haas (Don't buy if you're having the microwave enchilada for lunch on Sunday.)

Broccoli

Carrots, baby

Celery

Corn

Cucumbers

Dill

Garlic

Ginger

Lettuce (either a head of romaine or other leafy lettuce or a bag of mixed greens)

Parsley or basil

Peppers, green

Scallions

Spinach (For convenience, buy bags of prewashed spinach.)

Squash, butternut, or sweet potatoes (Don't buy if you're eating dinner out on Monday.)

Tomatoes, cherry and regular

Zucchini (Don't get if you're buying a pizza for Saturday.)

CANNED AND BOTTLED GOODS

Anchovy paste (Don't buy if you're eating lunch out on Tuesday or buying bottled Caesar dressing.)

Applesauce, unsweetened (such as Musselman's or Mott's Natural Style)

Beans, pinto or black, canned (Don't buy if you're eating lunch out or having a microwave burrito on Friday.)

Chickpeas, canned

Fruit, canned in its own juice or light syrup, with 50 to 60 calories per serving (such as Dole FruitBowls or Del Monte Fruit Naturals)

Honey

Hot-pepper sauce

Jam or jelly

Lemon juice

Mustard, Dijon

Oil, canola

Oil, olive

Pasta sauce, meatless

Peanut butter

Pizza sauce (Don't get if you're buying a pizza for Saturday.)

Salad dressing, Caesar (Don't buy if you're making your own or eating lunch out on Tuesday.)

Salad dressing, reduced-calorie Italian or vinaigrette

Salad dressing, regular Italian or vinaigrette (for 1,800-calorie plan only)

Salsa (Don't get if you're buying a burrito on Friday and having a microwave enchilada for lunch on Sunday.)

Soup, black bean (such as Progresso)

Soup, lentil (such as Progresso)

Soy sauce, reduced-sodium

Syrup, chocolate

Syrup, maple or maple-flavored

Tuna, water-packed

Vinegar, preferably balsamic (Don't buy if you're eating lunch out on Tuesday or buying bottled Caesar dressing.)

Worchestershire sauce (Don't buy if you're eating lunch out on Tuesday or buying bottled Caesar dressing.)

DRY GOODS AND BREAD

Almonds

Bagels, whole wheat or oat bran, such as Lender's (Don't buy if you're having breakfast at a deli or coffee shop on Wednesday.)

Bread, whole wheat, with no more than 90 calories and at least 2 grams of fiber per slice

Cereal, granola

Cereal, oat-based "O" cereal (such as Kashi Heart to Heart or Cheerios)

Cereal, oatmeal (plain)

Crackers, graham

Crackers, whole grain (such as Ak-Mak)

Fettuccine, whole wheat

Herbes de Provence, other mixed herbs, or poultry seasoning (Don't buy if you're eating dinner out on Monday.)

Muffins, bran (Don't buy if you're having breakfast at a deli on Friday.)

Pizza crust, such as Boboli Original, with about 1,100 calories (Don't get if you're buying a pizza for dinner on Saturday.)

Rice, brown (such as Texmati, basmati, or quick-cooking Uncle Ben's)

REFRIGERATED FOODS

Alfredo sauce, reduced-fat (such as Buitoni or DiGiorno)

Butter or trans-free margarine

Cheese, Parmesan

Cheese, part-skim mozzarella (Don't get if you're buying a pizza for Saturday.)

Cheese, reduced-fat (such as Cabot 50% Light Cheddar)

Cottage cheese, 1% or 2% (for 1,600- and 1,800-calorie plans)

Cream cheese, reduced-fat (Don't buy if you're having breakfast at a deli on Wednesday.)

Milk, fat-free

Tortellini, cheese-filled (such as Buitoni)

Tortillas, corn, 8-inch diameter (Don't buy if using flour tortillas for lunch on Sunday.)

Tortillas, flour (preferably whole wheat), 8-inch diameter (Don't get if you're buying a burrito on Friday and having the microwave enchilada for lunch on Sunday.)

Yogurt, low-fat fruit, with about 210 calories per 8 ounces (for 1,600- and 1,800-calorie plans)

Yogurt, low-fat plain

Yogurt, reduced-calorie flavored, with no more than 120 calories per 8 ounces

MEAT, POULTRY, AND FISH

Beef, lean, such as sirloin

Chicken, boneless and skinless breasts or precooked Perdue Short Cuts or Louis Rich strips

Chicken, boneless and skinless thighs

Chicken, whole (Don't buy if you're eating dinner out on Monday.)

Fish, fillets (such as salmon, tuna, or monkfish)

FROZEN FOODS

Bean burrito (Don't buy if you're going to Taco Bell on Friday or if you're making your own.)

Chicken enchilada entrée, with no more than 310 calories, such as Healthy Choice or Lean Cuisine Everyday Favorites (Don't buy if you're making your own for lunch on Sunday.)

Fruit bars, frozen, with no more than 80 calories (such as Frozfruit, Edy's, or Dreyer's)

Ice cream or frozen yogurt, light, with no more than 110 calories per ½ cup (such as Breyers, Edy's, or Dreyer's)

Pizza, vegetarian (Don't buy if you're getting pizza delivered or making your own on Saturday.)

Vegetables (such as a mixture of broccoli, carrots, and other vegetables)

Waffles, whole grain toaster, with about 170 calories for 2 (such as Nutri-Grain Multibran)

OPTIONAL

Beer, light

Cilantro

Treats (see Wednesday, Thursday, Friday, and Saturday)

Wine

MONDAY

1,400	1,600
BREAKFAST	
STRAWBERRY-BANANA SMOOTHIE: In a blender, process until smooth 1 small ripe banana, ½ cup strawberries, ½ cup fat-free milk, ½ cup low-fat plain yogurt, 2 teaspoons honey, and 1 or 2 ice cubes.	**STRAWBERRY-BANANA SMOOTHIE:** In a blender, process until smooth 1 small ripe banana, ½ cup strawberries, ½ cup fat-free milk, ½ cup low-fat plain yogurt, 2 teaspoons honey, and 1 or 2 ice cubes.
WHOLE WHEAT TOAST: 1 slice spread with 1 teaspoon trans-free margarine	**WHOLE WHEAT TOAST:** 2 slices spread with 2 teaspoons trans-free margarine

LUNCH

1,400	1,600
LENTIL SOUP: 1 cup soup (such as Progresso) with a spritz of lemon juice	**LENTIL SOUP:** 1 cup soup (such as Progresso) with a spritz of lemon juice
CHEESE AND TOMATO SANDWICH: Place 1 slice reduced-fat cheese on 1 slice whole wheat bread and spread with mustard, then add tomato slices.	**CHEESE AND TOMATO SANDWICH:** Place 2 slices reduced-fat cheese on 2 slices whole wheat bread and spread with mustard, then add tomato slices.
TOMATO: Remaining portion, sliced	**TOMATO:** Remaining portion, sliced

SNACK

1,400	1,600
LATTE: 1 cup fat-free milk with a shot of espresso coffee and 1 teaspoon sugar	**LATTE:** 1 cup fat-free milk with a shot of espresso coffee and 1 teaspoon sugar
ALMONDS: 2 tablespoons	**ALMONDS:** 2 tablespoons

DINNER

1,400	1,600
ROASTED CHICKEN: *At home,* make Roasted Chicken (recipe on page 384). *At Boston Market,* have either the ¼ white-meat chicken (no wing) or the ¼ dark-meat chicken, both without skin. *At other take-outs,* have either 1 leg or ½ breast (no wing), both without skin.	**ROASTED CHICKEN:** *At home,* make Roasted Chicken (recipe on page 384). *At Boston Market,* have either the ¼ white-meat chicken (no wing) or the ¼ dark-meat chicken, both without skin. *At other take-outs,* have either 1 leg or ½ breast (no wing), both without skin.
2 SIDE DISHES: *At home,* have 1 cup steamed vegetables and ¾ cup corn, boiled potatoes, sweet potatoes, or butternut squash. *At Boston Market,* order the steamed vegetables and either herbed buttered corn, butternut squash, or garlic-dill new potatoes. *At other takeouts,* have 1 cup steamed vegetables and ¾ cup of corn or boiled potatoes prepared with a *little* butter, sweet potatoes, or butternut squash.	**2 SIDE DISHES:** *At home,* have 1 cup steamed vegetables and ¾ cup corn, boiled potatoes, sweet potatoes, or butternut squash. *At Boston Market,* order the steamed vegetables and either herbed buttered corn, butternut squash, or garlic-dill new potatoes. *At other takeouts,* have 1 cup steamed vegetables and ¾ cup of corn or boiled potatoes prepared with a *little* butter, sweet potatoes, or butternut squash.

TREAT

1,400	1,600
LIGHT ICE CREAM OR FROZEN YOGURT: ¾ cup, with no more than 110 calories per ½ cup (such as Breyers or Dreyer's), topped with 1 tablespoon chocolate syrup	**LIGHT ICE CREAM OR FROZEN YOGURT:** ¾ cup, with no more than 110 calories per ½ cup (such as Breyers or Dreyer's), topped with 1 tablespoon chocolate syrup

1,800

BREAKFAST

STRAWBERRY-BANANA SMOOTHIE: In a blender, process until smooth 1 small ripe banana, ½ cup strawberries, ½ cup fat-free milk, ½ cup low-fat plain yogurt, 2 teaspoons honey, and 1 or 2 ice cubes.

WHOLE WHEAT TOAST: 2 slices spread with 2 teaspoons trans-free margarine

LUNCH

LENTIL SOUP: 1 cup soup (such as Progresso) with a spritz of lemon juice

CHEESE AND TOMATO SANDWICH: Place 2 slices reduced-fat cheese on 2 slices whole wheat bread and spread with mustard, then add tomato slices.

TOMATO: Remaining portion, sliced

SNACK

LATTE: 1 cup fat-free milk with a shot of espresso coffee and 1 teaspoon sugar

ALMONDS: 2 tablespoons

DINNER

ROASTED CHICKEN: *At home,* make Roasted Chicken (recipe on page 384). *At Boston Market,* have either the ¼ white-meat chicken (no wing) or the ¼ dark-meat chicken, both without skin. *At other takeouts,* have either 1 leg or ½ breast (no wing), both without skin.

3 SIDE DISHES: *At home,* have 1 cup steamed vegetables and ¾ cup corn, boiled potatoes, sweet potatoes, or butternut squash (3 total). *At Boston Market,* order the steamed vegetables and either herbed buttered corn, butternut squash, or garlic-dill new potatoes (3 total). *At other takeouts,* have 1 cup steamed vegetables and ¾ cup corn or boiled potatoes with a *little* butter, sweet potatoes, or butternut squash (3 total).

TREAT

LIGHT ICE CREAM OR FROZEN YOGURT: ¾ cup, with no more than 110 calories per ½ cup (such as Breyers or Dreyer's), topped with 1 tablespoon chocolate syrup

Nutrition Tallies

	1,400	1,600	1,800
CALORIES	1,363	1,609	1,786
FAT (G)	33	43	48
SATURATED FAT (G)	14.2	18.3	19.3
PROTEIN (G)	82	96	99
CARBOHYDRATES (G)	198	225	256
DIETARY FIBER (G)	23	27	30
CHOLESTEROL (MG)	155	170	170
SODIUM (MG)	2,266	2,781	3,208
CALCIUM (MG)	1,232	1,489	1,499

Nutrient Booster!

AFTER CHECKING THE LABEL for portion size, I look at the rest of the label, too: the grams of fat, carbs, and protein; sodium levels; and so forth. I compare labels, choosing brands lower in total fat, saturated fat, and sodium. I also check the ingredient list and try to buy foods without partially hydrogenated oil. This is a bad type of fat that contributes to heart disease.

TUESDAY

1,400	1,600
BREAKFAST	

CEREAL: 150 calories of oat-based "O" cereal (such as 1 cup Kashi Heart to Heart or 1⅓ cups Cheerios) topped with 1 cup fat-free milk, 1 small sliced apple or 1 cup berries, and 2 tablespoons granola

> **TIP** Check the label: The cereal should have at least 3 grams of fiber per serving.

CEREAL: 150 calories of oat-based "O" cereal (such as 1 cup Kashi Heart to Heart or 1⅓ cups Cheerios) topped with 1 cup fat-free milk, 1 small sliced apple or 1 cup berries, and 2 tablespoons granola

> **TIP** Check the label: The cereal should have at least 3 grams of fiber per serving.

LUNCH

CHICKEN CAESAR SALAD: 2½ or more cups romaine lettuce with ⅔ cup chicken (about the size of a deck of cards), and 2 tablespoons Caesar dressing

> **TIP** *If dining out*, ask for dressing on the side so that you can control the amount. *At home*, use leftover chicken from last night's dinner; see dressing recipe on page 385.

1 SMALL ROLL: Have this (2½-inch size) or 1 slice bread (preferably whole grain).

CHICKEN CAESAR SALAD: 2½ or more cups romaine lettuce with ⅔ cup chicken (about the size of a deck of cards), and 2 tablespoons Caesar dressing

> **TIP** *If dining out*, ask for dressing on the side so that you can control the amount. *At home*, use leftover chicken from last night's dinner; see dressing recipe on page 385.

1 SMALL ROLL: Have this (2½-inch size) or 1 slice bread (preferably whole grain).

SNACK

YOGURT: 8 ounces reduced-calorie flavored yogurt with no more than 120 calories

YOGURT: 8 ounces low-fat fruit yogurt with no more than 210 calories

DINNER

FETTUCCINE WITH TOMATO ALFREDO SAUCE: See recipe on page 385.

FROZEN MIXED VEGETABLES: 1 cup, microwaved or steamed and with a spritz of lemon juice

FETTUCCINE WITH TOMATO ALFREDO SAUCE: See recipe on page 385.

PARMESAN CHEESE: 1 tablespoon

FROZEN MIXED VEGETABLES: 1 cup, microwaved or steamed and with a spritz of lemon juice

TREAT

1 FROZEN FRUIT BAR: Choose one with no more than 80 calories (such as Frozfruit or Edy's).

1 FROZEN FRUIT BAR: Choose one with no more than 80 calories (such as Frozfruit or Edy's).

1,800

BREAKFAST

CEREAL: 150 calories of oat-based "O" cereal (such as 1 cup Kashi Heart to Heart or 1⅓ cups Cheerios) topped with 1 cup fat-free milk, 1 small sliced apple or 1 cup berries, and 3 tablespoons granola

TIP Check the label: The cereal should have at least 3 grams of fiber per serving.

LUNCH

CHICKEN CAESAR SALAD: 2½ or more cups romaine lettuce with ⅔ cup chicken (about the size of a deck of cards), and 2 tablespoons Caesar dressing

TIP *If dining out*, ask for dressing on the side so that you can control the amount. *At home*, use leftover chicken from last night's dinner; see dressing recipe on page 385.

1 SMALL ROLL: Have this (2½-inch size) or 1 slice bread (preferably whole grain) with 1 teaspoon butter or trans-free margarine

SNACK

YOGURT: 8 ounces low-fat fruit yogurt with no more than 210 calories

ALMONDS 2 tablespoons

DINNER

FETTUCCINE WITH TOMATO ALFREDO SAUCE: See recipe on page 385.

PARMESAN CHEESE: 1 tablespoon

FROZEN MIXED VEGETABLES: 1 cup, microwaved or steamed and with a spritz of lemon juice

TREAT

1 FROZEN FRUIT BAR: Choose one with no more than 80 calories (such as Frozfruit or Edy's).

Nutrition Tallies

	1,400	1,600	1,800
CALORIES	1,418	1,575	1,763
FAT (G)	33	37	53
SATURATED FAT (G)	8.9	10.7	14.4
PROTEIN (G)	76	81	87
CARBOHYDRATES (G)	213	241	249
DIETARY FIBER (G)	24	24	28
CHOLESTEROL (MG)	110	113	124
SODIUM (MG)	1,631	1,763	1,805
CALCIUM (MG)	825	981	1,039

WEDNESDAY

1,400	1,600
BREAKFAST	
BAGEL: *At home or at the bagel shop,* ½ large (3½- to 4-ounce) or 1 small (2-ounce) oat bran or whole wheat bagel with 2 tablespoons reduced-fat cream cheese	**BAGEL:** *At home or at the bagel shop,* 1 large (3½- to 4-ounce) oat bran or whole wheat bagel with 4 tablespoons reduced-fat cream cheese
FAT-FREE MILK: 1 cup	**FAT-FREE MILK:** 1 cup
FRUIT SALAD: 1 cup (your choice of fruit)	**FRUIT SALAD:** 1 cup (your choice of fruit)
LUNCH	
TUNA AND BEAN SALAD: See recipe on page 387.	**TUNA AND BEAN SALAD:** See recipe on page 387.
SNACK	
HOT OR COLD CHOCOLATE MILK: 1 cup fat-free milk with 2 teaspoons chocolate syrup	**HOT OR COLD CHOCOLATE MILK:** 1 cup fat-free milk with 2 teaspoons chocolate syrup
DINNER	
GRILLED HONEY-MUSTARD CHICKEN: See recipe on page 386.	**GRILLED HONEY-MUSTARD CHICKEN:** See recipe on page 386.
BROWN RICE: Serve with ⅔ cup cooked rice or have the other half of the breakfast bagel (toasted).	**BROWN RICE:** ⅔ cup, cooked
1 ORANGE	**1 ORANGE**
TREAT	
15 SUNCHIPS: Choose these or 200 calories' worth of another treat (see page 255 for more suggestions). **TIP** Check labels to confirm number of calories!	**15 SUNCHIPS:** Choose these or 200 calories' worth of another treat (see page 255 for more suggestions). **TIP** Check labels to confirm number of calories!

1,800

BREAKFAST

BAGEL: *At home or at the bagel shop,* 1 large (3½- to 4-ounce) oat bran or whole wheat bagel with 4 tablespoons reduced-fat cream cheese

FAT-FREE MILK: 1 cup

FRUIT SALAD: 1 cup (your choice of fruit)

LUNCH

TUNA AND BEAN SALAD: See recipe on page 387.

1 WHOLE WHEAT ROLL: Have this or 1 slice French bread.

SNACK

HOT OR COLD CHOCOLATE MILK: 1 cup fat-free milk with 2 teaspoons chocolate syrup

DINNER

GRILLED HONEY-MUSTARD CHICKEN: See recipe on page 386.

BROWN RICE: ⅔ cup, cooked

1 ORANGE

TREAT

15 SUNCHIPS: Choose these or 200 calories' worth of another treat (see page 255 for more suggestions).

TIP Check labels to confirm number of calories!

Nutrition Tallies

	1,400	1,600	1,800
CALORIES	1,423	1,607	1,828
FAT (G)	36	42	47
SATURATED FAT (G)	18.9	22.3	23.2
PROTEIN (G)	89	95	101
CARBOHYDRATES (G)	195	223	262
DIETARY FIBER (G)	23	25	29
CHOLESTEROL (MG)	157	174	174
SODIUM (MG)	1,881	2,259	2,273
CALCIUM (MG)	980	1,019	1,067

THURSDAY

1,400	1,600
BREAKFAST	
CEREAL: 150 calories of oat-based "O" cereal topped with 1 cup fat-free milk, 1 small sliced apple or 1 cup berries, and 2 tablespoons granola **TIP** Check the label: The cereal should have at least 3 grams of fiber per serving.	**CEREAL:** 150 calories of oat-based "O" cereal topped with 1 cup fat-free milk, 1 small sliced apple or 1 cup berries, and 2 tablespoons granola **TIP** Check the label: The cereal should have at least 3 grams of fiber per serving.
LUNCH	
PEANUT BUTTER AND JELLY SANDWICH: Spread 2 tablespoons peanut butter and 2 tablespoons jelly or jam on 2 slices whole wheat bread. **FAT-FREE MILK:** 1 cup **CELERY STICKS AND BABY CARROTS:** 1 cup	**PEANUT BUTTER AND JELLY SANDWICH:** Spread 2 tablespoons peanut butter and 2 tablespoons jelly or jam on 2 slices whole wheat bread. **FAT-FREE MILK:** 1 cup **CELERY STICKS AND BABY CARROTS:** 1 cup
SNACK	
FRUIT CUP: Choose fruit in its own syrup (such as Dole FruitBowls or Del Monte Fruit Naturals). **TIP** Check labels for 50 to 60 calories per container.	**FRUIT CUP:** Choose fruit in its own syrup (such as Dole FruitBowls or Del Monte Fruit Naturals). **TIP** Check labels for 50 to 60 calories per container. **LOW-FAT COTTAGE CHEESE:** ½ cup
DINNER	
BEEF AND BROCCOLI STIR-FRY: See recipe on page 387. **BROWN RICE:** ¾ cup, cooked (Quick-cooking Uncle Ben's is fine; if you have more time, try brown basmati or Texmati.) **TIP** Make extra rice for tomorrow night.	**BEEF AND BROCCOLI STIR-FRY:** See recipe on page 387. **BROWN RICE:** 1 cup, cooked (Quick-cooking Uncle Ben's is fine; if you have more time, try brown basmati or Texmati.) **TIP** Make extra rice for tomorrow night.
TREAT	
3 GINGERSNAPS: Choose these or 80 calories' worth of another treat (see page 254 for suggestions).	**3 OREO COOKIES:** Choose these or 160 calories' worth of another treat (see page 255 for suggestions).

1,800

BREAKFAST

CEREAL: 150 calories of oat-based "O" cereal topped with 1 cup fat-free milk, 1 small sliced apple or 1 cup berries, and 3 tablespoons granola

> **TIP** Check the label: The cereal should have at least 3 grams of fiber per serving.

PEANUT BUTTER AND JELLY SANDWICH: Spread 2 tablespoons peanut butter and 2 tablespoons jelly or jam on 2 slices whole wheat bread.

FAT-FREE MILK: 1 cup

CELERY STICKS AND BABY CARROTS: 1 cup

GRAPES: 1 cup

FRUIT CUP: Choose fruit in its own syrup (such as Dole FruitBowls or Del Monte Fruit Naturals).

> **TIP** Check labels for 50 to 60 calories per container.

LOW-FAT COTTAGE CHEESE: ½ cup

BEEF AND BROCCOLI STIR-FRY: See recipe on page 387.

BROWN RICE: 1 cup, cooked (Quick-cooking Uncle Ben's is fine; if you have more time, try brown basmati or Texmati.)

> **TIP** Make extra rice for tomorrow night.

3 OREO COOKIES: Choose these or 160 calories' worth of another treat (see page 255 for suggestions).

Nutrition Tallies

	1,400	1,600	1,800
CALORIES	1,403	1,635	1,783
FAT (G)	44	51	54
SATURATED FAT (G)	10.1	14.3	14.9
PROTEIN (G)	64	82	84
CARBOHYDRATES (G)	207	231	263
DIETARY FIBER (G)	24	26	28
CHOLESTEROL (MG)	64	77	77
SODIUM (MG)	1,426	1,900	1,904
CALCIUM (MG)	825	936	958

Nutrient Booster!

PEANUT BUTTER—ON A DIET?! Yup, as long as you budget fat (note Thursday's low-fat breakfast and dinner), peanut butter can certainly fit into a weight-loss plan. Sure, it's high in fat, but peanut butter has the good kinds of fat—monounsaturated and polyunsaturated—which don't raise blood cholesterol. In fact, in a famous ongoing Harvard study tracking thousands of women, those who ate 2 to 4 ounces of peanuts a week (the equivalent of 3½ to 7 tablespoons of peanut butter) cut their risk of heart attack by half compared with women who rarely ate peanuts.

FRIDAY

1,400	1,600

BREAKFAST

MUFFIN: ½ large or 1 small bran muffin

APPLESAUCE: ½ cup unsweetened (such as Musselman's Natural Style or Mott's Natural Style)

FAT-FREE MILK: 1 cup

MUFFIN: 1 large bran muffin

APPLESAUCE: ½ cup unsweetened (such as Musselman's Natural Style or Mott's Natural Style)

FAT-FREE MILK: 1 cup

LUNCH

1 BEAN BURRITO: *Dining out:* Order from Taco Bell. *Eating in:* Have a frozen microwave burrito (with no more than 370 calories and 12 grams fat) or make your own: Top a warmed 8-inch tortilla (preferably whole wheat) with ⅓ cup partly mashed canned pinto or black beans, 4 tablespoons shredded reduced-fat Cheddar (such as Kraft 2% Sharp Cheddar or Cabot 50% Light Cheddar), and 3 tablespoons salsa.

TIP If you make your own burrito, you can double your treat today.

1 MEDIUM PEAR

1 BEAN BURRITO: *Dining out:* Order from Taco Bell. *Eating in:* Have a frozen microwave burrito (with no more than 370 calories and 12 grams fat) or make your own: Top a warmed 8-inch tortilla (preferably whole wheat) with ⅓ cup partly mashed canned pinto or black beans, 4 tablespoons shredded reduced-fat Cheddar (such as Kraft 2% Sharp Cheddar or Cabot 50% Light Cheddar), and 3 tablespoons salsa.

TIP If you make your own burrito, you can double your treat today.

1 MEDIUM PEAR

SNACK

YOGURT: 8 ounces reduced-calorie flavored yogurt with no more than 120 calories

YOGURT: 8 ounces low-fat fruit yogurt with no more than 210 calories

DINNER

GRILLED FISH: See recipe on page 386.

SAUTÉED GREENS: ½ clove minced garlic and 2 cups spinach or other greens sautéed until just wilted in a teaspoon olive oil

BROWN RICE: ½ cup, cooked

TIP Reheat leftover rice that you made yesterday.

GRILLED FISH: See recipe on page 386.

SAUTÉED GREENS: ½ clove minced garlic and 2 cups spinach or other greens sautéed until just wilted in a teaspoon olive oil

BROWN RICE: ½ cup, cooked

TIP Reheat leftover rice that you made yesterday.

TREAT

LIGHT ICE CREAM OR FROZEN YOGURT: ½ cup, with no more than 110 calories per ½ cup

STRAWBERRIES: ½ cup unsweetened fresh or thawed frozen

WINE: 4 ounces (great with dinner) or another 80-calorie treat (see page 254 for suggestions)

LIGHT ICE CREAM OR FROZEN YOGURT: ½ cup, with no more than 110 calories per ½ cup

STRAWBERRIES: ½ cup unsweetened fresh or thawed frozen

WINE: 4 ounces (great with dinner) or another 80-calorie treat (see page 254 for suggestions)

BREAKFAST

MUFFIN: 1 large bran muffin

APPLESAUCE: ½ cup unsweetened (such as Musselman's Natural Style or Mott's Natural Style)

FAT-FREE MILK: 1 cup

LUNCH

1 BEAN BURRITO: *Dining out:* Order from Taco Bell. *Eating in:* Have a frozen microwave burrito (with no more than 370 calories and 12 grams fat) or make your own: Top a warmed 8-inch tortilla (preferably whole wheat) with ⅓ cup partly mashed canned pinto or black beans, 4 tablespoons shredded reduced-fat Cheddar (such as Kraft 2% Sharp Cheddar or Cabot 50% Light Cheddar), and 3 tablespoons salsa.

TIP If you make your own burrito, you can double your treat today.

1 MEDIUM PEAR

SNACK

YOGURT: 8 ounces low-fat fruit yogurt with no more than 210 calories

DINNER

GRILLED FISH: See recipe on page 386.

SAUTÉED GREENS: ½ clove minced garlic and 2 cups spinach or other greens sautéed until just wilted in a teaspoon olive oil

BROWN RICE: 1 cup, cooked

TIP Reheat leftover rice that you made yesterday.

TREAT

LIGHT ICE CREAM OR FROZEN YOGURT: ¾ cup, with no more than 110 calories per ½ cup

STRAWBERRIES: ½ cup unsweetened fresh or thawed frozen

WINE: 4 ounces (great with dinner) or another 80-calorie treat (see page 254 for suggestions)

Nutrition Tallies

	1,400	1,600	1,800
CALORIES	1,427	1,572	1,820
FAT (G)	33	39	43
SATURATED FAT (G)	10.5	12.2	14.1
PROTEIN (G)	72	78	83
CARBOHYDRATES (G)	202	225	274
DIETARY FIBER (G)	30	36	38
CHOLESTEROL (MG)	157	199	203
SODIUM (MG)	1,826	2,025	2,093
CALCIUM (MG)	1,150	1,270	1,414

people ask me . . .

"Is it okay to eat at fast-food restaurants?" Sure, as long as you don't do it more than once a week and as long as you order the smallest and least fatty items. For instance, the Taco Bell bean burrito has 370 calories and 12 grams of fat, low by fast-food standards. Small burgers are also in this range. Check out the calories and fat of fast foods by going to Web sites like www.burgerking.com, www.mcdonalds.com, www.tacobell.com, and www.wendys.com.

SATURDAY

1,400	1,600
BREAKFAST **OATMEAL:** 1 cup cooked unflavored oatmeal with 1 small chopped banana, 2 tablespoons almonds, and 1 teaspoon maple syrup **FAT-FREE MILK:** 1 cup	**OATMEAL:** 1 cup cooked unflavored oatmeal with 1 small chopped banana, 2 tablespoons almonds, and 1 teaspoon maple syrup **FAT-FREE MILK:** 1 cup
LUNCH **BLACK BEAN SOUP:** 1 cup soup (such as Progresso), simmered with 1 cup spinach **5 AK-MAK CRACKERS:** Have these or 115 calories' worth of another whole grain cracker.	**BLACK BEAN SOUP:** 1 cup soup (such as Progresso), simmered with 1 cup spinach **5 AK-MAK CRACKERS:** Have these or 115 calories' worth of another whole grain cracker.
SNACK **GRAHAM CRACKERS:** 1 rectangle **HOT OR COLD CHOCOLATE MILK:** 1 cup fat-free milk with 2 teaspoons chocolate syrup	**GRAHAM CRACKERS:** 2 rectangles **HOT OR COLD CHOCOLATE MILK:** 1 cup fat-free milk with 2 teaspoons chocolate syrup **1 ORANGE OR OTHER FRUIT**
DINNER **VEGETABLE PIZZA:** Quick Veggie Pizza (recipe on page 388), 2 slices of a large pizza topped with vegetables but not meat (2 of 8 slices of a 14-inch pizza, such as Domino's Hand-Tossed), or 525 calories' worth of frozen pizza **MIXED GREENS:** 2 to 3 cups, tossed with 1 tablespoon reduced-calorie dressing	**VEGETABLE PIZZA:** Quick Veggie Pizza (recipe on page 388), 2 slices of a large pizza topped with vegetables but not meat (2 of 8 slices of a 14-inch pizza, such as Domino's Hand-Tossed), or 525 calories' worth of frozen pizza **MIXED GREENS:** 2 to 3 cups, tossed with 1 tablespoon reduced-calorie dressing
TREAT **PRETZELS:** 1 ounce, or another 100-calorie treat, such as 12 ounces light beer (see page 254 for more suggestions)	**PRETZELS:** 1 ounce, or another 100-calorie treat, such as 12 ounces light beer (see page 254 for more suggestions)

1,800

BREAKFAST

OATMEAL: 1 cup cooked unflavored oatmeal with 1 small chopped banana, 2 tablespoons almonds, and 1 teaspoon maple syrup

FAT-FREE MILK: 1 cup

LUNCH

BLACK BEAN SOUP: 1 cup soup (such as Progresso), simmered with 1 cup spinach

5 AK-MAK CRACKERS: Have these or 115 calories' worth of another whole grain cracker.

SNACK

GRAHAM CRACKERS: 2 rectangles

PEANUT BUTTER: 2 teaspoons

HOT OR COLD CHOCOLATE MILK: 1 cup fat-free milk with 2 teaspoons chocolate syrup

1 ORANGE OR OTHER FRUIT

DINNER

VEGETABLE PIZZA: Quick Veggie Pizza (recipe on page 388), 2 slices of a large pizza topped with vegetables but not meat (2 of 8 slices of a 14-inch pizza, such as Domino's Hand-Tossed), or 525 calories' worth of frozen pizza

MIXED GREENS: 2 to 3 cups, tossed with 1 tablespoon regular dressing

TREAT

PRETZELS: 2 ounces, or another 200-calorie treat (see page 254 for more suggestions)

Nutrition Tallies

	1,400	1,600	1,800
CALORIES	1,402	1,608	1,788
FAT (G)	28	30	43
SATURATED FAT (G)	8.9	9.1	11.9
PROTEIN (G)	61	67	70
CARBOHYDRATES (G)	214	256	270
DIETARY FIBER (G)	31	39	40
CHOLESTEROL (MG)	38	38	46
SODIUM (MG)	2,402	2,852	2,891
CALCIUM (MG)	1,043	1,129	1,143

Fat Buster!

GET THIS: Calcium definitely keeps your bones strong, and it also helps you lose weight. Research studies show that people taking in the recommended 1,000 milligrams of calcium daily lose more weight than people who get less calcium. (On this plan, you get that much or more.) Low calcium levels send out an alarm in the body that a period of starvation is ahead. In response, you store more fat. Studies show calcium in dairy products is even more effective at lowering body fat than supplements. That's why, on this plan, you get at least two dairy servings daily.

SUNDAY

1,400	1,600

BREAKFAST

WAFFLES: 2 whole grain toaster waffles (such as Nutri-Grain Multibran) topped with 1 teaspoon trans-free margarine, ½ cup strawberries, and 1 teaspoon maple syrup.

TIP Look for waffles with about 170 calories and 4 grams of fiber for 2 waffles.

FAT-FREE MILK: 1 cup

WAFFLES: 2 whole grain toaster waffles (such as Nutri-Grain Multibran) topped with 1 teaspoon trans-free margarine, ½ cup strawberries, and 1 teaspoon maple syrup.

TIP Look for waffles with about 170 calories and 4 grams of fiber for 2 waffles.

FAT-FREE MILK: 1 cup

LUNCH

1 CHICKEN ENCHILADA: Have a microwave enchilada (such as Healthy Choice) with no more than 310 calories or make your own: Top a warmed 8-inch whole wheat or corn tortilla with ⅓ cup diced cooked chicken breast (no skin), 2 tablespoons shredded reduced-fat cheese, 2 to 4 tablespoons salsa, and ¼ sliced Haas (dark-skinned) avocado. Roll up.

TIP To save time, use precooked chicken (such as Perdue Short Cuts).

BABY CARROTS: ½ cup

1 CHICKEN ENCHILADA: Have a microwave enchilada (such as Healthy Choice) with no more than 310 calories or make your own: Top a warmed 8-inch whole wheat or corn tortilla with ⅓ cup diced cooked chicken breast (no skin), 2 tablespoons shredded reduced-fat cheese, 2 to 4 tablespoons salsa, and ¼ sliced Haas (dark-skinned) avocado. Roll up.

TIP To save time, use precooked chicken (such as Perdue Short Cuts).

BABY CARROTS: ½ cup

1 MANGO OR OTHER FRUIT

SNACK

MAPLE MILK: 1 cup fat-free milk with 1 teaspoon maple syrup

GRAHAM CRACKERS: 1 rectangle

MAPLE MILK: 1 cup fat-free milk with 1 teaspoon maple syrup

GRAHAM CRACKERS: 2 rectangles

DINNER

CHEESE TORTELLINI: ¾ cup (such as Buitoni) or 250 calories' worth of another tortellini

PASTA SAUCE: ¼ to ⅓ cup meatless pasta sauce and 1 tablespoon grated Parmesan cheese

SALAD: 2 cups mixed greens, ½ cup chopped vegetables (such as cucumber and tomato), and 1½ tablespoons reduced-calorie dressing

CHEESE TORTELLINI: 1 cup (such as Buitoni) or 330 calories' worth of another tortellini

PASTA SAUCE: ¼ to ⅓ cup meatless pasta sauce and 1 tablespoon grated Parmesan cheese

SALAD: 2 cups mixed greens, ½ cup chopped vegetables (such as cucumber and tomato), and 1½ tablespoons reduced-calorie dressing

TREAT

1 FROZEN FRUIT BAR: Choose one with no more than 80 calories.

1 FROZEN FRUIT BAR: Choose one with no more than 80 calories.

BREAKFAST

WAFFLES: 2 whole grain toaster waffles (such as Nutri-Grain Multibran) topped with 1 teaspoon trans-free margarine, ½ cup strawberries, and 1 teaspoon maple syrup.

> **TIP** Look for waffles with about 170 calories and 4 grams of fiber for 2 waffles.

FAT-FREE MILK: 1 cup

LUNCH

1 CHICKEN ENCHILADA: Have a microwave enchilada (such as Healthy Choice) with no more than 310 calories or make your own: Top a warmed 8-inch whole wheat or corn tortilla with ⅓ cup diced cooked chicken breast (no skin), 2 tablespoons shredded reduced-fat cheese, 2 to 4 tablespoons salsa, and ¼ sliced Haas (dark-skinned) avocado. Roll up.

> **TIP** To save time, use precooked chicken (such as Perdue Short Cuts).

BABY CARROTS: ½ cup

1 MANGO OR OTHER FRUIT

SNACK

MAPLE MILK: 1 cup fat-free milk with 1 teaspoon maple syrup

GRAHAM CRACKERS: 2 rectangles

PEANUT BUTTER: 2 teaspoons

DINNER

CHEESE TORTELLINI: 1 cup (such as Buitoni) or 330 calories' worth of another tortellini

PASTA SAUCE: ¼ to ⅓ cup meatless pasta sauce and 1 tablespoon grated Parmesan cheese

SALAD: 2 cups mixed greens, ½ cup chopped vegetables (such as cucumber and tomato), and 1½ tablespoons regular dressing

TREAT

15 JUNIOR MINTS: Choose these or another 150-calorie treat (see page 255 for suggestions).

Nutrition Tallies

	1,400	1,600	1,800
CALORIES	1,382	1,599	1,799
FAT (G)	44	47	59
SATURATED FAT (G)	11	12.3	14.7
PROTEIN (G)	65	70	74
CARBOHYDRATES (G)	199	247	269
DIETARY FIBER (G)	22	27	28
CHOLESTEROL (MG)	109	126	132
SODIUM (MG)	2,730	2,850	2,853
CALCIUM (MG)	1,351	1,405	1,420

Nutrient Booster!

COUNT ½ CUP of meatless tomato sauce as a vegetable serving. Concentrated tomato products such as sauces and salsas are loaded with one of the most powerful antioxidants: lycopene. Lycopene is what gives tomatoes their beautiful red color, and it's credited with cutting cancer risk in half for people who regularly eat tomatoes and tomato products.

CHAPTER 11

Fight Fat with Fiber

You might have heard that a high-fiber diet helps ward off cancer and other diseases. Yes, it can! But did you know that it also fights fat?

Isn't this great: Studies show that if you give people virtually the same diet—same calories, similar foods—except one diet is high in fiber and the other low in fiber, those on the high-fiber diet *will lose more weight*. And surveys show that thinner people do eat more fiber than heavier people.

How Fiber Works Its Magic

Also known as roughage, fiber is a multitasking marvel that fights fat in several ways.

▪ **Fiber helps you curb your appetite.** Besides helping you feel fuller longer on fewer calories, fiber also keeps blood sugar on an even keel. All carbs—fruit, vegetables, bread, grains, sugar—are made up of thousands of sugar strands. If you eat a low-fiber carb—like cornflakes, white bread, or sugar—the strands come apart quickly and easily. This sends your blood sugar (glucose) soaring, then it crashes, leaving you hungrier than before. But fiber puts the brakes on blood sugar surges. It takes more time and ef-

280

1,400 CALORIES: 22% calories from fat, 22% protein, 56% carbohydrates
1,600 CALORIES: 25% calories from fat, 21% protein, 54% carbohydrates
1,800 CALORIES: 26% calories from fat, 21% protein, 53% carbohydrates

fort to unravel sugar strands when fiber's in the way. So after you eat a high-fiber food like oatmeal, glucose makes its way into the blood in a nice even trickle, suppressing hunger. It's a natural appetite suppressant. Isn't that great?

▪ Fiber removes fat. Fiber carries wastes out of the body more quickly, taking some unabsorbed fat (and calories) with it. Fiber can remove up to an estimated 5 percent of the fat in a meal. Five percent adds up over months and years, which is also one of the ways fiber protects you against colon cancer, by whisking cancer-causing agents out of the gut.

▪ Fiber turns on the "burn fat" signal. Fiber lowers insulin levels. The hormone insulin is the blood glucose cleanup crew. When blood sugar rises, insulin rushes in, scooping up glucose and depositing it in cells to use for energy. If you eat a low-fiber diet, you'll be hit with lots of sugar rushes, making a lot of work for insulin. While insulin levels are high, you burn carbs for energy and store fat. But when insulin is low, the body switches into fat-burning mode. So a high-fiber diet lowers blood sugar, which lowers insulin levels and helps you burn more fat and store less.

Your 6-week plan brings you up to the daily 25 to 35 grams of fiber recommended by major health organizations, enough to fight disease and attack fat and more than double the fiber that the average American gets. An added plus to more fiber: It wards off constipation, particularly if you drink lots of water—at least eight glasses a day.

> **WEEKLY CHECK-IN:** Time to congratulate yourself for finishing a full week on the Shrink Your Female Fat Zones plan! Whether you get on the scale, try on that pair of pants, or use the measuring tape, make a note of how your body changed this week. Write your results in your daily log (page 408).

SHOPPING LIST

CHECK YOUR FRIDGE and cupboards. Much of this food might still be there from last week. And some of what you'll buy this week will carry over to the upcoming weeks. There are no portions listed, because these vary depending on how many people are in your family. So just go through the menu plan and note how much of everything you'll need.

If you don't like something, substitute with as close an equivalent as you can find. For instance, have a pear instead of an apple or pinto beans instead of black beans. But don't substitute white flour products (like white bread) when whole grain products (like whole wheat bread) are called for. Whole grains are important weight-loss tools.

FRESH FRUIT

Apples

Bananas

Berries, such as raspberries (Don't buy if you're using blueberries for breakfast on Monday and strawberries for breakfast on Sunday.)

Blueberries

Cantaloupe

Lemons

Nectarines (for 1,600- and 1,800-calorie plans)

Oranges

Peaches

Strawberries

FRESH VEGETABLES AND HERBS

Asparagus

Avocados, Haas

Basil

Broccoli

Carrots, baby and regular

Celery

Corn

Cucumber

Garlic

Greens, mixed, or spinach

Lettuce (You can use mixed greens instead.)

Mushrooms, portobello or white button

Onions

Peas or green beans

Peppers, green

Peppers, red

Tomatoes, cherry or grape and regular

CANNED AND BOTTLED GOODS

Beans, black, canned (Don't buy if you're using canned chili for dinner on Friday.)

Beans, kidney or pinto, canned (Don't buy if you're using canned chili for dinner on Friday.)

Beans, white (such as cannellini), canned

Capers

Chickpeas, canned (Don't buy if you're eating out at the salad bar on Tuesday.)

Chili, vegetarian (Don't buy if you're making chili for dinner on Friday.)

Honey

Hot-pepper sauce

Jam or jelly

Ketchup

Lemon juice

Mayonnaise, low-fat

Mustard, Dijon

Oil, olive

Olives, black, preferably Moroccan or kalamata

Pasta sauce, meatless

Peanut butter

Pickles

Preserves, apricot

Salad dressing, reduced-calorie Italian or vinaigrette

Salad dressing, regular Italian or vinaigrette (for 1,800-calorie plan only)

Syrup, chocolate

Syrup, maple or maple-flavored

Tomatoes, diced, canned (Don't buy if you're using canned chili for dinner on Friday.)

Tomatoes, whole, canned

Tuna, water-packed

Vinegar, red wine (Don't buy if you're using canned chili for dinner on Friday.)

DRY GOODS AND BREAD

Almonds (for 1,600- and 1,800-calorie plans only, unless you're using almonds instead of walnuts in the Chicken Waldorf Salad on Friday)

Bread, whole wheat sandwich loaf, with no more than 90 calories and at least 2 grams of fiber per slice

Buns, whole wheat hamburger

Cereal, granola

Cereal, high-fiber, with 5 to 8 grams of fiber per serving (such as Kellogg's Complete Wheat Bran Flakes or Kashi Good Friends)

Cereal, oatmeal (plain, unflavored)

Chili powder (Don't buy if you're using canned chili for dinner on Friday.)

Cinnamon

Cornbread or corn muffin

Couscous, whole wheat (found in bulk in natural food stores and in boxes, such as Fantastic Foods)

Crackers, graham

Crackers, whole rye (such as Wasa or Ryvita)

Cumin (Don't buy if you're using canned chili for dinner on Friday.)

Muffins, English, oat bran or whole wheat

Pasta, whole wheat noodles or short tubular type

Raisins

Rice, brown (such as Texmati, basmati, or quick-cooking Uncle Ben's)

Seeds, sunflower (for 1,800-calorie plan only; don't buy if you're eating out at a salad bar for lunch on Tuesday)

Walnuts

REFRIGERATED FOODS

Butter or trans-free margarine (will state "trans-free" on the label)

Cheese, Parmesan

Cheese, reduced-fat (such as Cabot 50% Light Cheddar, Tine 75% Jarlsberg, or Kraft or Borden 2% Singles)

Cheese sticks, with about 70 calories each (such as Polly-O or Sargento)

Cottage cheese, 1% or 2% (for 1,600- and 1,800-calorie plans)

Eggs or egg substitute (such as Egg Beaters)

Milk, fat-free (If you haven't adjusted to fat-free milk, buy 1% or mix equal parts 1% and 2%. Your calorie level will be a little higher, but you can gradually train your tastebuds to like fat-free. If you're lactose intolerant, try Lactaid milk. If you prefer soy milk—low-fat or fat-free—buy calcium-fortified with at least 25% of the Daily Value of calcium per cup.)

Yogurt, low-fat fruit, with about 210 calories per 8 ounces (for 1,600- and 1,800-calorie plans)

Yogurt, low-fat plain

Yogurt, reduced-calorie flavored, with no more than 120 calories per 8 ounces

MEAT, POULTRY, AND FISH

Beef, lean ground

Chicken, boneless and skinless breasts

Fish, white fillets (such as red snapper or tilapia)

Shrimp, large

Turkey, sliced breast

FROZEN FOODS

Fruit bars, frozen, with no more than 80 calories (such as Frozfruit, Edy's, or Dreyer's)

Ice cream or frozen yogurt, light, with no more than 110 calories per ½ cup (such as Breyers, Edy's, or Dreyer's)

Vegetable burgers, with about 120 calories (such as Gardenburgers)

Waffles, whole grain toaster waffles, with about 170 calories for 2 (such as Nutri-Grain Multibran)

OPTIONAL

Beer, light

Dill or parsley (for Shrimp and Vegetable Kebabs on Monday)

Garlic salt (for Friday night dinner)

Red-pepper flakes (for Pasta with Broccoli and Chicken on Tuesday)

Treats (see Monday, Saturday, and Sunday)

Wine

MONDAY

1,400	1,600

BREAKFAST

CEREAL: 150 calories of high-fiber cereal (such as 1¼ cups Kashi Good Friends or Kellogg's Complete Wheat Bran Flakes) topped with 1 cup fat-free milk, ½ cup blueberries or other berries, and 2 table-spoons granola

> **TIP** Check label for 5 to 8 grams of fiber per 30-gram serving.

CEREAL: 150 calories of high-fiber cereal (such as 1¼ cups Kashi Good Friends or Kellogg's Complete Wheat Bran Flakes) topped with 1 cup fat-free milk, ½ cup blueberries or other berries, and 2 table-spoons granola

> **TIP** Check label for 5 to 8 grams of fiber per 30-gram serving.

LUNCH

TURKEY AND CHEESE SANDWICH: Between 2 slices whole wheat bread, layer 2 slices turkey breast, 1 slice reduced-fat cheese, tomato slices, and lettuce. If desired, spread 1 slice of bread with 1 teaspoon low-fat mayo, the other with mustard.

RED PEPPER SLICES: 1 cup

1 ORANGE OR APPLE

TURKEY AND CHEESE SANDWICH: Between 2 slices whole wheat bread, layer 2 slices turkey breast, 1 slice reduced-fat cheese, tomato slices, and lettuce. If desired, spread 1 slice of bread with 1 teaspoon low-fat mayo, the other with mustard.

RED PEPPER SLICES: 1 cup

LOW-FAT COTTAGE CHEESE: ½ cup

1 ORANGE OR APPLE

SNACK

YOGURT: 8 ounces reduced-calorie flavored yogurt with no more than 120 calories

YOGURT: 8 ounces low-fat fruit yogurt with no more than 210 calories

ALMONDS: 2 tablespoons

DINNER

SHRIMP AND VEGETABLE KEBABS: See recipe on page 389.

BROWN RICE: 1 cup, cooked

> **TIP** Try brown Texmati or basmati rice.

SHRIMP AND VEGETABLE KEBABS: See recipe on page 389.

BROWN RICE: 1 cup, cooked

> **TIP** Try brown Texmati or basmati rice.

TREAT

2 KEEBLER SANDIES COOKIES: Choose these or another 160-calorie treat (see page 255 for more suggestions).

2 KEEBLER SANDIES COOKIES: Choose these or another 160-calorie treat (see page 255 for more suggestions).

BREAKFAST

CEREAL: 150 calories of high-fiber cereal (such as 1¼ cups Kashi Good Friends or Kellogg's Complete Wheat Bran Flakes) topped with 1 cup fat-free milk, ½ cup blueberries or other berries, and 3 tablespoons granola

TIP Check label for 5 to 8 grams of fiber per 30-gram serving.

LUNCH

TURKEY AND CHEESE SANDWICH: Between 2 slices whole wheat bread, layer 2 slices turkey breast, 2 slices reduced-fat cheese, tomato slices, and lettuce. If desired, spread 1 slice of bread with 1 teaspoon low-fat mayo, the other with mustard.

RED PEPPER SLICES: 1 cup

LOW-FAT COTTAGE CHEESE: ½ cup

1 ORANGE OR APPLE

SNACK

YOGURT: 8 ounces low-fat fruit yogurt with no more than 210 calories

ALMONDS: 2 tablespoons

DINNER

SHRIMP AND VEGETABLE KEBABS: See recipe on page 389.

BROWN RICE: 1 cup, cooked

TIP Try brown Texmati or basmati rice.

TREAT

2 KEEBLER SANDIES COOKIES: Choose these or another 160-calorie treat (see page 255 for more suggestions).

Nutrition Tallies

	1,400	1,600	1,800
CALORIES	1,397	1,613	1,773
FAT (G)	28	41	52
SATURATED FAT (G)	7.4	9.4	13.4
PROTEIN (G)	73	93	102
CARBOHYDRATES (G)	230	237	256
DIETARY FIBER (G)	29	31	31
CHOLESTEROL (MG)	167	168	190
SODIUM (MG)	1,978	2,464	2,641
CALCIUM (MG)	969	1,134	1,384

Fat Buster!

Thanks to fiber, the oatmeal and bran cereals on this plan may help you lose weight by suppressing your appetite. In two different studies, these champions squared off against cornflakes (which is virtually fiber-free). After eating the high-fiber cereals, people were able to make it to lunch without feeling hungry. Those who started the day with cornflakes listened to their stomachs growl.

TUESDAY

1,400	1,600
BREAKFAST	
ENGLISH MUFFIN: 1 oat bran or whole wheat English muffin, split and toasted, each half spread with 1 teaspoon trans-free margarine	**ENGLISH MUFFIN:** 1 oat bran or whole wheat English muffin, split and toasted, each half spread with 1 teaspoon trans-free margarine and 1 tablespoon jam or jelly
STRAWBERRIES: 1 cup of these or blueberries	**STRAWBERRIES:** 1 cup of these or blueberries
FAT-FREE MILK: 1 cup	**FAT-FREE MILK:** 1 cup
LUNCH	
SATISFYING VEGGIE SALAD: At home or the salad bar, toss 1 cup mixed greens or spinach with 1 cup other vegetables (such as carrot, tomato, cucumber), ½ cup canned chickpeas or other beans, 2 tablespoons chopped eggs or grated cheese, and 2 tablespoons reduced-calorie dressing.	**SATISFYING VEGGIE SALAD:** At home or the salad bar, toss 1 cup mixed greens or spinach with 1 cup other vegetables (such as carrot, tomato, cucumber), ½ cup canned chickpeas or other beans, 2 tablespoons chopped eggs or grated cheese, and 2 tablespoons reduced-calorie dressing.
1 SMALL ROLL: Have this or 1 slice bread (preferably whole grain).	**1 SMALL ROLL:** Have this or 1 slice bread (preferably whole grain).
	LOW-FAT COTTAGE CHEESE: ½ cup
SNACK	
CHOCOLATE MILK: 1 cup fat-free milk with 2 teaspoons chocolate syrup	**CHOCOLATE MILK:** 1 cup fat-free milk with 2 teaspoons chocolate syrup
GRAHAM CRACKERS: 1 rectangle	**GRAHAM CRACKERS:** 1 rectangle
DINNER	
PASTA WITH BROCCOLI AND CHICKEN: See recipe on page 390.	**PASTA WITH BROCCOLI AND CHICKEN:** See recipe on page 390.
TREAT	
1 FROZEN FRUIT BAR: Choose one with no more than 70 to 80 calories.	**1 FROZEN FRUIT BAR:** Choose one with no more than 70 to 80 calories.

BREAKFAST

ENGLISH MUFFIN: 1 oat bran or whole wheat English muffin, split and toasted, each half spread with 1 teaspoon trans-free margarine and 1 tablespoon jam or jelly

STRAWBERRIES: 1 cup of these or blueberries

FAT-FREE MILK: 1 cup

LUNCH

SATISFYING VEGGIE SALAD: At home or the salad bar, toss 1 cup mixed greens or spinach with 1 cup other vegetables (such as carrot, tomato, cucumber), ½ cup canned chickpeas or other beans, 2 tablespoons chopped eggs or grated cheese, 2 tablespoons reduced-calorie dressing, and 2 tablespoons sunflower seeds.

1 SMALL ROLL: Have this or 1 slice bread (preferably whole grain).

LOW-FAT COTTAGE CHEESE: ½ cup

SNACK

CHOCOLATE MILK: 1 cup fat-free milk with 2 teaspoons chocolate syrup

GRAHAM CRACKERS: 2 rectangles

DINNER

PASTA WITH BROCCOLI AND CHICKEN: See recipe on page 390.

TREAT

1 FROZEN FRUIT BAR: Choose one with no more than 70 to 80 calories.

Nutrition Tallies

	1,400	1,600	1,800
CALORIES	1,395	1,639	1,791
FAT (G)	36	38	48
SATURATED FAT (G)	8.6	10	11.1
PROTEIN (G)	80	99	104
CARBOHYDRATES (G)	205	242	256
DIETARY FIBER (G)	31	35	37
CHOLESTEROL (MG)	120	129	129
SODIUM (MG)	1,879	2,346	2,431
CALCIUM (MG)	1,121	1,213	1,228

Nutrient Booster!

BERRIES ARE CHOCK-FULL of amazing compounds. For instance, blueberries and cranberries both help stave off urinary tract infections, and blueberries contain more antioxidants—compounds that ward off cancer, heart disease, and other age-related ills—than nearly any other fruit. Maybe that's why feeding blueberry extracts to aging lab rats improved their memory and balance. A cup of strawberries offers nearly double your daily vitamin C requirement and also contains a potent anti-cancer agent called ellagic acid.

WEDNESDAY

1,400	1,600
BREAKFAST	
PEACH-BANANA SMOOTHIE: In a blender, process until smooth 1 small ripe banana, $\frac{1}{2}$ cup fresh or canned (in juice or light syrup) peaches, $\frac{1}{2}$ cup fat-free milk, $\frac{1}{2}$ cup low-fat plain yogurt, 2 teaspoons honey, and 1 or 2 ice cubes.	**PEACH-BANANA SMOOTHIE:** In a blender, process until smooth 1 small ripe banana, $\frac{1}{2}$ cup fresh or canned (in juice or light syrup) peaches, $\frac{1}{2}$ cup fat-free milk, $\frac{1}{2}$ cup low-fat plain yogurt, 2 teaspoons honey, and 1 or 2 ice cubes.
WHOLE WHEAT BREAD: 1 slice spread with 1 teaspoon trans-free margarine	**WHOLE WHEAT BREAD:** 2 slices spread with 2 teaspoons trans-free margarine

1,400	1,600
LUNCH	
TUNA SANDWICH: Mix 3 ounces water-packed tuna; 1 tablespoon finely chopped celery, carrots, or pickles; 1 teaspoon low-fat mayo; 1 teaspoon low-fat plain yogurt; and $\frac{1}{2}$ teaspoon Dijon mustard. Spread on 2 slices whole wheat bread.	**TUNA SANDWICH:** Mix 3 ounces water-packed tuna; 1 tablespoon finely chopped celery, carrots, or pickles; 1 teaspoon low-fat mayo; 1 teaspoon low-fat plain yogurt; and $\frac{1}{2}$ teaspoon Dijon mustard. Spread on 2 slices whole wheat bread.
CARROT AND CELERY STICKS: 1 cup	**CARROT AND CELERY STICKS:** 1 cup
	1 NECTARINE OR OTHER FRUIT

1,400	1,600
SNACK	
1 CHEESE STICK: Choose one with no more than 70 calories (such as Sargento or Polly-O).	**1 CHEESE STICK:** Choose one with no more than 70 calories (such as Sargento or Polly-O).
1 PICKLE	**1 PICKLE**

1,400	1,600
DINNER	
HAMBURGER: 1 small burger (broil or grill 4 ounces lean ground beef) on 1 whole wheat bun with ketchup and mustard	**HAMBURGER:** 1 small burger (broil or grill 4 ounces lean ground beef) on 1 whole wheat bun with ketchup and mustard
CORN ON THE COB: 1 ear	**CORN ON THE COB:** 1 ear
PEAS: Have $\frac{1}{2}$ cup of these or green beans with a spritz of lemon juice.	**PEAS:** Have $\frac{1}{2}$ cup of these or green beans with a spritz of lemon juice.

1,400	1,600
TREAT	
LIGHT ICE CREAM OR FROZEN YOGURT: 1 cup, with no more than 110 calories per $\frac{1}{2}$ cup	**LIGHT ICE CREAM OR FROZEN YOGURT:** 1 cup, with no more than 110 calories per $\frac{1}{2}$ cup

1,800

BREAKFAST

PEACH-BANANA SMOOTHIE: In a blender, process until smooth 1 small ripe banana, ½ cup fresh or canned (in juice or light syrup) peaches, ½ cup fat-free milk, ½ cup low-fat plain yogurt, 1 tablespoon honey, and 1 or 2 ice cubes.

WHOLE WHEAT BREAD: 2 slices spread with 2 teaspoons trans-free margarine

LUNCH

TUNA SANDWICH: Mix 3 ounces water-packed tuna; 1 tablespoon finely chopped celery, carrots, or pickles; 1 teaspoon low-fat mayo; 1 teaspoon low-fat plain yogurt; and ½ teaspoon Dijon mustard. Spread on 2 slices whole wheat bread.

CARROT AND CELERY STICKS: 1 cup

1 NECTARINE OR OTHER FRUIT

SNACK

1 CHEESE STICK: Choose one with no more than 70 calories (such as Sargento or Polly-O).

1 PICKLE

3 WASA FIBER RYE CRACKERS: Have these or 90 calories' worth of another whole grain rye cracker (such as Ryvita).

DINNER

HAMBURGER: 1 small burger (broil or grill 4 ounces lean ground beef) on 1 whole wheat bun with ketchup and mustard

CORN ON THE COB: 1 ear

PEAS: Have 1 cup of these or green beans with a spritz of lemon juice.

TREAT

LIGHT ICE CREAM OR FROZEN YOGURT: 1 cup, with no more than 110 calories per ½ cup

Nutrition Tallies

	1,400	1,600	1,800
CALORIES	1,441	1,619	1,750
FAT (G)	42	48	51
SATURATED FAT (G)	17.1	18.1	18.2
PROTEIN (G)	87	91	95
CARBOHYDRATES (G)	192	222	253
DIETARY FIBER (G)	22	27	35
CHOLESTEROL (MG)	148	148	148
SODIUM (MG)	2,678	2,897	2,903
CALCIUM (MG)	1,042	1,082	1,176

Nutrient Booster!

HIGH-FIBER CARBS are "good carbs," those that help you lose weight. You'll see that this week—and every week—I have you eating many of the foods on this list.

Barley

Beans (black, pinto, chickpeas, lentils, and all the others)

Bread (100% whole wheat)

Brown rice

Cereal (high-fiber, such as bran flakes)

Couscous (whole wheat)

Oatmeal

Pasta (whole wheat)

Rye crackers (such as Wasa or Ryvita)

Tortillas (whole wheat)

THURSDAY

1,400	1,600
BREAKFAST	
CINNAMON OATMEAL: Cook ½ cup rolled oats according to package directions, adding 1 small diced apple, 2 teaspoons maple syrup, and a dash of cinnamon.	**CINNAMON OATMEAL:** Cook ½ cup rolled oats according to package directions, adding 1 small diced apple, 2 teaspoons maple syrup, and a dash of cinnamon.
FAT-FREE MILK: 1 cup	**FAT-FREE MILK:** 1 cup
	WALNUTS: 2 tablespoons
LUNCH	
AVOCADO AND WHITE BEAN SALAD: See recipe on page 391.	**AVOCADO AND WHITE BEAN SALAD:** See recipe on page 391.
2 WASA FIBER RYE CRACKERS: Have these or 60 calories' worth of another whole grain cracker (such as Ryvita).	**5 WASA FIBER RYE CRACKERS:** Have these or 150 calories' worth of another whole grain cracker (such as Ryvita).
SNACK	
YOGURT: 8 ounces reduced-calorie flavored yogurt with no more than 120 calories	**YOGURT:** 8 ounces reduced-calorie flavored yogurt with no more than 120 calories
DINNER	
APRICOT-GLAZED CHICKEN: See recipe on page 390.	**APRICOT-GLAZED CHICKEN:** See recipe on page 390.
TIP Make an extra piece of chicken breast for tomorrow's Chicken Waldorf Salad.	**TIP** Make an extra piece of chicken breast for tomorrow's Chicken Waldorf Salad.
LEMON COUSCOUS: 1 cup (recipe on page 391)	**LEMON COUSCOUS:** 1 cup (recipe on page 391)
TIP If you can't find whole wheat couscous (such as Fantastic Foods), have brown rice or whole wheat pasta.	**TIP** If you can't find whole wheat couscous (such as Fantastic Foods), have brown rice or whole wheat pasta.
ASPARAGUS: 4 to 6 stalks steamed, with a spritz of lemon juice	**ASPARAGUS:** 4 to 6 stalks steamed, with a spritz of lemon juice
TREAT	
HOT CHOCOLATE: 1 cup hot fat-free milk mixed with 2 teaspoons chocolate syrup	**HOT CHOCOLATE:** 1 cup hot fat-free milk mixed with 2 teaspoons chocolate syrup

BREAKFAST

CINNAMON OATMEAL: Cook ½ cup rolled oats according to package directions, adding 1 small diced apple, 2 teaspoons maple syrup, and a dash of cinnamon.

FAT-FREE MILK: 1 cup

WALNUTS: 2 tablespoons

LUNCH

AVOCADO AND WHITE BEAN SALAD: See recipe on page 391.

5 WASA FIBER RYE CRACKERS: Have these or 150 calories' worth of another whole grain cracker (such as Ryvita).

REDUCED-FAT CHEESE: 1 ounce

SNACK

YOGURT: 8 ounces low-fat fruit yogurt with no more than 210 calories

DINNER

APRICOT-GLAZED CHICKEN: See recipe on page 390.

> **TIP** Make an extra piece of chicken breast for tomorrow's Chicken Waldorf Salad.

LEMON COUSCOUS: 1 cup (recipe on page 391)

> **TIP** If you can't find whole wheat couscous (such as Fantastic Foods), have brown rice or whole wheat pasta.

ASPARAGUS: 4 to 6 stalks steamed, with a spritz of lemon juice

TREAT

HOT CHOCOLATE: 1 cup hot fat-free milk mixed with 2 teaspoons chocolate syrup

Nutrition Tallies

	1,400	1,600	1,800
CALORIES	1,356	1,587	1,786
FAT (G)	16	36	47
SATURATED FAT (G)	3.4	4.8	9.3
PROTEIN (G)	88	93	102
CARBOHYDRATES (G)	227	251	270
DIETARY FIBER (G)	29	38	28
CHOLESTEROL (MG)	94	94	116
SODIUM (MG)	897	904	1,081
CALCIUM (MG)	1,053	1,167	1,417

people ask me . . .

"How many servings of beans should I eat?"

Have at least ½ cup four or more times a week. According to a huge government survey of more than 9,600 Americans, people who eat beans four times a week are 22 percent less likely to get heart disease than people who eat beans less than once a week. Beans lower blood cholesterol and blood sugar and are full of iron and B vitamins.

FRIDAY

1,400	1,600

BREAKFAST

YOGURT: 8 ounces low-fat plain yogurt mixed with 2 teaspoons maple syrup and served over ½ cup blueberries

2 WASA FIBER RYE CRACKERS: Have these or 60 calories' worth of another whole rye cracker (1 cracker spread with 1 teaspoon peanut butter).

YOGURT: 8 ounces low-fat plain yogurt mixed with 2 teaspoons maple syrup and served over ½ cup blueberries

2 WASA FIBER RYE CRACKERS: Have these or 60 calories' worth of another whole rye cracker (1 cracker spread with 1 teaspoon peanut butter).

LUNCH

CHICKEN WALDORF SALAD: See recipe on page 392.

5 WASA FIBER RYE CRACKERS: Have these or 150 calories' worth of another whole rye cracker.

CHICKEN WALDORF SALAD: See recipe on page 392.

5 WASA FIBER RYE CRACKERS: Have these or 150 calories' worth of another whole rye cracker.

SNACK

1 CHEESE STICK: Choose one with no more than 70 calories.

5 BABY CARROTS

1 CHEESE STICK: Choose one with no more than 70 calories.

5 BABY CARROTS

DINNER

VEGETARIAN CHILI: Choose either ¾ cup canned or Easy Homemade Chili (recipe on page 392).

CORNBREAD: 170 calories' worth of cornbread (2 × 4-inch piece) or corn muffin (2 ounces)

FAST GUACAMOLE: ¼ avocado left over from yesterday, mashed with a spritz of lemon juice and a dash of garlic salt (optional)

MIXED GREENS: 2 cups, tossed with 1 tablespoon reduced-calorie dressing

VEGETARIAN CHILI: Choose either ¾ cup canned or Easy Homemade Chili (recipe on page 392).

CORNBREAD: 170 calories' worth of cornbread (2 × 4-inch piece) or corn muffin (2 ounces)

FAST GUACAMOLE: ¼ avocado left over from yesterday, mashed with a spritz of lemon juice and a dash of garlic salt (optional)

MIXED GREENS: 2 cups, tossed with 1 tablespoon reduced-calorie dressing

TREAT

LIGHT ICE CREAM OR FROZEN YOGURT: ½ cup, with no more than 110 calories per ½ cup

LIGHT ICE CREAM OR FROZEN YOGURT: ¾ cup, with no more than 110 calories per ½ cup

BREAKFAST

YOGURT: 8 ounces low-fat plain yogurt mixed with 2 teaspoons maple syrup and served over ½ cup blueberries

2 WASA FIBER RYE CRACKERS: Have these or 60 calories' worth of another whole rye cracker (1 cracker spread with 1 teaspoon peanut butter).

LUNCH

CHICKEN WALDORF SALAD: See recipe on page 392.

5 WASA FIBER RYE CRACKERS: Have these or 150 calories' worth of another whole rye cracker.

1 ORANGE OR OTHER FRUIT

SNACK

1 CHEESE STICK: Choose one with no more than 70 calories.

5 BABY CARROTS

DINNER

VEGETARIAN CHILI: Choose either ¾ cup canned or Easy Homemade Chili (recipe on page 392).

CORNBREAD: 170 calories' worth of cornbread (2 × 4-inch piece) or corn muffin (2 ounces)

FAST GUACAMOLE: ½ avocado left over from yesterday, mashed with a spritz of lemon juice and a dash of garlic salt (optional)

MIXED GREENS: 2 cups, tossed with 2 tablespoons regular dressing

TREAT

LIGHT ICE CREAM OR FROZEN YOGURT: 1¼ cups, with no more than 110 calories per ½ cup

Nutrition Tallies

	1,400	1,600	1,800
CALORIES	1,453	1,566	1,802
FAT (G)	46	49	66
SATURATED FAT (G)	12.7	14.2	17.7
PROTEIN (G)	76	80	82
CARBOHYDRATES (G)	198	214	244
DIETARY FIBER (G)	28	30	37
CHOLESTEROL (MG)	141	146	156
SODIUM (MG)	1,922	1,979	2,400
CALCIUM (MG)	963	1,020	1,231

Nutrient Booster!

SEE HOW MUCH MORE FIBER you get when you make the following switches!

Cornflakes (0 gram fiber in 1 ounce) to **bran-based cereal** (5 to 15 grams)

White bread (1 gram per slice) to **whole wheat bread** (2 to 3 grams)

White couscous (2 grams in 1 cooked cup) to **whole wheat couscous** (7 grams)

White flour tortilla (1 to 2 grams in an 8-inch diameter) to **whole wheat tortilla** (5 grams)

White pasta (2 grams in 1 cooked cup) to **whole wheat pasta** (6 grams)

SATURDAY

1,400	1,600

BREAKFAST

SCRAMBLED EGGS: ½ cup egg substitute, such as Egg Beaters (or 1 egg and 1 egg white), scrambled in 1 teaspoon butter or trans-free margarine

ENGLISH MUFFIN: 1 oat bran or whole wheat English muffin, split and toasted

CANTALOUPE: 1 cup cubes

SCRAMBLED EGGS: ½ cup egg substitute, such as Egg Beaters (or 1 egg and 1 egg white), scrambled in 1 teaspoon butter or trans-free margarine

ENGLISH MUFFIN: 1 oat bran or whole wheat English muffin, split and toasted, each half spread with 1 teaspoon trans-free margarine and 1 teaspoon jam or jelly

CANTALOUPE: 1 cup cubes

LUNCH

PEANUT BUTTER AND JELLY SANDWICH: Spread 2 tablespoons peanut butter and 2 tablespoons jelly or jam on 2 slices whole wheat bread.

FAT-FREE MILK: 1 cup

BABY CARROTS: ½ cup

PEANUT BUTTER AND JELLY SANDWICH: Spread 2 tablespoons peanut butter and 2 tablespoons jelly or jam on 2 slices whole wheat bread.

FAT-FREE MILK: 1 cup

BABY CARROTS: ½ cup

SNACK

MUG OF GRANOLA: 2 tablespoons granola in ¼ cup fat-free milk

MUG OF GRANOLA: ¼ cup granola in ¼ cup fat-free milk

DINNER

SPAGHETTI: 1 cup whole wheat spaghetti, with ¼ cup meatless pasta sauce, 2 tablespoons Parmesan, and 2 teaspoons chopped basil

MIXED GREENS: 2 cups, with 1 tablespoon reduced-calorie dressing

---

SPAGHETTI: 1½ cups whole wheat spaghetti, with ¼ cup meatless pasta sauce, 2 tablespoons Parmesan, and 2 teaspoons chopped basil

MIXED GREENS: 2 cups, with 1 tablespoon reduced-calorie dressing

TREAT

3 GINGERSNAPS: Have these or another 85-calorie treat (see page 254 for more suggestions).

---

3 GINGERSNAPS: Have these or another 85-calorie treat (see page 254 for more suggestions).

BREAKFAST

SCRAMBLED EGGS: ½ cup egg substitute, such as Egg Beaters (or 1 egg and 1 egg white), scrambled in 1 teaspoon butter or trans-free margarine

ENGLISH MUFFIN: 1 oat bran or whole wheat English muffin, split and toasted, each half spread with 1 teaspoon trans-free margarine and 1 teaspoon jam or jelly

CANTALOUPE: 1 cup cubes

LUNCH

PEANUT BUTTER AND JELLY SANDWICH: Spread 2 tablespoons peanut butter and 2 tablespoons jelly or jam on 2 slices whole wheat bread.

FAT-FREE MILK: 1 cup

BABY CARROTS: ½ cup

SNACK

MUG OF GRANOLA: ¼ cup granola in ¼ cup fat-free milk

DINNER

SPAGHETTI: 1¾ cups whole wheat spaghetti, with ½ cup meatless pasta sauce, 3 tablespoons Parmesan, and 2 teaspoons chopped basil

MIXED GREENS: 2 cups, with 1 tablespoon regular dressing

TREAT

FIDDLE FADDLE: ⅔ cup, or another 125-calorie treat (see page 255 for more suggestions)

Nutrition Tallies

	1,400	1,600	1,800
CALORIES	1,440	1,591	1,786
FAT (G)	42	50	57
SATURATED FAT (G)	10	11.4	13.3
PROTEIN (G)	67	69	75
CARBOHYDRATES (G)	194	213	233
DIETARY FIBER (G)	26	28	31
CHOLESTEROL (MG)	230	230	234
SODIUM (MG)	1,793	1,906	2,010
CALCIUM (MG)	1,144	1,155	1,236

SUNDAY

1,400	1,600
BREAKFAST	
WAFFLES: 2 whole grain toaster waffles (with about 170 calories and 4 grams fiber for 2 waffles) topped with ½ cup strawberries or other berries and 1 teaspoon maple syrup **FAT-FREE MILK:** 1 cup	**WAFFLES:** 2 whole grain toaster waffles (with about 170 calories and 4 grams fiber for 2 waffles) topped with 2 teaspoons trans-free margarine, ½ cup strawberries or other berries, and 1 teaspoon maple syrup **FAT-FREE MILK:** 1 cup
LUNCH	
VEGGIE CHEESEBURGER: Cook 1 vegetable burger (about 120 calories, such as a Gardenburger) according to package directions. Melt 1 slice reduced-fat cheese on top and place in 1 whole wheat hamburger bun with 2 teaspoons low-fat mayo, mustard, tomato slices, and lettuce. **RED PEPPER SLICES:** 1 cup	**VEGGIE CHEESEBURGER:** Cook 1 vegetable burger (about 120 calories, such as a Gardenburger) according to package directions. Melt 1 slice reduced-fat cheese on top and place in 1 whole wheat hamburger bun with 2 teaspoons low-fat mayo, mustard, tomato slices, and lettuce. **RED PEPPER SLICES:** 1 cup
SNACK	
MAPLE MILK: 1 cup hot or cold fat-free milk with 1 teaspoon maple syrup	**MAPLE MILK:** 1 cup hot or cold fat-free milk with 1 teaspoon maple syrup **WALNUTS:** 2 tablespoons **RAISINS:** 2 tablespoons
DINNER	
FISH WITH OLIVES AND CAPERS: See recipe on page 393. **LEMON COUSCOUS:** 1 cup (recipe on page 391) TIP If you can't find whole wheat couscous, have brown rice or whole wheat pasta. **BROCCOLI:** ½ cup, steamed, with a spritz of lemon juice	**FISH WITH OLIVES AND CAPERS:** See recipe on page 393. **LEMON COUSCOUS:** 1 cup (recipe on page 391) TIP If you can't find whole wheat couscous, have brown rice or whole wheat pasta. **BROCCOLI:** ½ cup, steamed, with a spritz of lemon juice
TREAT	
5 CHIPS AHOY! COOKIES: Have these or another 220-calorie treat (see page 255 for more suggestions).	**5 CHIPS AHOY! COOKIES:** Have these or another 220-calorie treat (see page 255 for more suggestions).

1,800

BREAKFAST

WAFFLES: 2 whole grain toaster waffles (with about 170 calories and 4 grams fiber for 2 waffles) topped with 2 teaspoons trans-free margarine, ½ cup strawberries or other berries, and 1 teaspoon maple syrup

FAT-FREE MILK: 1 cup

LUNCH

VEGGIE CHEESEBURGER: Cook 1 vegetable burger (about 120 calories, such as a Gardenburger) according to package directions. Melt 1 slice reduced-fat cheese on top and place in 1 whole wheat hamburger bun with 2 teaspoons low-fat mayo, mustard, tomato slices, and lettuce.

RED PEPPER SLICES: 1 cup

LOW-FAT COTTAGE CHEESE: ½ cup

SNACK

MAPLE MILK: 1 cup hot or cold fat-free milk with 1 teaspoon maple syrup

WALNUTS: 2 tablespoons

RAISINS: 2 tablespoons

DINNER

FISH WITH OLIVES AND CAPERS: See recipe on page 393.

LEMON COUSCOUS: 1 cup (recipe on page 391)

> **TIP** If you can't find whole wheat couscous, have brown rice or whole wheat pasta.

BROCCOLI: 1 cup, steamed, with a spritz of lemon juice and 1 tablespoon Parmesan

TREAT

5 CHIPS AHOY! COOKIES: Have these or another 220-calorie treat (see page 255 for more suggestions).

Nutrition Tallies

	1,400	1,600	1,800
CALORIES	1,396	1,598	1,785
FAT (G)	33	48	53
SATURATED FAT (G)	6.7	8.9	11.2
PROTEIN (G)	77	80	100
CARBOHYDRATES (G)	215	231	250
DIETARY FIBER (G)	29	31	33
CHOLESTEROL (MG)	84	84	97
SODIUM (MG)	2,453	2,555	3,116
CALCIUM (MG)	1,264	1,289	1,457

CHAPTER 12

Savor Good Fats

How are you doing? By now, your habits are getting a lot healthier, and you've probably lost a little weight. Keep up the great work!

Do you want more energy . . . soft, supple skin . . . shiny, pretty hair? Then—believe it or not—you want some fat. Now, don't be afraid of fat, although it's no wonder if you are. For years, we've been given the low-fat, reduced-fat, and fat-free diet message. Thousands of fat-free and reduced-fat products flooded the market during the 1980s and 1990s, and what happened? Americans got even fatter! It's left many of us wondering if should we eat a low-fat diet or just chow down on burgers and steak every day.

Now that nutrition experts have had a few decades to ponder and research this message, it turns out that *moderately* low-fat diets are the key to successful weight loss and weight maintenance. If the diet's too low in fat—20 percent or less of calories from fat—people just can't hack it. Foods don't taste good. And if it's too high—much over 30 percent—it's very hard to keep calories in check because fat has more than twice the calories of carbohydrate and protein. (Also, if you're eating a lot of saturated fat, it sends blood cholesterol soaring and puts you in line for heart disease.)

What's ideal for weight loss? About 24 percent of calories from fat, according to the National Weight Loss Registry. This ongoing study tracks thousands of people who have kept off at least 30 pounds for 5 years or more. These "successful losers" average 23 to 24 percent of calories from fat. Another 19 to 20 percent of calories come from protein, and 56 percent from carbohydrates.

It's also okay to eat more fat—up to 30 percent of your total calories—if most of that fat comes from olive oil, nuts, and other foods rich in "good" fats. In fact, the traditional Mediterranean diet, which has kept people slim and with a very low risk of breast cancer and heart disease, is about 40 percent fat!

So, my plan averages about 25 percent fat. Because this is a real-life plan, your fat levels vary from day to day. One day, you'll eat more low-fat foods, so your fat will come to 20 percent of calories. Another day, you'll have peanut butter for lunch and a side of guacamole with your Mexican dinner, putting you at 28 percent fat. But rest assured that most of the fat on this plan is the type that doesn't raise cholesterol.

Good Fat Can Be Your Weight-Loss Friend

Good fat is the type found in olive oil, nuts, avocados, flaxseed, other plant foods, and fish. So how can it actually help you *lose* weight? The answer lies in using fat wisely. It's not about loading up on fast food and other fatty foods. (Sorry!) But if you eat good fat moderately, it will help you lose weight. Here's why.

- **Good fat helps slow your stomach from emptying.** This means you feel fuller, longer. So try to have some fat at each meal, even if it's just a few nuts.

- **Good fat entices you to eat your vegetables.** That 50 to 100 calories spent on salad dressing or on olive oil in your stir-fry is well-spent. Those veggies fill you up on relatively few calories.

> **WEEKLY CHECK-IN:** Now's the time to congratulate yourself for finishing another full week on the Shrink Your Female Fat Zones plan! Whether you're getting on the scale, trying on that pair of pants, or using the measuring tape, make a note of how your body changed this week. Write your results in your daily log (page 409).

- **Good fat allows for treats.** If the fat in your main meals is good, then there's room for little bits of saturated fat in ice cream, chips, chocolate, and other fatty treats. You need these foods—in moderation—to stave off deprivation. Deprivation is not what we're after here. It's not good for a healthy eating plan. It's what makes us drop out or, even worse, go through cycles of "being good" followed by bingeing. That's why I give you treats, so that you never feel deprived. Life is too short and food is too fabulous, with everything in moderation. I eat well 80 percent of the time and have my treats the other 20 percent.

A Little Fat Keeps the Doctor Away

There are certain fats that you should be eating *more* of to protect your health. Let's look at the good ones.

- **Fish oils.** These are the famous omega-3 fatty acids; the two types in fish are docosahexaenoic acid (DHA) and eicosapentaenoic acid (EPA). These fats have been linked to a lower risk of heart disease, less likelihood of having a second heart attack, alleviation of arthritis pain, smarter infants, and even the treatment and prevention of depression. Fattier fish like salmon, herring, lake trout, sturgeon, bluefish, anchovies, and sardines are highest in omega-3s. The American Heart Association now recommends that you eat fish twice a week. I do it, and I think you should—and can—too. So my menu plans reflect that.

  If you're pregnant or planning on getting pregnant, however, you shouldn't eat swordfish, tilefish, king mackerel, and shark. These fish accumulate high levels of methyl mercury, which can damage a fetus. Don't panic if you've been eating these fish; it takes a lot of fish to do damage. Just avoid them from now on.

- **Alpha-linolenic acid.** It's the plant form of omega-3, found in flaxseed and in canola and soybean oils. Like fish oils, this fat has also proven to be healthy for the heart.

Week 3 Daily Averages

1,400 CALORIES: 23% calories from fat, 23% protein, 54% carbohydrates
1,600 CALORIES: 24% calories from fat, 23% protein, 53% carbohydrates
1,800 CALORIES: 27% calories from fat, 21% protein, 52% carbohydrates

- **Monounsaturated fat.** It's found in olive oil, canola oil, nuts, and avocados—all foods regularly included in this 6-week plan. This fat is great for you; it's also linked to a healthier heart and reduced cancer risk.

  Note: High-poly/low-mono oils—such as safflower, sunflower, corn, and cottonseed oils—are high in polyunsaturated fats. While these fats are good for the heart, in high quantities they are linked to a slight increase in cancer risk. And they negate the effects of omega-3s.

Beware the Bad Fats

Here are the "bad fats," the ones I want you to stay away from. Well, a little is okay (and unavoidable), so do the best you can. Prevention is the key to good health. Just try to eat less of the following fats:

- **Saturated fat.** This is the artery-clogging fat found in fatty meats, chicken skin, whole milk, cream, regular cheese, and butter. While it's okay to have a little of this fat, too much raises blood cholesterol and promotes heart disease.

- **Trans fat.** This is found in the partially hydrogenated oils used in regular margarine and many processed foods. Trans fat may be even worse than saturated fat. While both types of fat raise blood levels of artery-clogging LDL cholesterol, only trans fat lowers levels of beneficial HDL cholesterol (which sweeps cholesterol out of the body). Fortunately, many margarine manufacturers have come out with trans-free margarines, the type recommended in this book. Also, see "Treat Yourself" on page 254, where you'll find cookies and snacks that don't use partially hydrogenated oils.

SHOPPING LIST

CHECK YOUR FRIDGE and cupboards. Much of this food might still be there from last week. And some of what you'll buy this week will carry over to the upcoming weeks. There are no portions listed, because these vary depending on how many people are in your family. So please go through the menu plan and note how much of everything you'll need.

If you don't like something, substitute with as close an equivalent as you can find. For instance, have strawberries instead of blueberries or mozzarella instead of Cheddar. But don't substitute white flour products (like white bread) when whole grain products (like whole wheat bread) are called for. Whole grains are important weight-loss tools.

FRESH FRUIT

Apples

Bananas

Blueberries (Don't buy if you're using strawberries for breakfast on Saturday.)

Cantaloupe

Lemons

Limes

Mangoes (for 1,600- and 1,800-calorie plans)

Oranges (for 1,600- and 1,800-calorie plans)

Peaches (If not in season, use those canned in juice or light syrup.)

Strawberries

FRESH VEGETABLES AND HERBS

Asparagus

Avocados, Haas

Basil

Broccoli (Don't buy if you're getting Chinese takeout for dinner on Friday.)

Carrots

Celery

Cilantro

Corn

Cucumbers

Dill

Garlic

Ginger (Don't buy if you're getting Chinese takeout for dinner on Friday.)

Greens, mixed, or spinach

Lettuce (You can use mixed greens instead.)

Mushrooms, portobello or other

Onions

Parsley

Peppers, green or red

Radishes

Scallions

Spinach (For convenience, buy bags of prewashed spinach.)

Tomatoes, cherry and regular

Zucchini

CANNED AND BOTTLED GOODS

Beans, black or pinto, canned, or all-bean chili, canned

Chickpeas, canned

Chutney

Honey

Hot-pepper sauce

Jam or jelly (for 1,800-calorie plan only)

Lemon juice

Mayonnaise, low-fat

Oil, canola

Oil, olive

Peanut butter

Pizza sauce (Don't get if you're buying a pizza for dinner on Saturday.)

Salad dressing, reduced-calorie Italian or vinaigrette

Salad dressing, regular Italian or vinaigrette (for 1,800-calorie plan only)

Salsa

Soup, lentil (such as Progresso)

Soy sauce, reduced-sodium (Don't buy if you're getting Chinese takeout for dinner on Friday.)

Syrup, chocolate

Syrup, maple or maple-flavored

Tuna, water-packed

Vinegar, preferably balsamic

Wine, dry white

DRY GOODS AND BREAD

Almonds

Bagels, whole wheat or oat bran (Don't buy if you're having breakfast at a deli on Sunday.)

Bread, whole wheat pita, 6-inch

Bread, whole wheat sandwich loaf, with no more than 90 calories and at least 2 grams of fiber per slice

Buns, whole wheat hamburger, with no more than 120 calories per bun

Cereal, high-fiber, with 5 to 8 grams of fiber and no more than 110 calories per 30-gram serving

Cereal, oatmeal (plain, unflavored)

Cinnamon

Cloves

Couscous, whole wheat (found in bulk in natural food stores and in boxes, such as Fantastic Foods)

Crackers, graham

Crackers, whole grain (such as Ak-Mak)

Curry powder

Flour, all-purpose

Herbs, mixed Italian (Don't buy if you're using fresh herbs for Monday night's chicken.)

Pasta, whole wheat noodles or short tubular type

Peppercorns

Pizza crust, Boboli Original, with about 1,100 calories for the whole crust (Don't buy if you're getting pizza delivered or buying a frozen one for dinner on Saturday.)

Raisins

Rice, brown (such as Texmati, basmati, or quick-cooking Uncle Ben's)

Walnuts (for 1,600- and 1,800-calorie plans)

REFRIGERATED FOODS

Butter or trans-free margarine

Cheese, Parmesan

Cheese, part-skim mozzarella (Don't get if you're buying a pizza for dinner on Saturday.)

Cheese, reduced-fat (such as Cabot 50% Light Cheddar, Tine 75% Jarlsberg, Kraft or Borden 2% Singles)

Cottage cheese, 1% or 2%

Cream cheese, reduced-fat (Don't buy if you're having breakfast at a deli on Sunday.)

Eggs or egg substitute (such as Egg Beaters)

Hummus

Milk, fat-free (If you haven't adjusted to fat-free milk, buy 1% or mix equal parts 1% and 2%. Your calorie level will be a little higher, but you can gradually train your tastebuds to like fat-free. If you're lactose intolerant, try Lactaid milk. If you prefer soy milk—low-fat or fat-free—buy calcium-fortified with at least 25% of the Daily Value of calcium per cup.)

Sour cream, reduced-fat

Tortillas, flour (preferably whole wheat), 8-inch diameter

Yogurt, low-fat fruit, with about 210 calories per 8 ounces (for 1,800-calorie plan only)

Yogurt, low-fat plain

Yogurt, reduced-calorie, flavored, with no more than 120 calories per 8 ounces

MEAT, POULTRY, AND FISH

Chicken, boneless and skinless breasts

Salmon, fillets

Salmon, smoked (Don't buy if you're having breakfast at a deli on Sunday.)

Shrimp (Don't buy if you're getting Chinese takeout for dinner on Friday.)

Turkey, sliced breast

FROZEN FOODS

Ice cream or frozen yogurt, light, with no more than 110 calories per ½ cup (such as Breyers, Edy's, or Dreyer's)

Pizza, vegetarian (Don't buy if you're having pizza delivered on Saturday or if you're making your own.)

OPTIONAL

Beer, light

Treats (see Monday, Tuesday, Thursday, Friday, Saturday, and Sunday)

Wine

MONDAY

1,400	1,600

BREAKFAST

CEREAL: 150 calories of high-fiber cereal topped with 1 cup fat-free milk, 10 almonds, and ½ medium banana

TIP Check label for 5 to 8 grams of fiber per 30-gram serving.

CEREAL: 150 calories of high-fiber cereal topped with 1 cup fat-free milk, 10 almonds, 1 tablespoon raisins, and 1 medium banana

TIP Check label for 5 to 8 grams of fiber per 30-gram serving.

LUNCH

BEAN BURRITO WITH AVOCADO: Top a warmed 8-inch tortilla (preferably whole wheat) with ½ cup canned pinto or black beans or all-bean chili. Add ¼ chopped Haas (dark-skinned) avocado, 2 tablespoons salsa, 2 tablespoons shredded reduced-fat cheese, and cilantro.

CARROT AND CELERY STICKS: 1 cup

BEAN BURRITO WITH AVOCADO: Top a warmed 8-inch tortilla (preferably whole wheat) with ½ cup canned pinto or black beans or all-bean chili. Add ½ chopped Haas (dark-skinned) avocado, 2 tablespoons salsa, 2 tablespoons shredded reduced-fat cheese, and cilantro.

CARROT AND CELERY STICKS: 1 cup

SNACK

BANANA: ½ medium-size

FAT-FREE MILK: 1 cup

1 SLICED PEACH OR OTHER FRUIT

FAT-FREE MILK: 1 cup

DINNER

OVEN-BAKED CHICKEN: See recipe on page 394.

AVOCADO, TOMATO, AND CORN SALAD: Combine ¼ chopped Haas avocado, ½ cup cherry tomatoes, and ½ cup fresh, frozen, or low-sodium canned corn, and then toss with juice of ½ lime.

OVEN-BAKED CHICKEN: See recipe on page 394.

AVOCADO, TOMATO, AND CORN SALAD: Combine ¼ chopped Haas avocado, ½ cup cherry tomatoes, and ½ cup fresh, frozen, or low-sodium canned corn, and then toss with juice of ½ lime.

TREAT

1 CREAMSICLE: Have this or another 70- to 75-calorie treat (see page 254 for more suggestions).

1 CREAMSICLE: Have this or another 70- to 75-calorie treat (see page 254 for more suggestions).

BREAKFAST

CEREAL: 150 calories of high-fiber cereal topped with 1 cup fat-free milk, 10 almonds, 1 tablespoon raisins, and 1 medium banana

> **TIP** Check label for 5 to 8 grams of fiber per 30-gram serving.

LUNCH

BEAN BURRITO WITH AVOCADO: Top a warmed 8-inch tortilla (preferably whole wheat) with ½ cup canned pinto or black beans or all-bean chili. Add ½ chopped Haas (dark-skinned) avocado, 2 tablespoons salsa, 2 tablespoons shredded reduced-fat cheese, and cilantro.

CARROT AND CELERY STICKS: 1 cup

SNACK

1 SLICED PEACH OR OTHER FRUIT

LOW-FAT FRUIT YOGURT: 1 cup

DINNER

OVEN-BAKED CHICKEN: See recipe on page 394.

AVOCADO, TOMATO, AND CORN SALAD: Combine ½ chopped Haas avocado, ½ cup cherry tomatoes, and ½ cup fresh, frozen, or low-sodium canned corn, and then toss with juice of ½ lime.

TREAT

1 CREAMSICLE: Have this or another 70- to 75-calorie treat (see page 254 for more suggestions).

Nutrition Tallies

	1,400	1,600	1,800
CALORIES	1,415	1,560	1,796
FAT (G)	40	48	58
SATURATED FAT (G)	8	9.1	12
PROTEIN (G)	85	87	91
CARBOHYDRATES (G)	200	221	252
DIETARY FIBER (G)	35	39	41
CHOLESTEROL (MG)	111	111	121
SODIUM (MG)	1,920	1,926	1,976
CALCIUM (MG)	1,026	1,040	1,095

Nutrient Booster!

ISN'T IT FANTASTIC when something that tastes so good is also good for you? That's what you get with avocados. Sure, they're full of fat, but it's the good kind: heart-healthy monounsaturated fat. They're also rich in phytosterols, which lower cholesterol. Further, avocados are an excellent source of yet another heart helper: the B vitamin folate, which helps keep down levels of homocysteine, a substance that increases heart disease risk. Folate also helps prevent birth defects.

TUESDAY

1,400	1,600

BREAKFAST

MELON SMOOTHIE: In a blender, process until smooth 1 cup cantaloupe slices, ½ cup fat-free milk, ½ cup low-fat plain yogurt, 2 teaspoons honey, and 1 or 2 ice cubes.

WHOLE WHEAT TOAST: 1 slice spread with 1 teaspoon peanut butter

MELON SMOOTHIE: In a blender, process until smooth 1 cup cantaloupe slices, ½ cup fat-free milk, ½ cup low-fat plain yogurt, 2 teaspoons honey, and 1 or 2 ice cubes.

WHOLE WHEAT TOAST: 2 slices spread with 2 teaspoons peanut butter

LUNCH

LENTIL SOUP: 1½ cups

5 AK-MAK CRACKERS: Have these or 115 calories' worth of another whole grain cracker.

TOMATO SLICES: 1 cup, tossed with 1 tablespoon chopped parsley and 1 tablespoon reduced-calorie dressing

LOW-FAT COTTAGE CHEESE: ½ cup

LENTIL SOUP: 1½ cups

5 AK-MAK CRACKERS: Have these or 115 calories' worth of another whole grain cracker.

TOMATO SLICES: 1 cup, tossed with 1 tablespoon chopped parsley and 1 tablespoon reduced-calorie dressing

LOW-FAT COTTAGE CHEESE: ½ cup

SNACK

DECAF LATTE: 12 ounces with 1 teaspoon sugar or 1 pump of flavored syrup

GRAHAM CRACKERS: 1 rectangle

DECAF LATTE: 12 ounces with 1 teaspoon sugar or 1 pump of flavored syrup

GRAHAM CRACKERS: 1 rectangle

DINNER

POACHED SALMON WITH HERB SAUCE: See recipe on page 395.

SAUTÉED SPINACH: See recipe on page 394.

WHOLE WHEAT COUSCOUS: ½ cup, cooked

POACHED SALMON WITH HERB SAUCE: See recipe on page 395.

SAUTÉED SPINACH: See recipe on page 394.

WHOLE WHEAT COUSCOUS: 1 cup, cooked

TREAT

1 WHOLE-FRUIT FROZEN FRUIT BAR: Have this or another 80-calorie treat, such as 4 ounces wine (see page 254 for more suggestions).

1 WHOLE-FRUIT FROZEN FRUIT BAR: Have this or another 80-calorie treat, such as 4 ounces wine (see page 254 for more suggestions).

BREAKFAST

MELON SMOOTHIE: In a blender, process until smooth 1 cup cantaloupe slices, ½ cup fat-free milk, ½ cup low-fat plain yogurt, 2 teaspoons honey, and 1 or 2 ice cubes.

WHOLE WHEAT TOAST: 2 slices spread with 2 teaspoons peanut butter

LUNCH

LENTIL SOUP: 1½ cups

5 AK-MAK CRACKERS: Have these or 115 calories' worth of another whole grain cracker.

TOMATO SLICES: 1 cup, tossed with 1 tablespoon chopped parsley and 1 tablespoon reduced-calorie dressing

LOW-FAT COTTAGE CHEESE: ½ cup

SNACK

DECAF LATTE: 12 ounces with 1 teaspoon sugar or 1 pump of flavored syrup

GRAHAM CRACKERS: 1 rectangle

ALMONDS: 2 tablespoons

DINNER

POACHED SALMON WITH HERB SAUCE: See recipe on page 395.

SAUTÉED SPINACH: See recipe on page 394.

WHOLE WHEAT COUSCOUS: 1 cup, cooked

TREAT

1 STARBUCKS FROZEN COFFEE BAR: Have this or another 125-calorie treat, such as 6 ounces wine (see page 255 for suggestions).

Nutrition Tallies

	1,400	1,600	1,800
CALORIES	1,392	1,609	1,770
FAT (G)	35	40	50
SATURATED FAT (G)	8.4	9.3	10.1
PROTEIN (G)	85	94	98
CARBOHYDRATES (G)	171	209	214
DIETARY FIBER (G)	24	30	32
CHOLESTEROL (MG)	91	91	91
SODIUM (MG)	1,940	2,136	2,141
CALCIUM (MG)	987	1,031	1,089

WEDNESDAY

1,400	1,600
BREAKFAST	
CINNAMON OATMEAL: Cook ½ cup rolled oats according to package directions, adding 1 small diced apple and a dash of cinnamon. **FAT-FREE MILK:** 1 cup	**CINNAMON OATMEAL:** Cook ½ cup rolled oats according to package directions, adding 1 small diced apple and a dash of cinnamon. **FAT-FREE MILK:** 1 cup **ALMONDS OR WALNUTS:** 2 tablespoons
LUNCH	
HUMMUS AND PITA SANDWICH: In a 6-inch whole wheat pita, layer ¼ cup hummus, ¼ cup tomatoes, 1 slice reduced-fat cheese, and ⅛ cup cucumber slices. **CUCUMBER:** Remaining portion, sliced and lightly salted	**HUMMUS AND PITA SANDWICH:** In a 6-inch whole wheat pita, layer ¼ cup hummus, ¼ cup tomatoes, 1 slice reduced-fat cheese, and ⅛ cup cucumber slices. **CUCUMBER:** Remaining portion, sliced and lightly salted
SNACK	
YOGURT: 8 ounces reduced-calorie flavored yogurt with no more than 120 calories	**YOGURT:** 8 ounces reduced-calorie flavored yogurt with no more than 120 calories
DINNER	
SALMON BURGER: See recipe on page 396. Place burger on whole wheat bun and season with lemon juice and Herb Sauce (recipe on page 395). Add tomato slices and lettuce. **TOMATO AND GREEN PEPPER SALAD:** Toss together ½ cup chopped tomato, ½ cup chopped green pepper, 1 chopped scallion, 1 tablespoon chopped parsley or basil, ½ teaspoon olive oil, ¼ teaspoon vinegar (preferably balsamic), and a few drops of lemon juice.	**SALMON BURGER:** See recipe on page 396. Place burger on whole wheat bun and season with lemon juice and Herb Sauce (recipe on page 395). Add tomato slices and lettuce. **TOMATO AND GREEN PEPPER SALAD:** Toss together ½ cup chopped tomato, ½ cup chopped green pepper, 1 chopped scallion, 1 tablespoon chopped parsley or basil, ½ teaspoon olive oil, ¼ teaspoon vinegar (preferably balsamic), and a few drops of lemon juice.
TREAT	
LIGHT ICE CREAM OR FROZEN YOGURT: ½ cup, topped with 2 teaspoons chocolate syrup and ½ cup strawberries	**LIGHT ICE CREAM OR FROZEN YOGURT:** ¾ cup, topped with 2 teaspoons chocolate syrup and ½ cup strawberries

BREAKFAST

CINNAMON OATMEAL: Cook ½ cup rolled oats according to package directions, adding 1 small diced apple and a dash of cinnamon.

FAT-FREE MILK: 1 cup

ALMONDS OR WALNUTS: 2 tablespoons

LUNCH

HUMMUS AND PITA SANDWICH: In a 6-inch whole wheat pita, layer ½ cup hummus, ¼ cup tomatoes, 1 slice reduced-fat cheese, and ⅛ cup cucumber slices.

CUCUMBER: Remaining portion, sliced and lightly salted

SNACK

YOGURT: 8 ounces low-fat fruit yogurt with no more than 210 calories

DINNER

SALMON BURGER: See recipe on page 396. Place burger on whole wheat bun and season with lemon juice and Herb Sauce (recipe on page 395). Add tomato slices and lettuce.

TOMATO AND GREEN PEPPER SALAD: Toss together ½ cup chopped tomato, ½ cup chopped green pepper, 1 chopped scallion, 1 tablespoon chopped parsley or basil, ½ teaspoon olive oil, ¼ teaspoon vinegar (preferably balsamic), and a few drops of lemon juice.

TREAT

LIGHT ICE CREAM OR FROZEN YOGURT: ¾ cup, topped with 2 teaspoons chocolate syrup and ½ cup strawberries

Nutrition Tallies

	1,400	1,600	1,800
CALORIES	1,404	1,648	1,808
FAT (G)	41	59	65
SATURATED FAT (G)	10.7	13.7	14.7
PROTEIN (G)	79	87	92
CARBOHYDRATES (G)	193	208	232
DIETARY FIBER (G)	24	28	30
CHOLESTEROL (MG)	206	216	223
SODIUM (MG)	1,510	1,570	1,741
CALCIUM (MG)	1,047	1,161	1,228

Nutrient Booster!

THAT HUMMUS YOU HAD FOR LUNCH gets its creamy taste from tahini, a paste made from ground sesame seeds. Tahini is loaded with nutrition. Just 1 tablespoon has 1½ grams of fiber and 12 percent of your daily calcium needs. Plus, it has flavor compounds that fight heart disease and cancer.

THURSDAY

1,400	1,600
BREAKFAST	
SALSA OMELET: Cook 1 egg and 1 egg white in a nonstick skillet with ½ teaspoon olive oil or canola oil. Fill with 2 tablespoons salsa.	**SALSA OMELET:** Cook 1 egg and 1 egg white in a nonstick skillet with ½ teaspoon olive oil or canola oil. Fill with 2 tablespoons salsa.
WHOLE WHEAT BREAD: 1 slice	**WHOLE WHEAT BREAD:** 1 slice
FAT-FREE MILK: 1 cup	**FAT-FREE MILK:** 1 cup
FRUIT SALAD: 1 cup (your choice of fruit)	**FRUIT SALAD:** 1½ cups (your choice of fruit)
LUNCH	
GRILLED CHICKEN SANDWICH: Try Wendy's Grilled Chicken, McDonald's Chicken McGrill, or KFC Honey BBQ—all without mayo. **TIP** Skip Burger King and Arby's; they're too high in calories. Dress bun with ketchup, mustard, lettuce, and tomato.	**GRILLED CHICKEN SANDWICH:** Try Wendy's Grilled Chicken, McDonald's Chicken McGrill, or KFC Honey BBQ—all without mayo. **TIP** Skip Burger King and Arby's; they're too high in calories. Dress bun with ketchup, mustard, lettuce, and tomato.
SIDE SALAD: Drizzle 1 tablespoon low-fat dressing (about ⅓ of most packets) over salad.	**SIDE SALAD:** Drizzle 1 tablespoon low-fat dressing (about ⅓ of most packets) over salad.
SNACK	
FAT-FREE MILK: 1 cup	**FAT-FREE MILK:** 1 cup
GRAHAM CRACKERS: 1 rectangle	**GRAHAM CRACKERS:** 2 rectangles, each spread with ½ tablespoon peanut butter
DINNER	
PASTA PRIMAVERA: See recipe on page 397.	**PASTA PRIMAVERA:** See recipe on page 397.
TREAT	
LIGHT ICE CREAM OR FROZEN YOGURT: ⅔ cup, or another 150-calorie treat (see page 255 for more suggestions)	**LIGHT ICE CREAM OR FROZEN YOGURT:** ⅔ cup, or another 150-calorie treat (see page 255 for more suggestions)

BREAKFAST

SALSA OMELET: Cook 1 egg and 1 egg white in a nonstick skillet with ½ teaspoon olive oil or canola oil. Fill with 2 tablespoons salsa.

WHOLE WHEAT BREAD: 2 slices, each spread with 1 teaspoon trans-free margarine and 1 teaspoon jam or jelly

FAT-FREE MILK: 1 cup

FRUIT SALAD: 1½ cups (your choice of fruit)

LUNCH

GRILLED CHICKEN SANDWICH: Try Wendy's Grilled Chicken, McDonald's Chicken McGrill, or KFC Honey BBQ—all without mayo.

TIP Skip Burger King and Arby's; they're too high in calories. Dress bun with ketchup, mustard, lettuce, and tomato.

SIDE SALAD: Drizzle 1 tablespoon low-fat dressing (about ⅓ of most packets) over salad.

1 ORANGE

SNACK

FAT-FREE MILK: 1 cup

GRAHAM CRACKERS: 2 rectangles, each spread with ½ tablespoon peanut butter

DINNER

PASTA PRIMAVERA: See recipe on page 397.

TREAT

LIGHT ICE CREAM OR FROZEN YOGURT: ⅔ cup, or another 150-calorie treat (see page 255 for more suggestions)

Nutrition Tallies

	1,400	1,600	1,800
CALORIES	1,394	1,580	1,818
FAT (G)	40	49	58
SATURATED FAT (G)	9.3	11.1	12.6
PROTEIN (G)	90	95	100
CARBOHYDRATES (G)	181	203	241
DIETARY FIBER (G)	24	26	32
CHOLESTEROL (MG)	317	317	317
SODIUM (MG)	2,085	2,251	2,485
CALCIUM (MG)	1,003	1,019	1,110

FRIDAY

1,400	1,600

BREAKFAST

CEREAL: 150 calories of high-fiber cereal topped with 1 cup fat-free milk and 1 tablespoon almonds

TIP Check label for 5 to 8 grams of fiber per 30-gram serving.

CANTALOUPE OR OTHER FRUIT: 1 cup

CEREAL: 150 calories of high-fiber cereal topped with 1 cup fat-free milk, 1 tablespoon almonds, and 1 tablespoon raisins

TIP Check label for 5 to 8 grams of fiber per 30-gram serving.

CANTALOUPE OR OTHER FRUIT: 1 cup

LUNCH

HEARTY SALAD: At home or at the salad bar, have 1 cup mixed greens or spinach, 1½ cups chopped vegetables (such as green or red pepper, tomato, carrot), and ½ cup canned chickpeas, with 2 tablespoons reduced-calorie dressing.

LOW-FAT COTTAGE CHEESE: ½ cup

1 SMALL ROLL: Have this or 1 slice bread (preferably whole wheat).

HEARTY SALAD: At home or at the salad bar, have 1 cup mixed greens or spinach, 1½ cups chopped vegetables (such as green or red pepper, tomato, carrot), and ½ cup canned chickpeas, with 2 tablespoons reduced-calorie dressing.

LOW-FAT COTTAGE CHEESE: ½ cup

WATER-PACKED TUNA: ½ cup

1 SMALL ROLL: Have this or 1 slice bread (preferably whole wheat).

SNACK

CHOCOLATE MILK: 1 cup fat-free milk with 2 teaspoons chocolate syrup

CHOCOLATE MILK: 1 cup fat-free milk with 2 teaspoons chocolate syrup

DINNER

BROCCOLI AND CHICKEN OR BROCCOLI AND SHRIMP STIR-FRY: For takeout Chinese, have 1½ cups broccoli and chicken or broccoli and shrimp stir-fry with ½ cup cooked rice. Ask for less oil plus brown rice. At home, make your own by substituting chicken or shrimp for the beef in Beef and Broccoli Stir-Fry (recipe on page 387). Serve with 1 cup brown rice.

BROCCOLI AND CHICKEN OR BROCCOLI AND SHRIMP STIR-FRY: For takeout Chinese, have 1½ cups broccoli and chicken or broccoli and shrimp stir-fry with ¾ cup cooked rice. Ask for less oil plus brown rice. At home, make your own by substituting chicken or shrimp for the beef in Beef and Broccoli Stir-Fry (recipe on page 387). Serve with 1½ cups brown rice.

TREAT

1 FROZEN FRUIT BAR: Have this or another 80-calorie treat (see page 254 for suggestions).

1 FROZEN FRUIT BAR: Have this or another 80-calorie treat (see page 254 for suggestions).

BREAKFAST

CEREAL: 150 calories of high-fiber cereal topped with 1 cup fat-free milk, 1 tablespoon almonds, and 1 tablespoon raisins

TIP Check label for 5 to 8 grams of fiber per 30-gram serving.

CANTALOUPE OR OTHER FRUIT: 1 cup

LUNCH

HEARTY SALAD: At home or at the salad bar, have 1 cup mixed greens or spinach, 1½ cups chopped vegetables (such as green or red pepper, tomato, carrot), and ½ cup canned chickpeas, with 2 tablespoons reduced-calorie dressing.

LOW-FAT COTTAGE CHEESE: ½ cup

WATER-PACKED TUNA: ½ cup

1 SMALL ROLL: Have this or 1 slice bread (preferably whole wheat).

SNACK

CHOCOLATE MILK: 1 cup fat-free milk with 2 teaspoons chocolate syrup

2 AK-MAK CRACKERS: Have these or 45 calories' worth of another whole grain cracker. Spread each cracker with 1 teaspoon peanut butter.

DINNER

BROCCOLI AND CHICKEN OR BROCCOLI AND SHRIMP STIR-FRY: For takeout Chinese, have 1½ cups broccoli and chicken or broccoli and shrimp stir-fry with 1 cup cooked rice. Ask for less oil plus brown rice. At home, make your own by substituting chicken or shrimp for the beef in Beef and Broccoli Stir-Fry (recipe on page 387). Serve with 2 cups brown rice.

TREAT

1 FROZEN FRUIT BAR: Have this or another 80-calorie treat (see page 254 for suggestions).

Nutrition Tallies

	1,400	1,600	1,800
CALORIES	1,423	1,582	1,752
FAT (G)	33	34	40
SATURATED FAT (G)	6.3	6.9	8.1
PROTEIN (G)	84	106	111
CARBOHYDRATES (G)	213	228	251
DIETARY FIBER (G)	28	28	29
CHOLESTEROL (MG)	129	155	155
SODIUM (MG)	3,055	3,315	3,319
CALCIUM (MG)	951	966	971

SATURDAY

1,400	1,600
BREAKFAST	
FRENCH TOAST AND BERRIES: Dip 2 slices whole wheat bread in ⅓ cup egg substitute (or 2 egg whites mixed with 2 tablespoons fat-free milk), then brown in a nonstick skillet with 1 teaspoon canola oil. Top each slice with 1 teaspoon maple syrup and ½ cup blueberries or strawberries.	**FRENCH TOAST AND BERRIES:** Dip 2 slices whole wheat bread in ⅓ cup egg substitute (or 2 egg whites mixed with 2 tablespoons fat-free milk), then brown in a nonstick skillet with 1 teaspoon canola oil. Top each slice with 1 teaspoon maple syrup and ½ cup blueberries or strawberries.
FAT-FREE MILK: 1 cup	**FAT-FREE MILK:** 1 cup
LUNCH	
CURRIED TUNA SALAD: Combine 3 ounces water-packed tuna, 2 tablespoons finely chopped carrot or celery, 2 teaspoons low-fat mayo, 2 teaspoons almonds, 1 teaspoon raisins, and ½ teaspoon curry powder.	**CURRIED TUNA SALAD:** Combine 3 ounces water-packed tuna, 2 tablespoons finely chopped carrot or celery, 2 teaspoons low-fat mayo, 2 teaspoons almonds, 1 teaspoon raisins, and ½ teaspoon curry powder.
CARROT AND CELERY STICKS: 1 cup	**CARROT AND CELERY STICKS:** 1 cup
4 AK-MAK CRACKERS: Have these or 95 calories' worth of another whole grain cracker.	**4 AK-MAK CRACKERS:** Have these or 95 calories' worth of another whole grain cracker.
	1 MANGO: Choose this, 2 oranges, or other piece of fruit.
SNACK	
YOGURT: 8 ounces reduced-calorie flavored yogurt with no more than 120 calories	**YOGURT:** 8 ounces reduced-calorie flavored yogurt with no more than 120 calories
	WALNUTS OR OTHER NUTS: 1 tablespoon
DINNER	
VEGETABLE PIZZA: Quick Veggie Pizza (recipe on page 388), 2 slices of a large pizza topped with vegetables but not meat (2 of 8 slices of a 14-inch pizza, such as Domino's Hand-Tossed), or 525 calories' worth of frozen pizza	**VEGETABLE PIZZA:** Quick Veggie Pizza (recipe on page 388), 2 slices of a large pizza topped with vegetables but not meat (2 of 8 slices of a 14-inch pizza, such as Domino's Hand-Tossed), or 525 calories' worth of frozen pizza
MIXED GREENS: 2 cups, tossed with 1 tablespoon reduced-calorie dressing	**MIXED GREENS:** 2 cups, tossed with 1 tablespoon reduced-calorie dressing
TREAT	
PRETZELS: 1 ounce, or another 100-calorie treat, such as 12 ounces light beer (see page 254 for more suggestions)	**PRETZELS:** 1 ounce, or another 100-calorie treat, such as 12 ounces light beer (see page 254 for more suggestions)

1,800

BREAKFAST

FRENCH TOAST AND BERRIES: Dip 2 slices whole wheat bread in ⅓ cup egg substitute (or 2 egg whites mixed with 2 tablespoons fat-free milk), then brown in a nonstick skillet with 1 teaspoon canola oil. Top each slice with 1 teaspoon maple syrup and ½ cup blueberries or strawberries.

FAT-FREE MILK: 1 cup

LUNCH

CURRIED TUNA SALAD: Combine 3 ounces water-packed tuna, 2 tablespoons finely chopped carrot or celery, 2 teaspoons low-fat mayo, 2 teaspoons almonds, 1 teaspoon raisins, and ½ teaspoon curry powder.

CARROT AND CELERY STICKS: 1 cup

6 AK-MAK CRACKERS: Have these or 140 calories' worth of another whole grain cracker.

1 MANGO: Choose this, 2 oranges, or other piece of fruit.

SNACK

YOGURT: 8 ounces low-fat fruit yogurt with no more than 210 calories

DINNER

VEGETABLE PIZZA: Quick Veggie Pizza (recipe on page 388), 2 slices of a large pizza topped with vegetables but not meat (2 of 8 slices of a 14-inch pizza, such as Domino's Hand-Tossed), or 525 calories' worth of frozen pizza

MIXED GREENS: 2 cups, tossed with 1 tablespoon regular dressing

TREAT

PRETZELS: 1 ounce, or another 100-calorie treat, such as 12 ounces light beer (see page 254 for more suggestions)

Nutrition Tallies

	1,400	1,600	1,800
CALORIES	1,432	1,608	1,812
FAT (G)	28	33	43
SATURATED FAT (G)	8.9	9.4	11.6
PROTEIN (G)	82	84	87
CARBOHYDRATES (G)	201	238	264
DIETARY FIBER (G)	21	25	27
CHOLESTEROL (MG)	66	66	73
SODIUM (MG)	2,222	2,226	2,348
CALCIUM (MG)	1,047	1,074	1,125

Nutrient Booster!

THAT CURRY IN YOUR TUNA SALAD is giving you more than just flavor. It's also dousing you with curcumin, the pigment that makes turmeric—curry's main ingredient—yellow. Curcumin is a powerful cancer fighter and is thought to contribute to the low cancer rates in India, where curry is a staple.

SUNDAY

1,400	1,600

BREAKFAST

BAGEL: ½ large (3½- to 4-ounce) oat bran or whole wheat bagel with 1 tablespoon reduced-fat cream cheese and 1½ ounces (1½ strips) smoked salmon

FAT-FREE MILK: 1 cup

FRUIT SALAD: 1 cup (your choice of fruit)

BAGEL: ½ large (3½- to 4-ounce) oat bran or whole wheat bagel with 2 tablespoons reduced-fat cream cheese and 1½ ounces (1½ strips) smoked salmon

FAT-FREE MILK: 1 cup

FRUIT SALAD: 1 cup (your choice of fruit)

LUNCH

TURKEY AND CHUTNEY ROLL-UP: On an 8-inch whole wheat tortilla, spread 2 tablespoons chutney, then add 2 slices turkey, 1 slice reduced-fat Cheddar, and lettuce. Roll up.

FRESH VEGETABLES: 1 cup, sliced, such as radishes or red pepper

TURKEY AND CHUTNEY ROLL-UP: On an 8-inch whole wheat tortilla, spread 2 tablespoons chutney, then add 2 slices turkey, 1 slice reduced-fat Cheddar, and lettuce. Roll up.

FRESH VEGETABLES: 1 cup, sliced, such as radishes or red pepper

SNACK

MINI PEACH SMOOTHIE: In a blender, process until smooth 1 peach (or 4 ounces peaches canned in juice), ¼ cup fat-free milk, ½ cup low-fat plain yogurt, 2 teaspoons honey, and 1 or 2 ice cubes.

MINI PEACH SMOOTHIE: In a blender, process until smooth 1 peach (or 4 ounces peaches canned in juice), ¼ cup fat-free milk, ½ cup low-fat plain yogurt, 2 teaspoons honey, and 1 or 2 ice cubes.

DINNER

SOUTHWESTERN SALAD: Combine ½ cup rinsed and drained canned black beans; ½ cup fresh, frozen, or low-sodium canned corn; and ½ cup cooked brown rice. Toss with salsa to taste, ½ chopped Haas avocado, and 1 tablespoon chopped cilantro.

SOUTHWESTERN SALAD: Combine ½ cup rinsed and drained canned black beans; ½ cup fresh, frozen, or low-sodium canned corn; and ½ cup cooked brown rice. Toss with salsa to taste, ½ chopped Haas avocado, and 1 tablespoon chopped cilantro.

TREAT

STRAWBERRIES DIPPED IN CHOCOLATE: Dip the tips of ½ cup strawberries in 2 teaspoons chocolate syrup.

STRAWBERRIES DIPPED IN CHOCOLATE: Dip the tips of ½ cup strawberries in 2 teaspoons chocolate syrup.

BREAKFAST

BAGEL: 1 large (3½- to 4-ounce) oat bran or whole wheat bagel with 2 tablespoons reduced-fat cream cheese and 2 ounces (2 strips) smoked salmon

FAT-FREE MILK: 1 cup

FRUIT SALAD: 1 cup (your choice of fruit)

LUNCH

TURKEY AND CHUTNEY ROLL-UP: On an 8-inch whole wheat tortilla, spread 2 tablespoons chutney and 1 teaspoon low-fat mayo, then add 2 slices turkey, 1 slice reduced-fat Cheddar, and lettuce. Roll up.

FRESH VEGETABLES: 1 cup, sliced, such as radishes or red pepper

SNACK

MINI PEACH SMOOTHIE: In a blender, process until smooth 1 peach (or 4 ounces peaches canned in juice), ¼ cup fat-free milk, ½ cup low-fat plain yogurt, 2 teaspoons honey, and 1 or 2 ice cubes.

DINNER

SOUTHWESTERN SALAD: Combine ½ cup rinsed and drained canned black beans; ½ cup fresh, frozen, or low-sodium canned corn; and ½ cup cooked brown rice. Toss with salsa to taste, ½ chopped Haas avocado, and 1 tablespoon chopped cilantro.

LOW-FAT COTTAGE CHEESE: ½ cup

TREAT

STRAWBERRIES DIPPED IN CHOCOLATE: Dip the tips of ½ cup strawberries in 2 teaspoons chocolate syrup.

2 PEPPERIDGE FARM BORDEAUX COOKIES: Have these or another 70-calorie treat (see page 254 for more suggestions).

Nutrition Tallies

	1,400	1,600	1,800
CALORIES	1,442	1,584	1,823
FAT (G)	36	45	48
SATURATED FAT (G)	11.2	15.6	17.1
PROTEIN (G)	74	77	104
CARBOHYDRATES (G)	225	239	264
DIETARY FIBER (G)	28	29	32
CHOLESTEROL (MG)	76	97	133
SODIUM (MG)	3,467	3,567	4,263
CALCIUM (MG)	998	1,021	1,090

Fat Buster!

Instead of slathering your bagel with cream cheese and adding a little lox, reverse that! Ounce for ounce, lox has one-third the calories of cream cheese. And instead of the artery-clogging saturated fat in cream cheese, lox is loaded with heart-healthy omega-3 fatty acids.

CHAPTER 13

THE SHRINK YOUR FEMALE FAT ZONES DIET
WEEK 4

Fill Up on Fruits and Vegetables

Can you believe you've been on the plan for almost a month? I'll bet you look great—and feel even better—already! You're almost there. I'm proud of you; keep it up!

I hope you've been enjoying all the fruits and vegetables on this plan, because they're doing *amazing* things for your body! When you get a bunch of fruits and vegetables under your belt, there's less room for fattening foods.

Just as important as their slimming effects is the proven disease-fighting ability of fruits and vegetables. In hundreds of research studies, people who eat the most fruits and vegetables have the lowest rates of cancer, heart disease, and other illnesses. I try to eat something citrus every day to keep healthy; citrus contains lots of vitamin C to fight colds. I have an orange, half a grapefruit, or a squeeze of lemon or lime in my water. It's refreshing, too.

Fruits and vegetables safeguard your health in literally thousands of ways! They have thousands of beneficial compounds—some familiar, like vitamin C and magnesium. Others have more exotic names like sulforaphane and zeaxanthin. Scientists call them phytochemicals or phytonutrients. In the same way these compounds protect plants from disease-causing substances or the sun's damaging rays, they also protect us. The "Nutrient Booster!" boxes sprin-

318

1,400 CALORIES: 27% calories from fat, 21% protein, 52% carbohydrates
1,600 CALORIES: 27% calories from fat, 21% protein, 52% carbohydrates
1,800 CALORIES: 28% calories from fat, 20% protein, 52% carbohydrates

kled throughout this 6-week eating plan describe how tomatoes, spinach, blueberries, and other fruits and vegetables boost your health.

Major health organizations like the National Cancer Institute, the Centers for Disease Control and Prevention, and others want you to reap the health benefits of fruits and vegetables. That's why they've been pushing the "five-a-day" message. Actually, five daily fruits and vegetables are just a starting point for good health. I try to encourage people to eat even more.

It's Easier Than You Think

I used to think it would be impossible to get five servings a day until I started to *really* try. And now I can actually get in seven a day, and you can, too. Over these 6 weeks, five a day is your minimum. On most days, it's seven—and sometimes we've squeezed in even more.

Sounds like a lot, but as you've probably noticed, it's not so hard to rack 'em up. In this plan, they're often the main ingredients in your meal. A smoothie: two easy fruit servings. Chicken Caesar salad: two to four vegetable servings down the hatch! I'm going to teach you how easy it is to eat your fruits and veggies every day and truly enjoy them. They are the key to losing weight, feeling great, and improving your health.

> **WEEKLY CHECK-IN:** Now's the time to congratulate yourself for finishing another full week on the Shrink Your Female Fat Zones plan! Whether you're getting on the scale, trying on that pair of pants, or using the measuring tape, make a note of how your body changed this week. Write your results in your daily log (page 410).

SHOPPING LIST

CHECK YOUR FRIDGE and cupboards. Much of this food might still be there from last week. And some of what you'll buy this week will carry over to the upcoming weeks. There are no portions listed, because these depend on how many people are in your family. So just go through the menu plan and note how much of everything you'll need.

If you don't like something, substitute with as close an equivalent as you can find. For instance, have cauliflower instead of broccoli or whole wheat toast instead of whole wheat English muffins. But don't substitute white flour products (like white bread) when whole grain products (like whole wheat bread) are called for. Whole grains are important weight-loss tools.

FRESH FRUIT

Bananas

Berries (such as blueberries, raspberries, strawberries, or blackberries)

Kiwifruit

Lemons (Don't buy if you're eating dinner out on Thursday.)

Oranges

Strawberries

Tangerines

Watermelon, if in season (for 1,800-calorie plan only)

FRESH VEGETABLES AND HERBS

Basil

Beans, green (If not in season, get frozen or no-sodium-added vacuum-packed canned.)

Broccoli

Carrots

Celery

Corn (If not in season, get frozen or no-sodium-added vacuum-packed canned.)

Dill or parsley (Don't buy if you're using basil in lunch on Sunday.)

Eggplant

Fennel

Garlic

Lettuce (either a head of romaine or other leafy lettuce or a bag of mixed greens)

Peppers, green and red

Spinach (For convenience, buy bags of prewashed spinach.)

Sprouts (Don't buy if you're eating lunch out on Saturday.)

Squash, butternut (Don't buy if you're eating out for dinner on Thursday.)

Sweet potatoes

Tomatoes, regular

CANNED AND BOTTLED GOODS

Anchovy paste (Don't buy if you're eating lunch out on Monday or buying bottled Caesar dressing.)

Barbecue sauce

Chickpeas, canned

Honey

Ketchup

Lemon juice

Marinara sauce

Mustard, Dijon

Oil, olive

Olives, black, preferably Moroccan or kalamata

Peanut butter (for 1,600- and 1,800-calorie plans)

Pickles (Don't buy if you're eating lunch out on Saturday.)

Salad dressing, Caesar (Don't buy if you're making your own or eating lunch out on Monday.)

Salad dressing, reduced-calorie Italian or vinaigrette

Salad dressing, regular Italian or vinaigrette (for 1,800-calorie plan only)

Salsa

Soup, lentil, black bean, or other bean (such as Progresso)

Syrup, chocolate

Syrup, maple or maple-flavored

Tuna, water-packed

Vinegar, preferably balsamic

Worchestershire sauce (Don't buy if you're eating lunch out on Monday or buying bottled Caesar dressing.)

DRY GOODS AND BREAD

Almonds

Apricots, dried (for 1,600- and 1,800-calorie plans)

Bread, whole wheat pita, 6-inch

Bread, whole wheat sandwich loaf, with no more than 90 calories and at least 2 grams of fiber per slice

Buns, whole wheat hamburger, with no more than 120 calories per bun

Cereal, high-fiber, with 5 to 8 grams of fiber per 30-gram serving (such as Kellogg's Complete Wheat Bran Flakes or Kashi Good Friends)

Crackers, graham

Crackers, whole grain (such as Ak-Mak)

Herbes de Provence, other mixed herbs, or poultry seasoning (Don't buy if you're eating dinner out on Thursday.)

Muffins, bran (Don't buy if you're having breakfast at a deli on Wednesday and Sunday.)

Muffins, English, whole wheat or oat bran

Pasta, whole wheat tubular type

Rice, brown (such as Texmati, basmati, or quick-cooking Uncle Ben's)

Seeds, sunflower

REFRIGERATED FOODS

Butter or trans-free margarine

Cheese, Parmesan

Cheese, part-skim mozzarella

Cheese, reduced-fat, such as Cabot 50% Light Cheddar or Kraft or Borden 2% Singles (Don't buy if you're getting a sandwich from Subway for lunch on Saturday.)

Coleslaw

Cottage cheese, 1% or 2% (for 1,600- and 1,800-calorie plans)

Eggs

Hummus

Milk, fat-free (If you haven't adjusted to fat-free milk, buy 1% or mix equal parts 1% and 2%. Your calorie level will be a little higher, but you can gradually train your tastebuds to like fat-free. If you're lactose intolerant, try Lactaid milk. If you prefer soy milk—low-fat or fat-free—buy calcium-fortified with at least 25% of the Daily Value of calcium per cup.)

Yogurt, low-fat fruit, with about 210 calories per 8 ounces (for 1,800-calorie plan only)

Yogurt, low-fat plain

Yogurt, reduced-calorie flavored, with no more than 120 calories per 8 ounces

MEAT, POULTRY, AND FISH

Beef, lean ground

Chicken, boneless and skinless breasts or precooked Perdue Short Cuts or Louis Rich strips (Don't buy if you're eating out for lunch on Monday.)

Chicken, boneless and skinless breasts or skinless legs and thighs

Chicken, whole (Don't buy if you're eating dinner out on Thursday.)

Salmon, fillets (If you're making the grilled salmon, this is all you need. If you're making the Poached Salmon with Herb Sauce, see page 395 for other ingredients.)

Shrimp, large

FROZEN FOODS

Bean burrito, with 350 to 370 calories (Don't buy if you're eating out for lunch on Tuesday.)

Ice cream or frozen yogurt, light, with no more than 110 calories per ½ cup (such as Breyers, Edy's, or Dreyer's)

Waffles, whole grain toaster waffles, with about 170 calories for 2 (such as Nutri-Grain Multibran)

OPTIONAL

Beer, light

Treats (see Monday, Tuesday, and Saturday)

Wine

MONDAY

1,400	1,600

BREAKFAST

CEREAL: 150 calories of high-fiber cereal topped with 1 cup fat-free milk, ½ cup strawberries or other fruit, and 2 tablespoons almonds

TIP Check label for 5 to 8 grams of fiber per 30-gram serving.

CEREAL: 150 calories of high-fiber cereal topped with 1 cup fat-free milk, ½ cup strawberries or other fruit, and 2 tablespoons almonds

TIP Check label for 5 to 8 grams of fiber per 30-gram serving.

LUNCH

CHICKEN CAESAR SALAD: 2 to 3 cups romaine lettuce and other vegetables with 3 ounces chicken strips (altogether, about the size of a deck of cards) and 2 tablespoons Caesar Salad Dressing (recipe on page 385).

TIP If dining out, ask for dressing on the side so that you can control the amount.

CHICKEN CAESAR SALAD: 2 to 3 cups romaine lettuce and other vegetables with 3 ounces chicken strips (altogether, about the size of a deck of cards) and 2 tablespoons Caesar Salad Dressing (recipe on page 385).

TIP If dining out, ask for dressing on the side so that you can control the amount.

1 ROLL: Have this or 1 slice bread (preferably whole grain).

SNACK

YOGURT: 8 ounces reduced-calorie flavored yogurt with no more than 120 calories

YOGURT: 8 ounces reduced-calorie flavored yogurt with no more than 120 calories

DINNER

EGGPLANT PASTA: See recipe on page 398.

FENNEL, ORANGE, AND OLIVE SALAD: See recipe on page 398.

EGGPLANT PASTA: See recipe on page 398.

FENNEL, ORANGE, AND OLIVE SALAD: See recipe on page 398.

TREAT

FIDDLE FADDLE: ⅔ cup, or another 125-calorie treat, such as 6 ounces wine (see page 255 for more suggestions)

FIDDLE FADDLE: ⅔ cup, or another 125-calorie treat, such as 6 ounces wine (see page 255 for more suggestions)

BREAKFAST

CEREAL: 150 calories of high-fiber cereal topped with 1 cup fat-free milk, ½ cup strawberries or other fruit, and 2 tablespoons almonds

TIP Check label for 5 to 8 grams of fiber per 30-gram serving.

LUNCH

CHICKEN CAESAR SALAD: 2 to 3 cups romaine lettuce and other vegetables with 3 ounces chicken strips (altogether, about the size of a deck of cards) and 2 tablespoons Caesar Salad Dressing (recipe on page 385).

TIP If dining out, ask for dressing on the side so that you can control the amount.

1 ROLL: Have this or 1 slice bread (preferably whole grain).

BUTTER OR TRANS-FREE MARGARINE: 1 teaspoon

SNACK

YOGURT: 8 ounces low-fat fruit yogurt with no more than 210 calories

DINNER

EGGPLANT PASTA: See recipe on page 398.

FENNEL, ORANGE, AND OLIVE SALAD: See recipe on page 398.

TREAT

FIDDLE FADDLE: ⅔ cup, or another 125-calorie treat, such as 6 ounces wine (see page 255 for more suggestions)

Nutrition Tallies

	1,400	1,600	1,800
CALORIES	1,405	1,602	1,765
FAT (G)	44	49	58
SATURATED FAT (G)	7.7	8.6	10.3
PROTEIN (G)	72	78	81
CARBOHYDRATES (G)	172	206	225
DIETARY FIBER (G)	37	40	42
CHOLESTEROL (MG)	88	100	100
SODIUM (MG)	1,964	2,111	2,198
CALCIUM (MG)	950	979	1,065

Fat Buster!

In a *Consumer Report* survey of 32,213 people who had lost weight (or were trying to), about 70 percent said that eating fruits and vegetables helped them lose weight and—better yet—keep it off!

TUESDAY

1,400	1,600
BREAKFAST	
STRAWBERRY-BANANA SMOOTHIE: In a blender, process until smooth 1 small ripe banana, $\frac{1}{2}$ cup strawberries, $\frac{1}{2}$ cup fat-free milk, $\frac{1}{2}$ cup low-fat plain yogurt, 2 teaspoons honey, and 1 or 2 ice cubes.	**STRAWBERRY-BANANA SMOOTHIE:** In a blender, process until smooth 1 small ripe banana, $\frac{1}{2}$ cup strawberries, $\frac{1}{2}$ cup fat-free milk, $\frac{1}{2}$ cup low-fat plain yogurt, 2 teaspoons honey, and 1 or 2 ice cubes.
WHOLE WHEAT TOAST: 1 slice spread with 1 teaspoon trans-free margarine	**WHOLE WHEAT TOAST:** 2 slices spread with 2 teaspoons trans-free margarine
LUNCH	
BURRITO: 1 Taco Bell bean burrito, 1 microwave bean burrito with 350 to 370 calories, or $\frac{1}{2}$ giant California-style burrito; no sour cream	**BURRITO:** 1 Taco Bell bean burrito, 1 microwave bean burrito with 350 to 370 calories, or $\frac{1}{2}$ giant California-style burrito; no sour cream
RED PEPPER SLICES: 1 cup, or other crudités, dipped in 2 to 3 tablespoons salsa	**RED PEPPER SLICES:** 1 cup, or other crudités, dipped in 2 to 3 tablespoons salsa
SNACK	
FAT-FREE LATTE: 12 ounces regular or decaf	**FAT-FREE LATTE:** 12 ounces regular or decaf
GRAHAM CRACKERS: 1 rectangle	**GRAHAM CRACKERS:** 1 rectangle
DINNER	
HAMBURGER: 1 small burger (broil or grill 3 ounces lean ground beef) on 1 whole wheat bun with ketchup, mustard, tomato slices, and mixed greens	**HAMBURGER:** 1 small burger (broil or grill 3 ounces lean ground beef) on 1 whole wheat bun with ketchup, mustard, tomato slices, and mixed greens
CORN: 1 ear or $\frac{1}{2}$ cup	**CORN:** 1 ear or $\frac{1}{2}$ cup
TOMATO: Remaining portion, sliced	**TOMATO:** Remaining portion, sliced
TREAT	
2 HERSHEY'S KISSES: Have these or another 50-calorie treat, such as 1 Fig Newton or 1 Oreo cookie.	**4 HERSHEY'S KISSES:** Have these or another 100-calorie treat (see page 254 for more suggestions).

BREAKFAST

STRAWBERRY-BANANA SMOOTHIE: In a blender, process until smooth 1 small ripe banana, ½ cup strawberries, ½ cup fat-free milk, ½ cup low-fat plain yogurt, 2 teaspoons honey, and 1 or 2 ice cubes.

WHOLE WHEAT TOAST: 2 slices spread with 2 teaspoons trans-free margarine

LUNCH

BURRITO: 1 Taco Bell bean burrito, 1 microwave bean burrito with 350 to 370 calories, or ½ giant California-style burrito; no sour cream

RED PEPPER SLICES: 1 cup, or other crudités, dipped in 2 to 3 tablespoons salsa

SNACK

FAT-FREE LATTE: 12 ounces regular or decaf

GRAHAM CRACKERS: 2 rectangles spread with 2 teaspoons peanut butter

DINNER

HAMBURGER: 1 small burger (broil or grill 3 ounces lean ground beef) on 1 whole wheat bun with ketchup, mustard, tomato slices, and mixed greens

CORN: 1 ear or ½ cup

TOMATO: Remaining portion, sliced

WATERMELON OR OTHER FRUIT: 2 cups

TREAT

4 HERSHEY'S KISSES: Have these or another 100-calorie treat (see page 254 for more suggestions).

Nutrition Tallies

	1,400	1,600	1,800
CALORIES	1,416	1,581	1,800
FAT (G)	44	52	60
SATURATED FAT (G)	15	17.7	19
PROTEIN (G)	68	72	77
CARBOHYDRATES (G)	200	221	255
DIETARY FIBER (G)	27	29	32
CHOLESTEROL (MG)	100	102	102
SODIUM (MG)	2,413	2,643	2,785
CALCIUM (MG)	975	1,027	1,059

Nutrient Booster!

EATING FRUIT not only helps ward off cancer and heart disease but also may protect your bones. A British study found that women who ate the most fruit as children had denser, stronger bones. Fruits (and vegetables) are rich in potassium, vitamin C, beta-carotene, and magnesium—all bone-strengthening nutrients.

WEDNESDAY

1,400	1,600
BREAKFAST	

BRAN MUFFIN: 1 small or ½ medium muffin

1 ORANGE

FAT-FREE MILK: 1 cup

BRAN MUFFIN: 1 small or ½ medium muffin

1 ORANGE

FAT-FREE MILK: 1 cup

LUNCH

MOZZARELLA AND TOMATO SANDWICH:
Between 2 slices whole grain bread, layer
2 slices part-skim mozzarella, 2 to 3
tomato slices, 3 chopped olives, and basil.
TIP This is great heated in the toaster
oven!

SPINACH: 2 cups, tossed with 1 tablespoon
reduced-calorie dressing

MOZZARELLA AND TOMATO SANDWICH:
Between 2 slices whole grain bread, layer
2 slices part-skim mozzarella, 2 to 3
tomato slices, 3 chopped olives, and basil.
TIP This is great heated in the toaster
oven!

SPINACH: 2 cups, tossed with 1 tablespoon
reduced-calorie dressing

SNACK

HOT OR COLD CHOCOLATE MILK: 1 cup fat-
free milk with 2 teaspoons chocolate
syrup

GRAHAM CRACKERS: 1 rectangle

HOT OR COLD CHOCOLATE MILK: 1 cup fat-
free milk with 2 teaspoons chocolate
syrup

GRAHAM CRACKERS: 1 rectangle

DINNER

PASTA WITH SHRIMP AND BROCCOLI: See
recipe on page 399.

1 KIWIFRUIT OR OTHER FRUIT

PASTA WITH SHRIMP AND BROCCOLI: See
recipe on page 399.

2 KIWIFRUIT OR OTHER FRUIT

TREAT

BANANA SPLIT: Slice 1 small banana in half
lengthwise and top with ½ cup light ice
cream or frozen yogurt and 2 teaspoons
chocolate syrup.

BANANA SPLIT: Slice 1 small banana in half
lengthwise and top with ½ cup light ice
cream or frozen yogurt and 2 teaspoons
chocolate syrup.

1,800

BREAKFAST

BRAN MUFFIN: 1 small or ½ medium muffin

1 ORANGE

FAT-FREE MILK: 1 cup

LOW-FAT COTTAGE CHEESE: 4 ounces

LUNCH

MOZZARELLA AND TOMATO SANDWICH:
Between 2 slices whole grain bread, layer 2 slices part-skim mozzarella, 2 to 3 tomato slices, 3 chopped olives, and basil. **TIP** This is great heated in the toaster oven!

SPINACH: 2 cups, tossed with 1 tablespoon regular dressing

SNACK

HOT OR COLD CHOCOLATE MILK: 1 cup fat-free milk with 2 teaspoons chocolate syrup

GRAHAM CRACKERS: 1 rectangle

DINNER

PASTA WITH SHRIMP AND BROCCOLI: See recipe on page 399.

2 KIWIFRUIT OR OTHER FRUIT

TREAT

BANANA SPLIT: Slice 1 small banana in half lengthwise and top with 1 cup light ice cream or frozen yogurt and 2 teaspoons chocolate syrup.

Nutrition Tallies

	1,400	1,600	1,800
CALORIES	1,456	1,602	1,813
FAT (G)	55	56	62
SATURATED FAT (G)	14.6	14.6	17.9
PROTEIN (G)	70	75	91
CARBOHYDRATES (G)	191	225	245
DIETARY FIBER (G)	26	32	32
CHOLESTEROL (MG)	197	197	211
SODIUM (MG)	3,036	3,041	3,512
CALCIUM (MG)	1,407	1,438	1,604

Nutrient Booster!

1 FRUIT SERVING EQUALS . . .
- 1 fruit, such as an apple, peach, pear, banana
- ½ cup cut-up raw, canned, or frozen fruit, such as berries, grapes, cantaloupe, apples
- 6 ounces (¾ cup) fruit juice
- ¼ cup dried fruit, such as raisins, apricots (To keep calories in check, we're using ⅛ cup as a serving on the 1,600- and 1,800-calorie plans.)

1 VEGETABLE SERVING EQUALS . . .
- ½ cup raw, canned, or frozen vegetables, such as green or red pepper, cauliflower, tomatoes
- ½ cup cooked vegetables, such as broccoli, spinach, tomatoes (Fried vegetables don't count on this plan!)
- 1 cup raw leafy salad greens, such as spinach, romaine, mixed greens
- 6 ounces (¾ cup) vegetable juice

THURSDAY

1,400	1,600

BREAKFAST

CEREAL: 150 calories of high-fiber cereal topped with 1 cup fat-free milk, ½ cup berries or other fruit, and 1 tablespoon almonds

TIP Check label for 5 to 8 grams of fiber per 30-gram serving.

CEREAL: 150 calories of high-fiber cereal topped with 1 cup fat-free milk, ½ cup berries or other fruit, and 2 tablespoons almonds

TIP Check label for 5 to 8 grams of fiber per 30-gram serving.

LUNCH

HUMMUS AND SPINACH SANDWICH: In 1 medium whole wheat pita, stuff ⅓ cup hummus and 1 cup spinach.

CARROT AND CELERY STICKS: 1 cup

1 ORANGE OR OTHER FRUIT

HUMMUS AND SPINACH SANDWICH: In 1 medium whole wheat pita, stuff ⅓ cup hummus and 1 cup spinach.

CARROT AND CELERY STICKS: 1 cup

1 ORANGE OR OTHER FRUIT

SNACK

GRAHAM CRACKERS: 1 rectangle

YOGURT: 8 ounces reduced-calorie flavored yogurt with no more than 120 calories

GRAHAM CRACKERS: 2 rectangles

YOGURT: 8 ounces reduced-calorie flavored yogurt with no more than 120 calories

DINNER

ROASTED CHICKEN: *At home*, make Roasted Chicken (recipe on page 384). *At Boston Market*, have either the ¼ white-meat chicken (no wing) or the ¼ dark-meat chicken, both without skin. *At other takeouts*, have either 1 leg or ½ breast (no wing), both without skin.

2 SIDE DISHES: *At home*, have 1 cup steamed vegetables, and ¾ cup corn, boiled potatoes, sweet potatoes, or butternut squash. *At Boston Market*, order the steamed vegetables and either herbed buttered corn, butternut squash, or garlic-dill new potatoes. *At other takeouts*, have 1 cup steamed vegetables and ¾ cup of corn or boiled potatoes prepared with a *little* butter, sweet potatoes, or butternut squash.

ROASTED CHICKEN: *At home*, make Roasted Chicken (recipe on page 384). *At Boston Market*, have either the ¼ white-meat chicken (no wing) or the ¼ dark-meat chicken, both without skin. *At other takeouts*, have either 1 leg or ½ breast (no wing), both without skin.

2 SIDE DISHES: *At home*, have 1 cup steamed vegetables, and ¾ cup corn, boiled potatoes, sweet potatoes, or butternut squash. *At Boston Market*, order the steamed vegetables and either herbed buttered corn, butternut squash, or garlic-dill new potatoes. *At other takeouts*, have 1 cup steamed vegetables and ¾ cup of corn or boiled potatoes prepared with a *little* butter, sweet potatoes, or butternut squash.

TREAT

LIGHT ICE CREAM OR FROZEN YOGURT: ⅔ cup, with no more than 110 calories per ½ cup

LIGHT ICE CREAM OR FROZEN YOGURT: 1 cup, with no more than 110 calories per ½ cup

BREAKFAST

CEREAL: 150 calories of high-fiber cereal topped with 1 cup fat-free milk, ½ cup berries or other fruit, and 2 tablespoons almonds

TIP Check label for 5 to 8 grams of fiber per 30-gram serving.

LUNCH

HUMMUS AND SPINACH SANDWICH: In 1 medium whole wheat pita, stuff ⅓ cup hummus and 1 cup spinach.

CARROT AND CELERY STICKS: 1 cup

1 ORANGE OR OTHER FRUIT

SNACK

GRAHAM CRACKERS: 2 rectangles

YOGURT: 8 ounces low-fat fruit yogurt with no more than 210 calories

DINNER

ROASTED CHICKEN: *At home*, make Roasted Chicken (recipe on page 384). *At Boston Market*, have either the ¼ white-meat chicken (no wing) or the ¼ dark-meat chicken, both without skin. *At other take-outs*, have either 1 leg or ½ breast (no wing), both without skin.

2 SIDE DISHES: *At home*, have 1 cup steamed vegetables, and ¾ cup corn, boiled potatoes, sweet potatoes, or butternut squash. *At Boston Market*, order the steamed vegetables and either herbed buttered corn, butternut squash, or garlic-dill new potatoes. *At other takeouts*, have 1 cup steamed vegetables and ¾ cup of corn or boiled potatoes prepared with a *little* butter, sweet potatoes, or butternut squash.

WHOLE GRAIN BREAD: 1 slice

TREAT

LIGHT ICE CREAM OR FROZEN YOGURT: 1 cup, with no more than 110 calories per ½ cup

Nutrition Tallies

	1,400	1,600	1,800
CALORIES	1,380	1,574	1,760
FAT (G)	33	41	45
SATURATED FAT (G)	6.9	8.9	10.2
PROTEIN (G)	77	83	87
CARBOHYDRATES (G)	218	243	280
DIETARY FIBER (G)	40	40	44
CHOLESTEROL (MG)	124	131	138
SODIUM (MG)	1,708	1,827	2,011
CALCIUM (MG)	962	1,061	1,144

people ask me . . .

"How do you get your kids to eat more vegetables?"

I sneak them in! I shred zucchini into pasta sauce (check out Wednesday night's dinner in week 5). I put tomatoes in low-fat Alfredo sauce— they *love* that (see Tuesday's dinner in week 1). And I top their pizza with loads of veggies.

FRIDAY

	1,400	**1,600**

BREAKFAST

SALSA SCRAMBLE: Scramble 1 egg and 1 egg white in a nonstick skillet with 1 teaspoon trans-free margarine or olive oil. When half-cooked, add 1 to 2 tablespoons salsa. Scramble until done.

ENGLISH MUFFIN: 1 whole wheat English muffin, split and toasted

FAT-FREE MILK: 1 cup

1 TANGERINE OR OTHER FRUIT

SALSA SCRAMBLE: Scramble 1 egg and 1 egg white in a nonstick skillet with 1 teaspoon trans-free margarine or olive oil. When half-cooked, add 1 to 2 tablespoons salsa. Scramble until done.

ENGLISH MUFFIN: 1 whole wheat English muffin, split and toasted

FAT-FREE MILK: 1 cup

1 TANGERINE OR OTHER FRUIT

LUNCH

SOUP: 1¼ cups lentil, black bean, or other bean soup

BREAD: 1 slice (preferably whole wheat)

SPINACH: 2 cups, tossed with 1 tablespoon reduced-calorie dressing

---

SOUP: 1¼ cups lentil, black bean, or other bean soup

BREAD: 1 slice (preferably whole wheat)

SPINACH: 2 cups, tossed with 1 tablespoon reduced-calorie dressing

LOW-FAT COTTAGE CHEESE: 4 ounces

SNACK

YOGURT: 8 ounces reduced-calorie flavored yogurt with no more than 120 calories

---

YOGURT: 8 ounces reduced-calorie flavored yogurt with no more than 120 calories

DINNER

SALMON: 4 ounces, grilled or poached

SAUTÉED VEGGIES: 1 cup green beans or other vegetable and a little garlic sautéed in 1 teaspoon butter, trans-free margarine, or olive oil

BROWN RICE: ½ cup, cooked

SALMON: 4 ounces, grilled or poached

SAUTÉED VEGGIES: 1 cup green beans or other vegetable and a little garlic sautéed in 1 teaspoon butter, trans-free margarine, or olive oil

BROWN RICE: ¾ cup, cooked

TREAT

REGULAR ICE CREAM: ½ cup (in case you're at a restaurant and can't get light ice cream or frozen yogurt)

REGULAR ICE CREAM: ½ cup (in case you're at a restaurant and can't get light ice cream or frozen yogurt)

BREAKFAST

SALSA SCRAMBLE: Scramble 1 egg and 1 egg white in a nonstick skillet with 1 teaspoon trans-free margarine or olive oil. When half-cooked, add 1 to 2 tablespoons salsa. Scramble until done.

ENGLISH MUFFIN: 1 whole wheat English muffin, split and toasted

FAT-FREE MILK: 1 cup

1 TANGERINE OR OTHER FRUIT

LUNCH

SOUP: 1¼ cups lentil, black bean, or other bean soup

BREAD: 1 slice (preferably whole wheat)

SPINACH: 2 cups, tossed with 1 tablespoon reduced-calorie dressing

LOW-FAT COTTAGE CHEESE: 4 ounces

SNACK

YOGURT: 8 ounces low-fat fruit yogurt with no more than 210 calories

DINNER

SALMON: 4 ounces, grilled or poached

SAUTÉED VEGGIES: 1 cup green beans or other vegetable and a little garlic sautéed in 1 teaspoon butter, trans-free margarine, or olive oil

BROWN RICE: ¾ cup, cooked

TREAT

REGULAR ICE CREAM: 1 cup (in case you're at a restaurant and can't get light ice cream or frozen yogurt)

Nutrition Tallies

	1,400	1,600	1,800
CALORIES	1,403	1,552	1,799
FAT (G)	39	40	51
SATURATED FAT (G)	10.8	11.9	17.8
PROTEIN (G)	81	97	100
CARBOHYDRATES (G)	168	184	221
DIETARY FIBER (G)	24	25	25
CHOLESTEROL (MG)	321	328	364
SODIUM (MG)	2,616	3,212	3,377
CALCIUM (MG)	958	1,037	1,167

Nutrient Booster!

IF YOU HAVEN'T had time to go grocery shopping, you're always saved by frozen fruits or vegetables waiting in your freezer. I use them all the time. It's so easy—I just open a package and with minimal preparation, they are ready to serve. And as far as nutrients go, frozen produce retains most of its vitamins and minerals. So it can actually be more nutritious than "fresh" that's been sitting in the supermarket for too long.

SATURDAY

1,400	1,600
BREAKFAST	
WAFFLES: 2 whole grain toaster waffles topped with 1 teaspoon trans-free margarine, ½ cup berries, and 1 teaspoon maple syrup. **TIP** Look for waffles with about 170 calories and 4 grams of fiber for 2 waffles. **FAT-FREE MILK:** 1 cup	**WAFFLES:** 2 whole grain toaster waffles topped with 1 teaspoon trans-free margarine, ½ cup berries, and 1 teaspoon maple syrup. **TIP** Look for waffles with about 170 calories and 4 grams of fiber for 2 waffles. **FAT-FREE MILK:** 1 cup
LUNCH	
VEGGIE SANDWICH WITH CHEESE: Get from Subway or make your own with a whole wheat hamburger bun stuffed with ½ cup vegetables (such as tomato, pickle, sprouts) and 1-ounce slice reduced-fat cheese **GREENS:** 2 cups, tossed with 1 tablespoon reduced-calorie dressing	**VEGGIE SANDWICH WITH CHEESE:** Get from Subway or make your own with a whole wheat hamburger bun stuffed with ½ cup vegetables (such as tomato, pickle, sprouts) and 2 slices (1 ounce each) reduced-fat cheese. **GREENS:** 2 cups, tossed with 1 tablespoon reduced-calorie dressing
SNACK	
YOGURT: 1 cup low-fat plain yogurt mixed with 1 tablespoon sunflower seeds and 2 teaspoons maple syrup	**YOGURT:** 1 cup low-fat plain yogurt mixed with 1 tablespoon sunflower seeds, 2 teaspoons maple syrup, and 6 dried apricot halves
DINNER	
BARBECUED CHICKEN: Coat a 4-ounce piece of skinless chicken breast or skinless leg and thigh with barbecue sauce. Bake at 425°F or grill outdoors, turning once, for 25 to 30 minutes, or until the juices run clear when the meat is pierced with a sharp knife. **COLESLAW:** ½ cup (look for a less creamy type or drain some of the dressing) **1 SWEET POTATO:** Bake then dollop with a few tablespoons low-fat plain yogurt. **1 ORANGE**	**BARBECUED CHICKEN:** Coat a 4-ounce piece of skinless chicken breast or skinless leg and thigh with barbecue sauce. Bake at 425°F or grill outdoors, turning once, for 25 to 30 minutes, or until the juices run clear when the meat is pierced with a sharp knife. **COLESLAW:** ½ cup (look for a less creamy type or drain some of the dressing) **1 SWEET POTATO:** Bake then dollop with a few tablespoons low-fat plain yogurt. **1 ORANGE**
TREAT	
PRETZELS: 1 ounce, or another 100-calorie treat (see page 254 for more suggestions)	**PRETZELS:** 1 ounce, or another 100-calorie treat (see page 254 for more suggestions)

BREAKFAST

WAFFLES: 2 whole grain toaster waffles topped with 1 teaspoon trans-free margarine, ½ cup berries, and 1 teaspoon maple syrup.

> **TIP** Look for waffles with about 170 calories and 4 grams of fiber for 2 waffles.

FAT-FREE MILK: 1 cup

LUNCH

VEGGIE SANDWICH WITH CHEESE: Get from Subway or make your own with a whole wheat hamburger bun stuffed with ½ cup vegetables (such as tomato, pickle, sprouts) and 2 slices (1 ounce each) reduced-fat cheese.

GREENS: 2 cups, tossed with 1 tablespoon regular dressing

SNACK

YOGURT: 1 cup low-fat plain yogurt mixed with 1 tablespoon sunflower seeds, 2 teaspoons maple syrup, and 6 dried apricot halves

GRAHAM CRACKERS: 1 rectangle

DINNER

BARBECUED CHICKEN: Coat a 4-ounce piece of skinless chicken breast or skinless leg and thigh with barbecue sauce. Bake at 425°F or grill outdoors, turning once, for 25 to 30 minutes, or until the juices run clear when the meat is pierced with a sharp knife.

COLESLAW: ½ cup (look for a less creamy type or drain some of the dressing)

1 SWEET POTATO: Bake then dollop with a few tablespoons low-fat plain yogurt.

1 ORANGE

TREAT

PRETZELS: 2 ounces, or another 200-calorie treat (see page 255 for more suggestions)

Nutrition Tallies

	1,400	1,600	1,800
CALORIES	1,448	1,623	1,806
FAT (G)	44	54	65
SATURATED FAT (G)	12.8	18.1	22.8
PROTEIN (G)	75	83	85
CARBOHYDRATES (G)	179	194	215
DIETARY FIBER (G)	23	24	25
CHOLESTEROL (MG)	144	178	178
SODIUM (MG)	1,827	2,017	2,034
CALCIUM (MG)	1,338	1,602	1,639

Nutrient Booster!

COLESLAW MAY NOT SEEM like something you'd eat when you're trying to lose weight, but it's actually not all that bad. Depending on how it's made, it ranges from 45 to 100 calories per ½ cup. And it's worth it for disease-fighting compounds in cabbage called indoles. Indoles boost your body's own cancer-fighting enzymes, which destroy chemicals before they can do damage. Indoles also halt the cancer process once it's begun. And there's more: Cabbage is high in vitamin C and certain B vitamins.

SUNDAY

1,400	1,600
BREAKFAST	

BREAKFAST

1,400	1,600
BRAN MUFFIN: $\frac{1}{2}$ large or 1 small muffin **YOGURT:** 8 ounces reduced-calorie flavored yogurt with no more than 120 calories **1 ORANGE**	**BRAN MUFFIN:** 1 large muffin **YOGURT:** 8 ounces reduced-calorie flavored yogurt with no more than 120 calories **1 ORANGE**

LUNCH

1,400	1,600
TUNA AND CHICKPEA SALAD: Combine 3 ounces water-packed tuna, 1 cup chopped vegetables (such as tomato and green pepper), $\frac{1}{2}$ cup canned chickpeas, juice of $\frac{1}{2}$ lemon, 1 teaspoon olive oil, and fresh or dried parsley, dill, or basil. **3 AK-MAK CRACKERS:** Have these or 70 calories' worth of another whole grain cracker.	**TUNA AND CHICKPEA SALAD:** Combine 3 ounces water-packed tuna, 1 cup chopped vegetables (such as tomato and green pepper), $\frac{1}{2}$ cup canned chickpeas, juice of $\frac{1}{2}$ lemon, 1 teaspoon olive oil, and fresh or dried parsley, dill, or basil. **3 AK-MAK CRACKERS:** Have these or 70 calories' worth of another whole grain cracker.

SNACK

1,400	1,600
FAT-FREE MILK: 1 cup **GRAHAM CRACKERS:** 1 rectangle	**FAT-FREE MILK:** 1 cup **GRAHAM CRACKERS:** 1 rectangle spread with 1 tablespoon peanut butter

DINNER

1,400	1,600
PASTA WITH BROCCOLI AND CHEESE: Toss $1\frac{1}{4}$ cups whole wheat pasta with 1 cup steamed broccoli, 2 tablespoons Parmesan or mozzarella, 1 tablespoon chopped basil, and 2 teaspoons olive oil.	**PASTA WITH BROCCOLI AND CHEESE:** Toss $1\frac{1}{4}$ cups whole wheat pasta with 1 cup steamed broccoli, 2 tablespoons Parmesan or mozzarella, 1 tablespoon chopped basil, and 2 teaspoons olive oil.

TREAT

1,400	1,600
LIGHT ICE CREAM OR FROZEN YOGURT: $\frac{1}{2}$ cup, topped with $\frac{1}{2}$ cup strawberries	**LIGHT ICE CREAM OR FROZEN YOGURT:** $\frac{1}{2}$ cup, topped with $\frac{1}{2}$ cup strawberries

BREAKFAST

BRAN MUFFIN: 1 large muffin

YOGURT: 8 ounces low-fat fruit yogurt with no more than 210 calories

1 ORANGE

LUNCH

TUNA AND CHICKPEA SALAD: Combine 3 ounces water-packed tuna, 1 cup chopped vegetables (such as tomato and green pepper), ½ cup canned chickpeas, juice of ½ lemon, 1 teaspoon olive oil, and fresh or dried parsley, dill, or basil.

5 AK-MAK CRACKERS: Have these or 115 calories' worth of another whole grain cracker.

SNACK

FAT-FREE MILK: 1 cup

GRAHAM CRACKERS: 1 rectangle spread with 1 tablespoon peanut butter

DINNER

PASTA WITH BROCCOLI AND CHEESE: Toss 1½ cups whole wheat pasta with 1 cup steamed broccoli, 2 tablespoons Parmesan or mozzarella, 1 tablespoon chopped basil, and 2 teaspoons olive oil.

TREAT

LIGHT ICE CREAM OR FROZEN YOGURT: ½ cup, topped with ½ cup strawberries

Nutrition Tallies

	1,400	1,600	1,800
CALORIES	1,351	1,572	1,752
FAT (G)	31	44	47
SATURATED FAT (G)	8.4	11.4	12.7
PROTEIN (G)	75	83	88
CARBOHYDRATES (G)	206	230	265
DIETARY FIBER (G)	32	38	41
CHOLESTEROL (MG)	88	126	133
SODIUM (MG)	1,606	1,860	1,871
CALCIUM (MG)	1,089	1,201	1,256

Nutrient Booster!

BROCCOLI IS A HEALTHY FOOD for many reasons. Broccoli is perhaps the richest source of sulforaphane, a compound that stimulates the body to make more cancer-zapping enzymes. A University of California study found that men and women who ate the most broccoli (2 cups a week) had half the risk of colon cancer of those who didn't eat broccoli. And in a study from Harvard University, researchers found that men who ate 1 cup of broccoli weekly had half the risk of bladder cancer of men who ate less than 1 cup. From a nutrition standpoint, a cup of cooked broccoli has 6 grams of fiber, the entire daily recommended level of vitamin C, and 25 percent of the recommended levels of vitamin A and folate.

CHAPTER 14

Home In on Hunger

If you're like most women, you've been on diets before, lost weight, then gained it all back. What happened? One explanation I often hear: "Cravings take over, and I just can't shake the urge to overeat!"

The truth is, these cravings we experience often have very little to do with hunger. If we eat to numb, obliterate, or avoid bad feelings or situations—or even to cope with good feelings—we'll have a very hard time losing weight and keeping it off.

I love to eat, just for the joy of it. At times I eat—or overeat—for different reasons. Often, it's because I'm happy, just happy to be with my family for dinner. I eat when I get together with my sisters and brother . . . I mean *really* eat! That's my favorite time to pig out and enjoy all the comfort foods we had together growing up. Like the Danish from our favorite hometown bakery. No one makes a raspberry Danish like Pollyanne's. When I go home to visit my entire family, I love to dine at our favorite Mexican restaurant, Arturo's. The food is so good that I sometimes eat more than I normally would.

And now, 4 weeks into a super-healthy eating plan, overeating and cravings may start creeping back into your life. But this time, you're going to confront the problem and begin to conquer it. We'll be spending these next 2 weeks tackling it so that you can learn to deal with cravings like a pro and reap a lifetime of a healthier, slimmer you.

This week, begin your attack on overeating by focusing on hunger. Eating in response to hunger is the opposite of eating for emotional reasons. When you eat to hunger—and not beyond—you lose weight and keep it off. You're giving your body just the right amount of calories. It's good to hear your stomach growl once in a while—that means you're truly hungry. But many of us have lost touch with hunger. Some of us rarely experience hunger because we're eating all the time. Others punish themselves for bouts of overeating by starving, ignoring their hunger as long as they can hold out (often culminating in a spectacular binge).

To learn how to separate "hunger eating" from eating for other reasons, we're going to keep a Hunger Record this week. Your Hunger Record will show you how often you come to a meal hungry. It will also point out patterns. For instance, when you skip breakfast or lunch, are you ravenous later in the day? You'll also record foods *not* on the plan and how hungry you were when you ate them.

Some women use this tool for a few days and learn what they need to do to make changes. Others of us may like to use it more regularly, to stay in touch with what's holding us back from achieving our weight-loss goals. Next week, you'll take it one step further and track both hunger and emotions.

Chart Your Hunger

Take out a journal or notebook and copy down the headings on the sample table on page 338. (You'll also find a condensed version on page 411 of your Fat Zone Workbook.) Here's how to fill out your Hunger Record.

> **WEEKLY CHECK-IN:** Now's the time to congratulate yourself for finishing another full week on the Shrink Your Female Fat Zones plan! Whether you're getting on the scale, trying on that pair of pants, or using the measuring tape, make a note of how your body changed this week. Write your results in your daily log (page 411).

1. Write down *everything* you ate, both meals and snacks. If you ate pretty much what was on the plan, you can just scribble down: breakfast, lunch, dinner, snack, treat. But please write down all the foods *not* on the plan; this is valuable information for attacking emotional eating. Also, if you skipped part of the meal, write that down, too.

2. Write down the time you ate, as precisely as possible.

3. At each meal, rate your hunger from 1 to 5 (1 = not at all hungry; 2 = a little hungry; 3 = hungry; 4 = very hungry; 5 = ravenous).

4. Record immediately after eating; the longer you wait, the more inaccurate your report.

Here's a sample day.

Your Hunger Record (sample)		
MONDAY		
MEAL	TIME OF DAY	HUNGER RATING
Breakfast, minus the fruit	7:30 A.M.	2
Lunch	12:00 NOON	4
Snack, candy bar	1:30 P.M.	1
Snack	3:00 P.M.	2
Dinner	7:30 P.M.	3
Treat	9:00 P.M.	3

Interpreting Hunger Ratings

Look over your hunger ratings for the past week. Add up how many times you got a 1, a 2, and so forth.

What 1 means: A 1 is a red flag. You're eating when you're not hungry, and this could very well mean eating for other reasons, like stress, fatigue,

1,400 CALORIES: 23% of calories from fat, 21% protein, 56% carbohydrates
1,600 CALORIES: 24% of calories from fat, 20% protein, 56% carbohydrates
1,800 CALORIES: 26% of calories from fat, 20% protein, 54% carbohydrates

or even happiness. Don't worry if you got just one or two 1s. But if you got more than that, you have to question why you ate when you weren't hungry. Next week, you should discover the answer to that question when you take this process a step further.

What 2, 3, and 4 mean: Ideally, you should eat when you're hungry but not starving, which corresponds to a 3 rating. Ratings of 2 and 4 aren't so bad either. You're in great shape if most of your meals got a 3. If you recorded lots of 2s and 4s, check out the "Time of Day" column. You should eat every 3 to 4 hours. Perhaps you're leaving too much—or too little—time between meals. Also, you may be grabbing snacks or second helpings that you don't really need—which translates to a 2 at the next meal. Or are you skipping foods? Maybe you ran out of almonds for breakfast, so by the time lunch arrived, you were at a stomach-growling 4.

What 5 means: A 5 rating signifies that you've gone way too long without food and let yourself get too hungry. The danger here is scarfing up everything in sight once you do eat. While one or two 5s a week is okay, more might mean calorie overload. On the days with 5s, check out the "Time of Day" column for the preceding meals. You should eat something every 3 to 4 hours. Are you waiting too long before the next meal?

Also, check out the meal column for foods that you skipped. While it might seem virtuous to have just one waffle instead of two, you can't fool your body! It knows that it didn't get enough calories for breakfast, and that's why you're starving at lunchtime.

SHOPPING LIST

CHECK YOUR FRIDGE and cupboards. Much of this food might still be there from last week. And some of what you'll buy this week will carry over to the upcoming weeks. There are no portions listed, because these depend on how many people are in your family. So just go through the menu plan and note how much of everything you'll need.

If you don't like something, substitute with as close an equivalent as you can find. For instance, have reduced-calorie ranch dressing instead of reduced-calorie Italian dressing. But don't substitute white flour products (like white bread) when whole grain products (like whole wheat bread) are called for. Whole grains are important weight-loss tools.

FRESH FRUIT

Apples

Bananas

Blueberries

Grapes

Mangoes

Oranges

Peaches, fresh or canned in juice or light syrup (for 1,800-calorie plan only)

Strawberries

Tangerines (for 1,600- and 1,800-calorie plans)

FRESH VEGETABLES AND HERBS

Basil

Carrots

Celery

Cucumbers

Garlic

Greens, mixed

Lettuce (You can use mixed greens instead.)

Parsley

Peppers, green and red

Potatoes, new or other little potatoes

Radishes

Scallions

Spinach (For convenience, buy bags of prewashed spinach.)

Tomatoes

Zucchini

CANNED AND BOTTLED GOODS

Beans, pinto, canned (Don't buy if you're eating out for dinner on Friday.)

Chickpeas, canned

Chutney

Coconut milk, reduced-calorie (such as Thai Kitchen or Trader Joe's)

Curry paste, Thai red

Fish sauce (such as Thai Kitchen)

Honey

Jam or jelly

Lemon juice

Mayonnaise, low-fat

Mustard, Dijon

Oil, olive

Peanut butter

Pickles

Salad dressing, reduced-calorie Italian or vinaigrette

Salad dressing, regular Italian or vinaigrette (for 1,600- and 1,800-calorie plan)

Salsa

Soup, lentil, black bean, or other bean (such as Progresso)

Spaghetti sauce, meatless

Syrup, chocolate

Syrup, maple or maple-flavored

Tuna, water-packed

Vinegar, preferably balsamic

DRY GOODS AND BREAD

Almonds

Bagel, whole wheat or oat bran (Don't buy if you're eating breakfast out on Saturday.)

Bread, crusty Italian-type, preferably whole grain (for 1,800-calorie plan only)

Bread, whole wheat, sandwich loaf, with no more than 90 calories and at least 2 grams of fiber per slice

Buns, whole wheat

Cereal, high-fiber, with 5 to 8 grams of fiber per 30-gram serving (such as Kellogg's Complete Wheat Bran Flakes or Kashi Good Friends)

Cereal, oatmeal (plain, unflavored)

Cinnamon

Crackers, graham

Crackers, whole grain (such as Ak-Mak)

Cranberries, dried (such as Ocean Spray Craisins)

Muffins, bran (Don't buy if you're having breakfast at a deli on Tuesday.)

Muffins, English, whole wheat

Pasta, whole wheat

Pistachios

Raisins

Rice, brown (such as Texmati, basmati, or quick-cooking Uncle Ben's)

Rice, white jasmine or white basmati

Sugar

Tortillas, flour (preferably whole wheat), 8-inch

Trail mix

Walnuts (Don't buy if you're using almonds in lunch for Tuesday.)

REFRIGERATED FOODS

Butter or trans-free margarine

Cheese, Parmesan

Cheese, reduced-fat (such as Cabot 50% Light Cheddar, Tine 75% Jarlsberg, or Kraft or Borden 2% Singles)

Cottage cheese, 1% or 2% (for 1,800-calorie plan only)

Eggs or egg substitute (such as Egg Beaters)

Guacamole (Don't buy if you're eating out for dinner on Friday.)

Milk fat-free (If you haven't adjusted to fat-free milk, buy 1% or mix equal parts 1% and 2%. Your calorie level will be a little higher, but you can gradually train your tastebuds to like fat-free. If you're lactose intolerant, try Lactaid milk. If you prefer soy milk—low-fat or fat-free—buy calcium-fortified with at least 25% of the Daily Value of calcium per cup.)

Yogurt, low-fat fruit, with about 210 calories per 8 ounces (for 1,800-calorie plan only)

Yogurt, low-fat plain

Yogurt, reduced-calorie, flavored, with no more than 120 calories per 8 ounces

MEAT, POULTRY, AND FISH

Chicken, boneless and skinless breasts

Pork tenderloin

Salmon, fillets

Turkey, sliced breast

FROZEN FOODS

Chicken enchiladas (Don't buy if you're eating out for dinner on Friday.)

Ice cream or frozen yogurt, light, with no more than 110 calories per ½ cup (such as Breyers, Edy's, or Dreyer's)

Peas

Pound cake (such as Sara Lee)

Vegetable burgers, with about 120 calories (such as Gardenburgers)

OPTIONAL

Bacon (for dinner recipe on Thursday)

Beer, light

Treats (see Monday, Tuesday, Thursday, Friday, and Sunday)

Wine

MONDAY

1,400	1,600
BREAKFAST	

BREAKFAST

1,400	1,600
CINNAMON OATMEAL: Cook ½ cup rolled oats according to package directions, adding 1 small diced apple, 1 teaspoon maple syrup, and a dash of cinnamon. **FAT-FREE MILK:** 1 cup **ALMONDS:** 1 tablespoon	**CINNAMON OATMEAL:** Cook ½ cup rolled oats according to package directions, adding 1 small diced apple, 1 teaspoon maple syrup, and a dash of cinnamon. **FAT-FREE MILK:** 1 cup **ALMONDS:** 2 tablespoons
LUNCH	
TURKEY AND CHUTNEY ROLL-UP: Spread 1 whole wheat tortilla with 1 to 2 tablespoons chutney, then add 2 slices turkey and 1 slice reduced-fat cheese. Roll up. **SPINACH:** 2 cups, tossed with 1 to 2 tablespoons reduced-calorie dressing **1 ORANGE**	**TURKEY AND CHUTNEY ROLL-UP:** Spread 1 whole wheat tortilla with 1 to 2 tablespoons chutney, then add 2 slices turkey and 1 slice reduced-fat cheese. Roll up. **SPINACH:** 2 cups, tossed with 1 to 2 tablespoons reduced-calorie dressing **1 ORANGE**
SNACK	
HOT OR COLD CHOCOLATE MILK: 1 cup fat-free milk with 2 teaspoons chocolate syrup **2 AK-MAK CRACKERS:** Have these or 45 calories' worth of another whole grain cracker. Spread each cracker with ½ teaspoon peanut butter.	**HOT OR COLD CHOCOLATE MILK:** 1 cup fat-free milk with 2 teaspoons chocolate syrup **2 AK-MAK CRACKERS:** Have these or 45 calories' worth of another whole grain cracker. Spread each cracker with ½ teaspoon peanut butter.
DINNER	
SPICY ORANGE PORK TENDERLOIN WITH MANGO RICE: See recipes on page 400. **COOL CUCUMBER SALAD:** Mix 1 teaspoon vinegar and ½ teaspoon sugar. Toss with 1 cup thinly sliced cucumber.	**SPICY ORANGE PORK TENDERLOIN WITH MANGO RICE:** See recipes on page 400. **COOL CUCUMBER SALAD:** Mix 1 teaspoon vinegar and ½ teaspoon sugar. Toss with 1 cup thinly sliced cucumber.
TREAT	
1 CREAMSICLE FROZEN BAR: Have this or another 70-calorie snack (see page 254 for more suggestions).	**1 DOVE CHOCOLATE BAR:** Have this or another 200-calorie snack (see page 255 for more suggestions).

BREAKFAST

CINNAMON OATMEAL: Cook ½ cup rolled oats according to package directions, adding 1 small diced apple, 1 teaspoon maple syrup, and a dash of cinnamon.

FAT-FREE MILK: 1 cup

ALMONDS: 2 tablespoons

LUNCH

TURKEY AND CHUTNEY ROLL-UP: Spread 1 whole wheat tortilla with 1 to 2 tablespoons chutney, then add 2 slices turkey and 1 slice reduced-fat cheese. Roll up.

SPINACH: 2 cups, tossed with 1 tablespoon regular dressing

1 ORANGE

SNACK

HOT OR COLD CHOCOLATE MILK: 1 cup fat-free milk with 2 teaspoons chocolate syrup

5 AK-MAK CRACKERS: Have these or 115 calories' worth of another whole grain cracker, spread with a total of 1 tablespoon peanut butter.

LOW-FAT COTTAGE CHEESE: ½ cup, topped with 1 sliced fresh peach or ½ cup peaches canned in light syrup or juice

DINNER

SPICY ORANGE PORK TENDERLOIN WITH MANGO RICE: See recipes on page 400.

COOL CUCUMBER SALAD: Mix 1 teaspoon vinegar and ½ teaspoon sugar. Toss with 1 cup thinly sliced cucumber.

TREAT

1 DOVE CHOCOLATE BAR: Have this or another 200-calorie snack (see page 255 for more suggestions).

Nutrition Tallies

	1,400	1,600	1,800
CALORIES	1,413	1,554	1,813
FAT (G)	36	41	55
SATURATED FAT (G)	8.7	8.7	12.2
PROTEIN (G)	88	91	111
CARBOHYDRATES (G)	196	218	236
DIETARY FIBER (G)	24	25	28
CHOLESTEROL (MG)	121	121	124
SODIUM (MG)	2,107	2,331	2,829
CALCIUM (MG)	1,021	1,051	1,133

Fat Buster!

It takes about 15 to 20 minutes—sometimes more—after eating for the brain to register "full." So before you take seconds or give in to a giant dessert, wait. If you're still hungry half an hour later, then you truly didn't eat enough and need more food. But chances are you'll be full—and it'll be a lot easier to pass up those extra calories.

TUESDAY

1,400	1,600
BREAKFAST	
BRAN MUFFIN: ½ large or 1 small muffin (great for carpooling or eating at your desk)	**BRAN MUFFIN:** ½ large or 1 small muffin (great for carpooling or eating at your desk)
YOGURT: 8 ounces reduced-calorie flavored yogurt with no more than 120 calories	**YOGURT:** 8 ounces reduced-calorie flavored yogurt with no more than 120 calories
GRAPES: ¾ cup	**GRAPES:** ¾ cup
LUNCH	
SOUP: 1¼ cups black bean, lentil, or other bean soup	**SOUP:** 1¼ cups black bean, lentil, or other bean soup
WHOLE WHEAT BREAD: 2 slices	**WHOLE WHEAT BREAD:** 2 slices, each spread with 1 teaspoon butter or trans-free margarine
CARROT AND CELERY STICKS: 1 cup	**CARROT AND CELERY STICKS:** 1 cup
SNACK	
BLUEBERRIES OR OTHER FRUIT: ½ cup	**BLUEBERRIES OR OTHER FRUIT:** ½ cup
DINNER	
PORK TENDERLOIN SANDWICH: On 1 whole grain roll or 2 slices whole grain bread, layer 4 slices roasted pork tenderloin (about 3 ounces), a few thin slices of apple, and 1 slice of reduced-fat Cheddar.	**PORK TENDERLOIN SANDWICH:** On 1 whole grain roll or 2 slices whole grain bread, layer 4 slices roasted pork tenderloin (about 3 ounces), a few thin slices of apple, and 1 slice of reduced-fat Cheddar.
WALDORF SALAD: See Chicken Waldorf Salad recipe on page 392. Omit chicken and make with remaining apple.	**WALDORF SALAD:** See Chicken Waldorf Salad recipe on page 392. Omit chicken and make with remaining apple.
TREAT	
1 GOOD HUMOR CREAMSICLE: Have this or another 100-calorie treat (see page 254 for more suggestions).	**1 GOOD HUMOR CREAMSICLE:** Have this or another 100-calorie treat (see page 254 for more suggestions).

1,800

BREAKFAST

BRAN MUFFIN: ½ large or 1 small muffin (great for carpooling or eating at your desk)

YOGURT: 8 ounces low-fat fruit yogurt with no more than 210 calories

GRAPES: ¾ cup

LUNCH

SOUP: 1¼ cups black bean, lentil, or other bean soup

WHOLE WHEAT BREAD: 2 slices, each spread with 1 teaspoon butter or trans-free margarine

CARROT AND CELERY STICKS: 1 cup

SNACK

BLUEBERRIES OR OTHER FRUIT: ½ cup

ALMONDS: 2 tablespoons

DINNER

PORK TENDERLOIN SANDWICH: On 1 whole grain roll or 2 slices whole grain bread, layer 4 slices roasted pork tenderloin (about 3 ounces), a few thin slices of apple, and 1 slice of reduced-fat Cheddar.

WALDORF SALAD: See Chicken Waldorf Salad recipe on page 392. Omit chicken and make with remaining apple.

TREAT

1 GOOD HUMOR CREAMSICLE: Have this or another 100-calorie treat (see page 254 for more suggestions).

Nutrition Tallies

	1,400	1,600	1,800
CALORIES	1,380	1,547	1,783
FAT (G)	31	44	56
SATURATED FAT (G)	9.4	12.2	14
PROTEIN (G)	69	74	79
CARBOHYDRATES (G)	224	244	266
DIETARY FIBER (G)	35	40	43
CHOLESTEROL (MG)	115	153	160
SODIUM (MG)	2,020	2,296	2,306
CALCIUM (MG)	926	1,034	1,137

WEDNESDAY

1,400	1,600
BREAKFAST	
CEREAL: 150 calories of high-fiber cereal topped with 1 cup fat-free milk, ½ sliced medium banana, and 2 tablespoons trail mix	**CEREAL:** 150 calories of high-fiber cereal topped with 1 cup fat-free milk and 2 tablespoons trail mix
TIP Check label for 5 to 8 grams of fiber per 30-gram serving.	**TIP** Check label for 5 to 8 grams of fiber per 30-gram serving.
	2 TANGERINES
LUNCH	
TUNA SANDWICH: Mix 3 ounces water-packed tuna; 2 tablespoons finely chopped celery, carrot, green pepper, or pickle; 1 tablespoon low-fat plain yogurt; ½ tablespoon low-fat mayo; ½ teaspoon Dijon mustard; and black pepper. Spread on 2 slices whole wheat bread with tomato slices and lettuce.	**TUNA SANDWICH:** Mix 3 ounces water-packed tuna; 2 tablespoons finely chopped celery, carrot, green pepper, or pickle; 1 tablespoon low-fat plain yogurt; ½ tablespoon low-fat mayo; ½ teaspoon Dijon mustard; and black pepper. Spread on 2 slices whole wheat bread with tomato slices and lettuce.
GRAPES OR OTHER FRUIT: ¾ cup	**GRAPES OR OTHER FRUIT:** ¾ cup
SNACK	
REDUCED-FAT CHEDDAR: 1 ounce, on 1 whole grain cracker	**REDUCED-FAT CHEDDAR:** 1 ounce, on 1 whole grain cracker
1 PICKLE	**1 PICKLE**
DINNER	
PASTA WITH ZUCCHINI SAUCE: Heat ⅓ cup meatless spaghetti sauce and ½ cup shredded zucchini until zucchini softens. Serve over 1¼ cups whole wheat pasta and top with 1 tablespoon Parmesan cheese.	**PASTA WITH ZUCCHINI SAUCE:** Heat ⅓ cup meatless spaghetti sauce and ½ cup shredded zucchini until zucchini softens. Serve over 1½ cups whole wheat pasta and top with 2 tablespoons Parmesan cheese.
	SALAD: 2 cups spinach or mixed greens with 1 tablespoon regular dressing
TREAT	
BANANA SPLIT: Slice the remaining ½ breakfast banana and top with ¾ cup light ice cream or frozen yogurt and 2 teaspoons chocolate syrup.	**BANANA SPLIT:** Slice 1 banana and top with ¾ cup light ice cream or frozen yogurt and 2 teaspoons chocolate syrup.

BREAKFAST

CEREAL: 150 calories of high-fiber cereal topped with 1 cup fat-free milk and 2 tablespoons trail mix

TIP Check label for 5 to 8 grams of fiber per 30-gram serving.

2 TANGERINES

LUNCH

TUNA SANDWICH: Mix 3 ounces water-packed tuna; 2 tablespoons finely chopped celery, carrot, green pepper, or pickle; 1 tablespoon low-fat plain yogurt; ½ tablespoon low-fat mayo; ½ teaspoon Dijon mustard; and black pepper. Spread on 2 slices whole wheat bread with tomato slices and lettuce.

GRAPES OR OTHER FRUIT: ¾ cup

SNACK

REDUCED-FAT CHEDDAR: 1 ounce, on 1 whole grain cracker

1 PICKLE

DINNER

PASTA WITH ZUCCHINI SAUCE: Heat ⅓ cup meatless spaghetti sauce and ½ cup shredded zucchini until zucchini softens. Serve over 1½ cups whole wheat pasta and top with 2 tablespoons Parmesan cheese.

SALAD: 2 cups spinach or mixed greens with 1 tablespoon regular dressing

GARLIC BREAD: Mix 2 teaspoons olive oil, 1 teaspoon Parmesan, and ¼ teaspoon minced garlic or a dash of garlic powder. Spread on 1 medium slice crusty bread (preferably whole wheat) and sprinkle with pepper. Heat until crispy.

TREAT

BANANA SPLIT: Slice 1 banana and top with 1 cup light ice cream or frozen yogurt and 1 tablespoon chocolate syrup.

Nutrition Tallies

	1,400	1,600	1,800
CALORIES	1,417	1,571	1,816
FAT (G)	30	32	48
SATURATED FAT (G)	11.2	12.3	15.5
PROTEIN (G)	75	80	86
CARBOHYDRATES (G)	234	266	288
DIETARY FIBER (G)	28	34	36
CHOLESTEROL (MG)	67	71	77
SODIUM (MG)	1,912	2,014	2,444
CALCIUM (MG)	947	1,046	1,193

THURSDAY

1,400	1,600
BREAKFAST	

BREAKFAST

1,400

ENGLISH MUFFIN: 1 whole wheat English muffin, split and toasted, each half spread with 1 teaspoon butter or trans-free margarine and 1 teaspoon jam or jelly

STRAWBERRIES OR OTHER BERRIES: 1 cup

FAT-FREE MILK: 1 cup

1,600

ENGLISH MUFFIN: 1 whole wheat English muffin, split and toasted, each half spread with 1 teaspoon butter or trans-free margarine and 1 teaspoon jam or jelly

STRAWBERRIES OR OTHER BERRIES: 1 cup

FAT-FREE MILK: 1 cup

LUNCH

1,400

GRILLED CHICKEN SANDWICH: Try Wendy's Grilled Chicken, McDonald's Chicken McGrill, or KFC Honey BBQ—all without mayo. TIP Skip Burger King and Arby's; they're too high in calories.) Dress bun with ketchup, mustard, lettuce, and tomato.

SIDE SALAD: Drizzle 1 tablespoon low-fat dressing (about ⅓ of most packets) over salad.

1 ORANGE OR OTHER FRUIT

1,600

GRILLED CHICKEN SANDWICH: Try Wendy's Grilled Chicken, McDonald's Chicken McGrill, or KFC Honey BBQ—all without mayo. TIP Skip Burger King and Arby's; they're too high in calories. Dress bun with ketchup, mustard, lettuce, and tomato.

SIDE SALAD: Drizzle 1 tablespoon low-fat dressing (about ⅓ of most packets) over salad.

1 ORANGE OR OTHER FRUIT

SNACK

1,400

FAT-FREE LATTE: 12 ounces regular or decaf

GRAHAM CRACKERS: 1 rectangle

1,600

FAT-FREE LATTE: 12 ounces regular or decaf

GRAHAM CRACKERS: 1 rectangle

GRAPES: 1 cup

ALMONDS OR OTHER NUTS: 1 tablespoon

DINNER

1,400

SPINACH SALAD: Mix 2 cups spinach, 1 sliced hard-cooked egg, ⅓ cup canned chickpeas, 1 tablespoon dried cranberries, 1 tablespoon pistachio nuts, and 1 crumbled bacon slice (optional). Toss with a mix of ½ tablespoon olive oil, 1 teaspoon lemon juice, and ½ teaspoon Dijon mustard.

WHOLE WHEAT BREAD: 2 slices

1,600

SPINACH SALAD: Mix 2 cups spinach, 1 sliced hard-cooked egg, ⅓ cup canned chickpeas, 1 tablespoon dried cranberries, 1 tablespoon pistachio nuts, and 1 crumbled bacon slice (optional). Toss with a mix of ½ tablespoon olive oil, 1 teaspoon lemon juice, and ½ teaspoon Dijon mustard.

WHOLE WHEAT BREAD: 2 slices

TREAT

1,400

TORTILLA CHIPS: 1 ounce, or another 150-calorie treat (see page 255 for more suggestions)

1,600

TORTILLA CHIPS: 1 ounce, or another 150-calorie treat (see page 255 for more suggestions)

BREAKFAST

ENGLISH MUFFIN: 1 whole wheat English muffin, split and toasted, each half spread with 1 teaspoon butter or trans-free margarine and 1 teaspoon jam or jelly

STRAWBERRIES OR OTHER BERRIES: 1 cup

FAT-FREE MILK: 1 cup

LUNCH

GRILLED CHICKEN SANDWICH: Try Wendy's Grilled Chicken, McDonald's Chicken McGrill, or KFC Honey BBQ—all without mayo.

TIP Skip Burger King and Arby's; they're too high in calories. Dress bun with ketchup, mustard, lettuce, and tomato.

SIDE SALAD: Drizzle 1 tablespoon low-fat dressing (about ⅓ of most packets) over salad.

1 ORANGE OR OTHER FRUIT

SNACK

FAT-FREE LATTE: 12 ounces regular or decaf

GRAHAM CRACKERS: 2 rectangles

GRAPES: 1 cup

ALMONDS OR OTHER NUTS: 2 tablespoons

DINNER

SPINACH SALAD: Mix 2 cups spinach, 1 sliced hard-cooked egg, ½ cup canned chickpeas, 1 tablespoon dried cranberries, 1 table-spoon pistachio nuts, and 1 crumbled bacon slice (optional). Toss with a mix of ½ tablespoon olive oil, 1 teaspoon lemon juice, and ½ teaspoon Dijon mustard.

WHOLE WHEAT BREAD: 2 slices

TREAT

TORTILLA CHIPS: 1 ounce, or another 150-calorie treat (see page 255 for more suggestions)

Nutrition Tallies

	1,400	1,600	1,800
CALORIES	1,409	1,582	1,762
FAT (G)	47	53	60
SATURATED FAT (G)	10.6	11.3	12
PROTEIN (G)	65	68	73
CARBOHYDRATES (G)	194	224	253
DIETARY FIBER (G)	28	31	35
CHOLESTEROL (MG)	262	262	262
SODIUM (MG)	2,116	2,119	2,204
CALCIUM (MG)	948	992	1,077

Fat Buster!

Retire this bad, old dieting motto: "If only I had more willpower, I could go hungry more often." Replace it with a kinder, gentler—and more effective—one: "Great, I'm hungry, a clear signal that it *is* time to eat." Remind yourself that attempting to override or defeat your body's hunger signals is a terrible misuse of willpower. In fact, eating to hunger is a critical component of weight control.

FRIDAY

1,400	1,600
BREAKFAST	
CEREAL: 150 calories of high-fiber cereal topped with 1 cup fat-free milk, 1 cup strawberries or other fruit, and 2 table-spoons trail mix	**CEREAL:** 150 calories of high-fiber cereal topped with 1 cup fat-free milk, 1 cup strawberries or other fruit, and 2 table-spoons trail mix
TIP Check label for 5 to 8 grams of fiber per 30-gram serving.	**TIP** Check label for 5 to 8 grams of fiber per 30-gram serving.

LUNCH	
VEGGIE ROLL-UP: On an 8-inch whole wheat tortilla, place 2 slices (1 ounce each) re-duced-fat cheese, ½ cup chopped vegeta-bles (such as green pepper, radish, tomato), and 2 teaspoons reduced-calorie salad dressing. Roll up.	**VEGGIE ROLL-UP:** On an 8-inch whole wheat tortilla, place 2 slices (1 ounce each) re-duced-fat cheese, ½ cup chopped vegeta-bles (such as green pepper, radish, tomato), and 2 teaspoons reduced-calorie salad dressing. Roll up.
SALAD: 2 cups spinach and 1 cup sliced red pepper tossed with 1 tablespoon reduced-calorie dressing	**SALAD:** 2 cups spinach and 1 cup sliced red pepper tossed with 1 tablespoon reduced-calorie dressing

SNACK	
YOGURT: 8 ounces reduced-calorie flavored yogurt with no more than 120 calories	**YOGURT:** 8 ounces reduced-calorie flavored yogurt with no more than 120 calories

DINNER	
ENCHILADAS: *At Mexican restaurant,* order 1 chicken enchilada topped with a little cheese. *At home,* have 1 frozen chicken en-chilada with no more than 240 calories.	**ENCHILADAS:** *At Mexican restaurant,* order 1 chicken enchilada topped with a little cheese. *At home,* have 1 frozen chicken en-chilada with no more than 240 calories.
RICE: *At restaurant,* have ½ cup Mexican rice. *At home,* have brown rice with a little salsa mixed in.	**RICE:** *At restaurant,* have 1 cup Mexican rice. *At home,* have brown rice with a little salsa mixed in.
BEANS: *At restaurant,* have ¼ cup beans. *At home,* heat canned pinto beans and a little chopped garlic or garlic salt; mash about half of the beans.	**BEANS:** *At restaurant,* have ½ cup beans. *At home,* heat canned pinto beans and a little chopped garlic or garlic salt; mash about half of the beans.
SALAD: 2 cups mixed greens with 2 tea-spoons dressing	**SALAD:** 2 cups mixed greens with 2 tea-spoons dressing
	GUACAMOLE: 2 tablespoons

TREAT	
LIGHT POPCORN: 5 cups, or another 100- to 110-calorie treat (see page 254 for sugges-tions)	**LIGHT POPCORN:** 5 cups, or another 100- to 110-calorie treat (see page 254 for sugges-tions)

1,800

BREAKFAST

CEREAL: 150 calories of high-fiber cereal topped with 1 cup fat-free milk, 1 cup strawberries or other fruit, and 2 tablespoons trail mix

TIP Check label for 5 to 8 grams of fiber per 30-gram serving.

LUNCH

VEGGIE ROLL-UP: On an 8-inch whole wheat tortilla, place 2 slices (1 ounce each) reduced-fat cheese, ½ cup chopped vegetables (such as green pepper, radish, tomato), and 2 teaspoons reduced-calorie salad dressing. Roll up.

SALAD: 2 cups spinach and 1 cup sliced red pepper tossed with 1 tablespoon reduced-calorie dressing

SNACK

YOGURT: 8 ounces reduced-calorie flavored yogurt with no more than 120 calories

DINNER

ENCHILADAS: *At Mexican restaurant,* order 2 chicken enchiladas topped with a little cheese. *At home,* have 2 frozen chicken enchiladas with no more than 240 calories each.

RICE: *At restaurant,* have 1 cup Mexican rice. *At home,* have brown rice with a little salsa mixed in.

BEANS: *At restaurant,* have ½ cup beans. *At home,* heat canned pinto beans and a little chopped garlic or garlic salt; mash about half of the beans.

SALAD: 2 cups mixed greens with 2 teaspoons dressing

GUACAMOLE: 2 tablespoons

TREAT

LIGHT POPCORN: 5 cups, or another 100- to 110-calorie treat (see page 254 for suggestions)

Nutrition Tallies

	1,400	1,600	1,800
CALORIES	1,370	1,577	1,817
FAT (G)	37	42	53
SATURATED FAT (G)	12.4	13.2	17.7
PROTEIN (G)	68	74	87
CARBOHYDRATES (G)	196	231	255
DIETARY FIBER (G)	35	39	43
CHOLESTEROL (MG)	78	78	114
SODIUM (MG)	2,227	2,668	2,930
CALCIUM (MG)	1,372	1,404	1,611

Nutrient Booster!

THAT BAG OF SPINACH you're chomping through this week is doing wonders for your body. It has powerful antioxidants called lutein and zeaxanthin. They help protect your eyes from cataracts and macular degeneration, which is the leading cause of blindness. Spinach is also rich in folate, a B vitamin that helps prevent birth defects and may also guard against heart disease.

SATURDAY

1,400	1,600
BREAKFAST	
BAGEL: ½ large (3½- to 4-ounce) oat bran or whole wheat bagel with 1 teaspoon butter or trans-free margarine and 2 teaspoons jam or jelly	**BAGEL:** 1 large (3½- to 4-ounce) oat bran or whole wheat bagel with 1 tablespoon butter or trans-free margarine and 2 teaspoons jam or jelly
FRUIT SALAD: 1 cup (your choice of fruit)	**FRUIT SALAD:** 1 cup (your choice of fruit)
FAT-FREE MILK: 1 cup	**FAT-FREE MILK:** 1 cup
LUNCH	
VEGGIE BURGER: Cook 1 vegetable burger (about 120 calories) according to package directions. Place in a whole wheat bun with 1 teaspoon low-fat mayo, 1 teaspoon mustard, tomato slices, and lettuce.	**VEGGIE BURGER:** Cook 1 vegetable burger (about 120 calories) according to package directions. Place in a whole wheat bun with 1 teaspoon low-fat mayo, 1 teaspoon mustard, tomato slices, and lettuce.
CRUDITÉS: 1 cup (such as radishes, green or red peppers, carrots)	**CRUDITÉS:** 1 cup (such as radishes, green or red peppers, carrots)
SNACK	
HOT OR COLD CHOCOLATE MILK: 1 cup fat-free milk with 2 teaspoons chocolate syrup	**HOT OR COLD CHOCOLATE MILK:** 1 cup fat-free milk with 2 teaspoons chocolate syrup
DINNER	
GRILLED SALMON: 4 ounces	**GRILLED SALMON:** 4 ounces
NEW POTATOES: ½ cup, with 1 teaspoon butter or trans-free margarine, 1 teaspoon chopped parsley, salt, and pepper	**NEW POTATOES:** ½ cup, with 1 teaspoon butter or trans-free margarine, 1 teaspoon chopped parsley, salt, and pepper
SAUTÉED SPINACH: See recipe on page 394.	**SAUTÉED SPINACH:** See recipe on page 394.
WINE: 4 ounces or another ½ cup potatoes	**WINE:** 4 ounces or another ½ cup potatoes
TREAT	
STRAWBERRY SHORTCAKE: Top a thin slice of pound cake (¹⁄₁₀ of a 10½-ounce loaf such as Sara Lee frozen pound cake) with ¼ cup vanilla light ice cream or frozen yogurt and ½ cup strawberries.	**STRAWBERRY SHORTCAKE:** Top a thin slice of pound cake (¹⁄₁₀ of a 10½-ounce loaf such as Sara Lee frozen pound cake) with ¼ cup vanilla light ice cream or frozen yogurt and ½ cup strawberries.

1,800

BREAKFAST

BAGEL: 1 large (3½- to 4-ounce) oat bran or whole wheat bagel with 1 tablespoon butter or trans-free margarine and 2 teaspoons jam or jelly

FRUIT SALAD: 1 cup (your choice of fruit)

FAT-FREE MILK: 1 cup

LUNCH

VEGGIE BURGER: Cook 1 vegetable burger (about 120 calories) according to package directions. Melt 1 slice reduced-fat Cheddar on burger and place in a whole wheat bun with 1 teaspoon low-fat mayo, 1 teaspoon mustard, tomato slices, and lettuce.

CRUDITÉS: 1 cup (such as radishes, green or red peppers, carrots)

SNACK

HOT OR COLD CHOCOLATE MILK: 1 cup fat-free milk with 2 teaspoons chocolate syrup

DINNER

GRILLED SALMON: 4 ounces

NEW POTATOES: ½ cup, with 1 teaspoon butter or trans-free margarine, 1 teaspoon chopped parsley, salt, and pepper

SAUTÉED SPINACH: See recipe on page 394.

WINE: 4 ounces or another ½ cup potatoes

TREAT

STRAWBERRY SHORTCAKE: Top a thin slice of pound cake (⅒ of a 10½-ounce loaf such as Sara Lee frozen pound cake) with ¾ cup vanilla light ice cream or frozen yogurt and ½ cup strawberries.

Nutrition Tallies

	1,400	1,600	1,800
CALORIES	1,419	1,631	1,811
FAT (G)	43	52	60
SATURATED FAT (G)	13.1	16	21
PROTEIN (G)	69	75	86
CARBOHYDRATES (G)	181	211	230
DIETARY FIBER (G)	18	20	20
CHOLESTEROL (MG)	180	189	214
SODIUM (MG)	1,749	2,118	2,335
CALCIUM (MG)	946	956	1,256

SUNDAY

1,400	1,600
BREAKFAST	
EGG BURRITO: Scramble ½ cup egg substitute (or 1 egg and 1 egg white) in a non-stick skillet with 1 teaspoon trans-free margarine, butter, canola oil, or olive oil. Place in a warm tortilla (preferably whole wheat) with 2 tablespoons shredded reduced-fat Cheddar and 1 to 2 tablespoons salsa.	**EGG BURRITO:** Scramble ½ cup egg substitute (or 1 egg and 1 egg white) in a non-stick skillet with 1 teaspoon trans-free margarine, butter, canola oil, or olive oil. Place in a warm tortilla (preferably whole wheat) with 2 tablespoons shredded reduced-fat Cheddar and 1 to 2 tablespoons salsa.
FAT-FREE MILK: 1 cup	**FAT-FREE MILK:** 1 cup
	1 ORANGE
LUNCH	
SOUP: 1¼ cups lentil, black bean, or other bean soup cooked with 2 cups spinach just until the spinach wilts	**SOUP:** 1¼ cups lentil, black bean, or other bean soup cooked with 2 cups spinach just until the spinach wilts
WHOLE GRAIN BREAD: 1 slice	**WHOLE GRAIN BREAD:** 1 slice
SNACK	
STRAWBERRY-BANANA SMOOTHIE: In a blender, process until smooth 1 small ripe banana, ½ cup strawberries, ½ cup fat-free milk, ½ cup low-fat plain yogurt, 2 teaspoons honey, and 1 or 2 ice cubes.	**STRAWBERRY-BANANA SMOOTHIE:** In a blender, process until smooth 1 small ripe banana, ½ cup strawberries, ½ cup fat-free milk, ½ cup low-fat plain yogurt, 2 teaspoons honey, and 1 or 2 ice cubes.
DINNER	
THAI CHICKEN CURRY: See recipe on page 401.	**THAI CHICKEN CURRY:** See recipe on page 401.
RICE: ½ cup cooked brown or white jasmine or basmati rice	**RICE:** ½ cup cooked brown or white jasmine or basmati rice
COOL CUCUMBER SALAD: Mix ½ teaspoon vinegar and a pinch of sugar. Toss with ½ cup thinly sliced cucumber.	**COOL CUCUMBER SALAD:** Mix ½ teaspoon vinegar and a pinch of sugar. Toss with ½ cup thinly sliced cucumber.
TREAT	
JELL-O: ¾ cup, or another 100-calorie treat, such as 12 ounces light beer (see page 254 for more suggestions)	**JELL-O:** ¾ cup, or another 100-calorie treat, such as 12 ounces light beer (see page 254 for more suggestions)

BREAKFAST

EGG BURRITO: Scramble ½ cup egg substitute (or 1 egg and 1 egg white) in a nonstick skillet with 1 teaspoon trans-free margarine, butter, canola oil, or olive oil. Place in a warm tortilla (preferably whole wheat) with 2 tablespoons shredded reduced-fat Cheddar and 1 to 2 tablespoons salsa.

FAT-FREE MILK: 1 cup

1 ORANGE

LUNCH

SOUP: 1¼ cups lentil, black bean, or other bean soup cooked with 2 cups spinach just until the spinach wilts

WHOLE GRAIN BREAD: 1 slice

SNACK

STRAWBERRY-BANANA SMOOTHIE: In a blender, process until smooth 1 small ripe banana, ½ cup strawberries, ½ cup fat-free milk, ½ cup low-fat plain yogurt, 1 tablespoon honey, and 1 or 2 ice cubes.

DINNER

THAI CHICKEN CURRY: See recipe on page 401.

RICE: 1 cup cooked brown or white jasmine or basmati rice

COOL CUCUMBER SALAD: Mix ½ teaspoon vinegar and a pinch of sugar. Toss with ½ cup thinly sliced cucumber.

TREAT

JELL-O: ¾ cup, or another 100-calorie treat, such as 12 ounces light beer (see page 254 for more suggestions)

Nutrition Tallies

	1,400	1,600	1,800
CALORIES	1,425	1,627	1,751
FAT (G)	27	36	37
SATURATED FAT (G)	10.8	12.4	12.4
PROTEIN (G)	87	90	93
CARBOHYDRATES (G)	193	222	250
DIETARY FIBER (G)	25	29	30
CHOLESTEROL (MG)	194	194	194
SODIUM (MG)	2,515	2,775	2,776
CALCIUM (MG)	1,058	1,132	1,140

Nutrient Booster!

HOT CHILE PEPPER is what gives Thai curry paste—an ingredient in tonight's curry—its heat. A compound called capsaicin makes hot peppers sizzle. This compound reduces inflammation, which helps out people with arthritis, and it also helps prevent clogged arteries. By making the blood less sticky, it lowers the risk for dangerous blood clots.

CHAPTER 15

THE SHRINK YOUR FEMALE FAT ZONES DIET
WEEK 6

Identify and Change Behaviors

You come in from work and head straight to the freezer. Before you know it, you've polished off the entire pint of ice cream. (Don't worry; I do it, too— once in a while.) Or you told yourself you'd have just one slice of pizza but ended up eating three slices.

What makes us do it? For me, personally, it's all about soothing myself, when I'm busy traveling or working hard. When I finally get a chance to sit down to a meal, I feel like overeating, telling myself, "I deserve this."

What we need to do is switch this around. We *deserve* to give ourselves a 10-minute walk around the block, something that supports all the hard work we're doing to stay healthy and slim. Let's treat ourselves better.

This week, you'll find out why you may overeat, and how you can stop that feeling in its tracks and tell yourself, "I've been good, and now this healthy meal (or walk or thought) is just for *me*."

Why You Eat When You're Not Hungry

Overeating and bingeing are often a response to stress, anxiety, and even elation. Food is soothing, calming, and—at least in the short term—a way to cope. And once we find an easy coping mechanism, it becomes hard to part with it. Often, we don't understand the source of our stress or anxiety. We usually don't stop before bingeing and ask ourselves, "Why am I heading for the ice cream?"

But this week, you're going to do just that. You're going to ask yourself a few questions before—and after—you overeat. You may not figure it out every time, but you'll notice some interesting patterns. Your tool: the Feelings Log.

As you'll see, this looks just like last week's Hunger Record, with one important addition: a column to record feelings, thoughts, and situations surrounding the overeating. You'll also be tracking hunger again, to make sure that the overeating didn't spring from "overhunger." After filling out the Feelings Log, you'll get a handle on the mindless eating that can sabotage all the hard work—and very mind*ful* eating and exercising—you're doing.

Stress and Belly Fat

Is your belly your fat zone? If so, you need to pay particular attention to any stressful situations recorded in this week's Feelings Log. Studies show that women who are most affected by stress have bigger bellies. In a series of fascinating studies at the University of California at San Francisco, researchers exposed women to various stressful situations, like impossibly time-pressured tests and public speaking. Women—both thin and overweight—with more abdominal fat had a much tougher time coping with the stressful situations than women with other types of body shapes. Women with more belly fat also reported more work and financial stress, scored lower in self-esteem questionnaires, and had more pessimistic outlooks.

> **WEEKLY CHECK-IN:** Now it's really time to celebrate! You can congratulate yourself for finishing another full week on the Shrink Your Female Fat Zones plan—with only one to go! Whether you're getting on the scale, trying on that pair of pants, or using the measuring tape, make a note of how your body changed this week. Write your results in your daily log (page 412).

How does stress go to your gut? It's probably because of the stress hormone cortisol. In the University of California experiments, bigger-bellied women secreted lots more cortisol than women with flatter stomachs. Cortisol triggers the body to deposit abdominal fat.

Cortisol may also trigger overeating, especially of sweets. In other experiments, the same University of California researchers found that "cortisol reactors"—those women whose cortisol shot up when exposed to a stressful situation—ate more after the experiments than women who didn't secrete much cortisol. The favorite type of snack? Sweets!

Belly fat isn't just a cosmetic issue. It puts you at risk for heart disease and diabetes. To find out if your belly is putting you at risk, get out a measuring tape. If your waist is more than 35 inches, you may be at risk.

We all know that mental health is very important for physical health. And now we know, without a doubt, that *feeling* good can be very good for you—and your waistline. After you fill out your Feelings Log this week, I'll give you instruction on how to pinpoint—and remove—stress from your life.

Pay Attention to Your Feelings

Just as you did last week, you'll keep track of meals, the time you ate, and your hunger rating. Take out your notebook from last week. (You'll also find a condensed version on page 412 of your Fat Zone Workbook.) This time, you'll fill out one more column: Feelings/Situation. Here's how.

1. Count all food—both meals and snacks. If you ate pretty much what was on the plan, you can just scribble down: breakfast, lunch, dinner, snack, and treat. But please write down all the foods not on the plan. This is valuable information for attacking emotional eating. Also, if you skipped part of the meal, write that down as well.

2. Record the time you ate, as precisely as possible.

3. At each meal, rate your hunger from 1 to 5 (1 = not at all hungry; 2 = a little hungry; 3 = hungry; 4 = very hungry; 5 = ravenous).

4. Before or after each meal or snack, write down how you're feeling. Sometimes, it's hard to name a feeling. Here are some descriptions that might help: uncomfortable, angry, helpless, overburdened, unappreciated, unattractive, bored, stressed-out, in pain, numb, frustrated, depressed, lonely, out of control, guilty, happy, overjoyed, hopeful, passionate, excited, in love, peaceful. Notice that both happy and unhappy emotions can trigger overeating!

5. Write down the place and situation surrounding the meal or snack. For instance: at your desk, at a meeting, in the kitchen, after the bus picked up your child, on the phone in the kitchen, after speaking to your mother, after your boss came into your office. Even if you can't always identify the emotion, you can link certain situations with overeating.

Here's a sample day.

Your Feelings Log (sample)			
FRIDAY			
MEAL	TIME OF DAY	HUNGER RATING	FEELINGS/SITUATION
Breakfast, minus the fruit	7:30 A.M.	2	Rushed/in the kitchen
Lunch	12:00 noon	4	Happy/at the deli
Snack, candy bar	1:30 P.M.	1	Frustrated/on a conference call for an hour, behind on my work
Snack	3:00 P.M.	2	Okay/at Starbucks
Dinner	7:30 P.M.	3	Rushed but happy/at home
Treat, 2 cups of ice cream instead of 1	9:00 P.M.	3	On the phone with a friend/ in the kitchen
Treat, another cup of ice cream	11:00 P.M.	1	Lonely/watching the news on TV

Now create your own Feelings Log.

Make Overeating Connections

Your record holds important clues to why you overeat. Here's how to put the pieces together.

1. Go through the records and circle each time you overate when your hunger rating was 3 or below (not very hungry).

2. For each circled meal or snack, look at the Feelings/Situation column. What was going on?

3. Identify patterns. Do you tend to overeat in the evenings? When you're stressed-out at work? Whenever you feel bored, lonely, or any other type of emotion?

4. Go back over week 5's hunger record and circle each time you overate with hunger ratings of 3 or below. Do you see any correlations with this week? For instance, was night bingeing a problem both weeks?

Conquer Cravings and Overeating

Now that you've identified certain situations or emotions that trigger overeating, you can work on changing them. Some changes will be easy, like talking on the phone in your bedroom instead of in the kitchen. But if you're stuffing yourself to numb the pain of a divorce, to quell the frustration of an abusive boss, or to deal with other deeper issues, you have more work ahead. Here's how to start.

1. Identify what you *really* need. Before you take a third helping or head to the vending machine when you're really not hungry, take a minute to ask yourself: "What do I really need right now?" Maybe it's someone to talk to, a short break from work, to face something you've been putting off, or any number of other things. Even if you wind up eating, you've helped yourself by learning something about your needs.

2. Deal with one issue at a time. For instance, if you're putting away a few candy bars at work and overeating in the evening, pick either the candy bar problem *or* the night eating. Give yourself weeks or months to deal with it before moving on to the next issue. Since problems are often related, solving one may get rid of the other.

3. Don't go hungry. Remember, skipping meals or skimping on food triggers overeating and bingeing, particularly at night.

> "When **tension hits,** take a **stretch** break—you deserve to feel good!"

1,400 CALORIES: 24% calories from fat, 21% protein, 55% carbohydrates
1,600 CALORIES: 25% calories from fat, 21% protein, 54% carbohydrates
1,800 CALORIES: 27% calories from fat, 20% protein, 53% carbohydrates

4. Reduce stress. Here are some of the ways I've found that work for me.

- Start pinpointing specific causes of stress: a long commute, high rent, an overly demanding person, or any other sources.

- Think of ways of changing or alleviating the situation, such as ending a relationship that's negative. Be around more positive people; it helps.

- Keep exercising. Tons of research shows that exercise is a great stress buster. And if your stress is depression-linked, a number of studies show exercise to be about as effective as antidepressant medication.

- Learn to relax. Most yoga classes and my yoga videos teach you how to completely relax your body and mind. Set the stage for your relaxation by creating a quiet environment. Turn off the TV and radio, unplug the phone, and play soothing music from artists such as Enya. Dim or turn off the lights.

> "Whenever I feel the urge to binge, I try to remember that nothing tastes as good as being fit feels."

■ Set aside time for a vacation and for activities that bring you joy.

■ Tune in to your negative thoughts and start replacing them with positive ones. Replace a thought like "This project is too overwhelming . . . I'll never get through it" with "I'll tackle this project one step at a time and complete it successfully."

■ Keep a sense of humor. Did you know that laughing is a great way to tone your ab muscles? There is nothing better than a good laugh. That's one of the best things about my husband—he's funny and keeps us laughing. So enjoy someone's sense of humor—even if it's your own. I chuckle at myself all the time. Life is fun; enjoy it. Put a smile on your face!

5. Tackle emotional issues. Many people overeat as a distraction from unpleasant or painful feelings, some dating back to childhood traumas. If you're in emotional pain or very anxious, don't hesitate to get counseling. Sometimes, even a few sessions can help tremendously. Or do what I do—call up a friend or family member. I call my sisters and brother whenever I get the slightest bit down, especially to talk about Mom, who passed away 2 years ago. Losing someone is a perfect example of a time when you need support. I talk to one of my three sisters or my brother every day. It's been so therapeutic . . . and much better for me than reaching for the chips!

SHOPPING LIST

CHECK YOUR FRIDGE and cupboards. Much of this food might still be there from last week. There are no portions listed, because these depend on how many people are in your family. So just go through the menu plan and note how much of everything you'll need.

If you don't like something, substitute with as close an equivalent as you can find. For instance, have plums instead of peaches or a skinless chicken thigh instead of a chicken breast. But don't substitute white flour products (like white bread) when whole grain products (like whole wheat bread) are called for. Whole grains are important weight-loss tools.

FRESH FRUIT

Apples

Bananas

Berries (such as blueberries, raspberries, strawberries, or blackberries)

Kiwifruit or other fruit

Lemons

Mangoes (for 1,600- and 1,800-calorie plans)

Melon, cantaloupe or honeydew

Oranges

Peaches (If not in season, use those canned in juice or light syrup.)

Plums (for 1,600- and 1,800-calorie plans)

FRESH VEGETABLES AND HERBS

Basil or dill (Don't buy if you're using parsley in dinner on Thursday.)

Broccoli

Carrots

Cauliflower

Celery

Cucumbers

Garlic

Greens, mixed

Lettuce (You can use mixed greens instead.)

Mushrooms, portobello and white button, cremini, or shiitake

Onions

Parsley

Potatoes, new, red, or Yukon Gold

Scallions

Spinach (For convenience, buy bags of prewashed spinach.)

Tarragon (If fresh herb is unavailable, use dried.)

Tomatoes

Zucchini (Don't buy if you're getting pizza delivered or buying a frozen one for dinner on Friday.)

CANNED AND BOTTLED GOODS

Beans, chili (unflavored) or pinto, canned, with about 150 milligrams or less of sodium per ½ cup (such as Westbrae brand)

Chicken broth, reduced-sodium, canned

Chickpeas, canned (Don't buy if you're going to a salad bar for lunch on Tuesday.)

Enchilada sauce

Honey

Jam or jelly

Lemon juice

Marinara sauce

Mayonnaise, low-fat

Mustard, Dijon

Oil, olive

Peanut butter

Pickles (Don't buy if you're eating lunch out on Monday.)

Pizza sauce (Don't buy if you're getting pizza delivered or buying a frozen one for dinner on Friday.)

Salad dressing, reduced-calorie Italian or vinaigrette

Salad dressing, regular Italian or vinaigrette (for 1,800-calorie plan only)

Salsa

Soup, lentil (such as Progresso)

Syrup, chocolate

Syrup, maple or maple-flavored

Tomatoes, diced, canned

Tuna, water-packed (Don't buy if you're going to a salad bar for lunch on Tuesday.)

Vinegar, balsamic

DRY GOODS AND BREAD

Almonds

Bread, whole wheat sandwich loaf, with no more than 90

calories and at least 2 grams of fiber per slice

Brownies

Buns, whole wheat hamburger, with no more than 120 calories per bun

Cereal, high-fiber, with 5 to 8 grams of fiber per 30-gram serving (such as Kellogg's Complete Wheat Bran Flakes or Kashi Good Friends)

Cereal, oatmeal (plain, unflavored)

Chili powder

Cinnamon

Couscous, whole wheat (found in bulk in natural food stores and in boxes, such as Fantastic Foods)

Crackers, graham (for 1,600- and 1,800-calorie plans)

Muffins, bran (Don't buy if you're having breakfast at a deli on Thursday.)

Muffins, English, whole wheat or oat bran

Pine nuts

Pizza crust, Boboli Original (Don't buy if you're getting pizza delivered or buying a frozen one for dinner on Friday.)

Rice, brown (such as Texmati, basmati, or quick-cooking Uncle Ben's)

Rice, wild

Rosemary

Seeds, sunflower (for 1,600- and 1,800-calorie plans)

Trail mix

REFRIGERATED FOODS

Butter or trans-free margarine

Cheese, Parmesan

Cheese, part-skim mozzarella (Don't buy if you're getting pizza delivered or buying a frozen one for dinner on Friday.)

Cheese, reduced-fat (such as Cabot 50% Light Cheddar, Tine 75% Jarlsberg, or Kraft or Borden 2% Singles)

Cottage cheese, 1% or 2% (for 1,800-calorie plan only)

Eggs (Don't buy if you're going to a salad bar for lunch on Tuesday.)

Milk, fat-free (If you haven't adjusted to fat-free milk, buy 1% or mix equal parts 1% and 2%. Your calorie level will be a little higher, but you can gradually train your tastebuds to like fat-free. If you're lactose intolerant, try Lactaid milk. If you prefer soy milk—low-fat or fat-free—buy calcium-fortified with at least 25% of the Daily Value of calcium per cup.)

Tofu, firm

Tortellini, cheese (such as Buitoni)

Tortillas, corn, 6-inch diameter, with about 84 calories for 2

Yogurt, low-fat fruit, with about 210 calories per 8 ounces (for 1,800-calorie plan only)

Yogurt, low-fat plain

Yogurt, reduced-calorie flavored, with no more than 120 calories per 8 ounces

MEAT, POULTRY, AND FISH

Chicken, boneless and skinless breasts or precooked Perdue Short Cuts or Louis Rich strips

Ham, lean

Tuna, steaks

Turkey, breast, lean (Don't buy if you're going to Subway or getting ham for lunch on Monday.)

Turkey, ground

FROZEN FOODS

Ice cream or frozen yogurt, light, with no more than 110 calories per ½ cup (such as Breyers, Edy's, or Dreyer's)

Peas

Pizza, vegetarian (Don't buy if you're getting takeout pizza or making your own on Friday.)

Vegetable burgers, with about 120 calories per burger (such as Gardenburgers)

Waffles, whole grain toaster waffles, with about 170 calories for 2 (such as Nutri-Grain Multibran)

OPTIONAL

Beer, light

Treats (see Tuesday, Wednesday, Friday, Saturday, and Sunday)

Wine

MONDAY

1,400	1,600

BREAKFAST

CEREAL: 150 calories of high-fiber cereal topped with 1 cup fat-free milk, 1 cup berries or sliced fruit, and 2 tablespoons trail mix

> **TIP** Check label for 5 to 8 grams of fiber per 30-gram serving.

CEREAL: 150 calories of high-fiber cereal topped with 1 cup fat-free milk, 1 cup berries or sliced fruit, and 2 tablespoons trail mix

> **TIP** Check label for 5 to 8 grams of fiber per 30-gram serving.

LUNCH

HAM AND CHEESE (OR TURKEY AND CHEESE) SUB: *At Subway:* Choose any of these Subway 6-inch "7 Under 6" sandwiches: ham, turkey breast, or turkey breast and ham, with cheese, lettuce, tomato, pickles, or other vegetables. *At home:* Stuff a whole wheat hamburger bun with 2 slices lean ham or turkey breast and 1 slice reduced-fat cheese. Add lettuce, tomato, pickles, and any other vegetables.

SALAD: *At Subway:* Have the Veggie Delight salad. *At home:* Have 2 cups mixed greens with 1 tablespoon reduced-calorie dressing.

HAM AND CHEESE (OR TURKEY AND CHEESE) SUB: *At Subway:* Choose any of these Subway 6-inch "7 Under 6" sandwiches: ham, turkey breast, or turkey breast and ham, with cheese, lettuce, tomato, pickles, or other vegetables. *At home:* Stuff a whole wheat hamburger bun with 2 slices lean ham or turkey breast and 1 slice reduced-fat cheese. Add lettuce, tomato, pickles, and any other vegetables.

SALAD: *At Subway:* Have the Veggie Delight salad. *At home:* Have 2 cups mixed greens with 1 tablespoon reduced-calorie dressing.

1 ORANGE OR OTHER FRUIT

SNACK

YOGURT: 8 ounces reduced-calorie flavored yogurt with no more than 120 calories

YOGURT: 8 ounces reduced-calorie flavored yogurt with no more than 120 calories

10 ALMONDS: Have this or 1 tablespoon other nut.

DINNER

CHEESE TORTELLINI WITH MARINARA SAUCE: ¾ cup cheese-filled tortellini topped with ⅓ to ½ cup marinara sauce

BROCCOLI: 1 cup, steamed, with a spritz of lemon juice

CHEESE TORTELLINI WITH MARINARA SAUCE: 1 cup cheese-filled tortellini topped with ⅓ to ½ cup marinara sauce

BROCCOLI: 1 cup, steamed, with a spritz of lemon juice

TREAT

BROWNIE SUNDAE: Top 1 small (2 × 3-inch) brownie with ½ cup light ice cream or frozen yogurt and 1 to 2 teaspoons chocolate syrup.

BROWNIE SUNDAE: Top 1 small (2 × 3-inch) brownie with ½ cup light ice cream or frozen yogurt and 1 to 2 teaspoons chocolate syrup.

BREAKFAST

CEREAL: 150 calories of high-fiber cereal topped with 1 cup fat-free milk, 1 cup berries or sliced fruit, and 2 tablespoons trail mix

TIP Check label for 5 to 8 grams of fiber per 30-gram serving.

LUNCH

HAM AND CHEESE (OR TURKEY AND CHEESE) SUB: *At Subway:* Choose any of these Subway 6-inch "7 Under 6" sandwiches: ham, turkey breast, or turkey breast and ham, with cheese, lettuce, tomato, pickles, or other vegetables. *At home:* Stuff a whole wheat hamburger bun with 2 slices lean ham or turkey breast and 1 slice reduced-fat cheese. Add lettuce, tomato, pickles, and any other vegetables.

SALAD: *At Subway:* Have the Veggie Delight salad. *At home:* Have 2 cups mixed greens with 1 tablespoon reduced-calorie dressing.

1 ORANGE OR OTHER FRUIT

SNACK

YOGURT: 8 ounces low-fat fruit yogurt with no more than 210 calories

20 ALMONDS: Have this or 2 tablespoons other nut.

DINNER

CHEESE TORTELLINI WITH MARINARA SAUCE: 1 cup cheese-filled tortellini topped with $\frac{1}{3}$ to $\frac{1}{2}$ cup marinara sauce

BROCCOLI: 1 cup, steamed, with a spritz of lemon juice

TREAT

BROWNIE SUNDAE: Top 1 small (2 × 3-inch) brownie with $\frac{1}{2}$ cup light ice cream or frozen yogurt and 1 to 2 teaspoons chocolate syrup.

Nutrition Tallies

	1,400	1,600	1,800
CALORIES	1,428	1,632	1,781
FAT (G)	38	45	52
SATURATED FAT (G)	12.7	14.1	15.5
PROTEIN (G)	66	73	77
CARBOHYDRATES (G)	226	256	276
DIETARY FIBER (G)	27	32	34
CHOLESTEROL (MG)	120	137	145
SODIUM (MG)	2,761	2,876	2,886
CALCIUM (MG)	1,075	1,187	1,264

people ask me . . .

"Why am I good all day, then overeat at night?"

You're not alone. Nighttime is prime time for bingeing. One culprit: skipping breakfast. Your body demands those calories later on, when you're too tired to make yourself a proper meal. Instead, you grab crackers, cookies, ice cream, and other foods.

You're still digesting that food in the morning, so you're not hungry for breakfast, setting up a vicious cycle. So eat breakfast, eat enough the rest of the day, and get out of the kitchen after dinner! If you're truly hungry, have a piece of fruit and 4 ounces of yogurt or fat-free milk.

Also, new research shows that eating in dim light encourages overeating in dieters. So if you do eat at night, turn up the lights.

TUESDAY

	1,400	1,600
BREAKFAST	**ENGLISH MUFFIN:** 1 whole wheat or oat bran English muffin, split and toasted, spread with 2 teaspoons butter or trans-free margarine and 1 tablespoon jam or jelly **FAT-FREE MILK:** 1 cup **1 ORANGE OR OTHER FRUIT**	**ENGLISH MUFFIN:** 1 whole wheat or oat bran English muffin, split and toasted, spread with 2 teaspoons butter or trans-free margarine and 1 tablespoon jam or jelly **FAT-FREE MILK:** 1 cup **1 ORANGE OR OTHER FRUIT**
LUNCH	**SUPER SPINACH SALAD:** At home or the salad bar, combine 2 cups spinach or other salad greens, 1 cup sliced vegetables or grated carrots, ½ cup canned chick-peas, ¼ cup water-packed tuna, 2 tablespoons chopped egg, and 2 tablespoons reduced-calorie dressing. **WHOLE GRAIN BREAD:** 1 slice	**SUPER SPINACH SALAD:** At home or the salad bar, combine 2 cups spinach or other salad greens, 1 cup sliced vegetables or grated carrots, ½ cup canned chick-peas, ¼ cup water-packed tuna, 2 tablespoons chopped egg, and 2 tablespoons reduced-calorie dressing **SUNFLOWER SEEDS:** 2 tablespoons **WHOLE GRAIN BREAD:** 2 slices
SNACK	**FAT-FREE LATTE:** 8 ounces regular or decaf	**FAT-FREE LATTE:** 8 ounces regular or decaf **GRAHAM CRACKERS:** 1 rectangle
DINNER	**WILD RICE, PEAS, AND CHICKEN:** See recipe on page 402.	**WILD RICE, PEAS, AND CHICKEN:** See recipe on page 402.
TREAT	**JELL-O:** ¾ cup, or another 100-calorie treat (see page 254 for more suggestions)	**JELL-O:** ¾ cup, or another 100-calorie treat (see page 254 for more suggestions)

1,800

BREAKFAST

ENGLISH MUFFIN: 1 whole wheat or oat bran English muffin, split and toasted, spread with 2 teaspoons butter or trans-free margarine and 1 tablespoon jam or jelly

FAT-FREE MILK: 1 cup

1 ORANGE OR OTHER FRUIT

LUNCH

SUPER SPINACH SALAD: At home or the salad bar, combine 2 cups spinach or other salad greens, 1 cup sliced vegetables or grated carrots, ½ cup canned chickpeas, ¼ cup water-packed tuna, 2 tablespoons chopped egg, and 2 tablespoons reduced-calorie dressing

SUNFLOWER SEEDS: 2 tablespoons

WHOLE GRAIN BREAD: 2 slices

SNACK

FAT-FREE LATTE: 8 ounces regular or decaf with 2 teaspoons sugar or 1 pump of flavored syrup

GRAHAM CRACKERS: 2 rectangles

DINNER

WILD RICE, PEAS, AND CHICKEN: See recipe on page 402.

TREAT

JELL-O: ¾ cup, or another 100-calorie treat (see page 254 for more suggestions)

Nutrition Tallies

	1,400	1,600	1,800
CALORIES	1,354	1,570	1,795
FAT (G)	33	44	50
SATURATED FAT (G)	7.7	9	10
PROTEIN (G)	87	94	106
CARBOHYDRATES (G)	187	214	245
DIETARY FIBER (G)	27	31	34
CHOLESTEROL (MG)	162	162	182
SODIUM (MG)	1,794	2,016	2,236
CALCIUM (MG)	947	988	1,012

Nutrient Booster!

THANKS TO THE ORANGE, spinach, and chickpeas, Tuesday is absolutely *loaded* with folate (also known as folic acid), a B vitamin that's especially important for women. Getting enough folate before and during pregnancy helps prevent birth defects. And keep well-supplied the rest of the time, because folate lowers blood levels of homocysteine. This substance, like cholesterol, puts you at risk for heart disease. Folate also helps protect you against colon cancer. Other folate-rich foods are asparagus, beets, broccoli, brussels sprouts, cauliflower, peanuts, strawberries, sunflower seeds, wheat germ, and legumes such as black beans, pinto beans, and other beans.

WEDNESDAY

1,400	1,600
BREAKFAST	
CINNAMON OATMEAL: Cook ½ cup rolled oats according to package directions, adding 1 small diced apple, 1 teaspoon maple syrup, and a dash of cinnamon. **FAT-FREE MILK:** 1 cup	**CINNAMON OATMEAL:** Cook ½ cup rolled oats according to package directions, adding 1 teaspoon butter or trans-free margarine, 1 small diced apple, 1 teaspoon maple syrup, and a dash of cinnamon. **FAT-FREE MILK:** 1 cup
LUNCH	
PEANUT BUTTER AND JELLY SANDWICH: Spread 2 tablespoons peanut butter and 2 tablespoons jelly or jam on 2 slices whole wheat bread. **FAT-FREE MILK:** 1 cup **CARROT AND CELERY STICKS:** 1 cup	**PEANUT BUTTER AND JELLY SANDWICH:** Spread 2 tablespoons peanut butter and 2 tablespoons jelly or jam on 2 slices whole wheat bread. **FAT-FREE MILK:** 1 cup **CARROT AND CELERY STICKS:** 1 cup
SNACK	
1 SMALL BANANA **10 ALMONDS**	**1 SMALL BANANA** **20 ALMONDS**
DINNER	
MEXICAN LASAGNA: ⅛ of casserole (recipe on page 403) **MIXED GREENS:** 2 cups, tossed with 1 tablespoon reduced-calorie dressing	**MEXICAN LASAGNA:** ⅛ of casserole (recipe on page 403) **MIXED GREENS:** 2 cups, tossed with 1 tablespoon reduced-calorie dressing
TREAT	
1 FROZEN FRUIT BAR: Have this or another 70-calorie treat (see page 254 for suggestions).	**1 FROZEN FRUIT BAR:** Have this or another 70-calorie treat (see page 254 for suggestions).

BREAKFAST

CINNAMON OATMEAL: Cook ½ cup rolled oats according to package directions, adding 1 teaspoon butter or trans-free margarine, 1 small diced apple, 1 teaspoon maple syrup, and a dash of cinnamon.

FAT-FREE MILK: 1 cup

LOW-FAT COTTAGE CHEESE: ½ cup

LUNCH

PEANUT BUTTER AND JELLY SANDWICH: Spread 2 tablespoons peanut butter and 2 tablespoons jelly or jam on 2 slices whole wheat bread.

FAT-FREE MILK: 1 cup

CARROT AND CELERY STICKS: 1 cup

SNACK

1 SMALL BANANA

20 ALMONDS

DINNER

MEXICAN LASAGNA: ⅛ of casserole (recipe on page 403)

MIXED GREENS: 2 cups, tossed with 1 tablespoon reduced-calorie dressing

TREAT

15 JUNIOR MINTS: Have these or another 150-calorie treat (see page 255 for suggestions).

Nutrition Tallies

	1,400	1,600	1,800
CALORIES	1,419	1,572	1,785
FAT (G)	42	55	66
SATURATED FAT (G)	9.5	10.8	15.4
PROTEIN (G)	61	66	82
CARBOHYDRATES (G)	215	220	233
DIETARY FIBER (G)	29	32	32
CHOLESTEROL (MG)	61	61	71
SODIUM (MG)	1,559	1,560	2,035
CALCIUM (MG)	833	871	970

people ask me . . .

"What should I do if I binge?"

Don't beat yourself up over it. Instead, use it as a valuable learning experience. Ask yourself: "Why did I overeat? What was going on in my life that triggered it? What can I do next time to avoid that situation?" Then just get up the next day and go back to your healthy eating plan. The binge is not the end of the world— it's what you do afterward that really counts!

THURSDAY

1,400	1,600

BREAKFAST

BRAN MUFFIN: 1 small or ½ large muffin

FAT-FREE MILK: 1 cup

1 ORANGE: Have this or 2 kiwifruit or other fruit

BRAN MUFFIN: 1 small or ½ large muffin

FAT-FREE MILK: 1 cup

1 ORANGE: Have this or 2 kiwifruit or other fruit

LUNCH

CHEESE AND TOMATO SANDWICH: Place 2 slices reduced-fat cheese (such as Cabot 50% Light Cheddar or part-skim mozzarella) and tomato slices on 2 slices whole wheat bread.

TIP This tastes great heated in the toaster oven.

TOMATO: Remaining portion, sliced

LENTIL SOUP: 1 cup, cooked with 1 cup spinach just until the spinach wilts

CHEESE AND TOMATO SANDWICH: Place 2 slices reduced-fat cheese (such as Cabot 50% Light Cheddar or part-skim mozzarella) and tomato slices on 2 slices whole wheat bread.

TIP This tastes great heated in the toaster oven.

TOMATO: Remaining portion, sliced

LENTIL SOUP: 1¼ cups, cooked with 1 cup spinach just until the spinach wilts

SNACK

YOGURT: 8 ounces reduced-calorie flavored yogurt with no more than 120 calories

YOGURT: 8 ounces reduced-calorie flavored yogurt with no more than 120 calories

DINNER

TOFU, MUSHROOM, AND CHICKEN RISOTTO: See recipe on page 404.

TIP Make extra plain rice for tomorrow's salad.

TOFU, MUSHROOM, AND CHICKEN RISOTTO: See recipe on page 404.

TIP Make extra plain rice for tomorrow's salad.

TREAT

LIGHT ICE CREAM OR FROZEN YOGURT: ½ cup

LIGHT ICE CREAM OR FROZEN YOGURT: ½ cup

BREAKFAST

BRAN MUFFIN: 1 small or ½ large muffin

FAT-FREE MILK: 1 cup

1 ORANGE: Have this or 2 kiwifruit or other fruit

LUNCH

CHEESE AND TOMATO SANDWICH: Place 2 slices reduced-fat cheese (such as Cabot 50% Light Cheddar or part-skim mozzarella) and tomato slices on 2 slices whole wheat bread.

> **TIP** This tastes great heated in the toaster oven.

TOMATO: Remaining portion, sliced

LENTIL SOUP: 1¼ cups, cooked with 1 cup spinach just until the spinach wilts

SNACK

YOGURT: 8 ounces low-fat fruit yogurt with no more than 210 calories

TRAIL MIX: 2 tablespoons

DINNER

TOFU, MUSHROOM, AND CHICKEN RISOTTO: See recipe on page 404.

> **TIP** Make extra plain rice for tomorrow's salad.

TREAT

LIGHT ICE CREAM OR FROZEN YOGURT: ¾ cup

Nutrition Tallies

	1,400	1,600	1,800
CALORIES	1,426	1,585	1,817
FAT (G)	39	44	53
SATURATED FAT (G)	14.8	16.3	19
PROTEIN (G)	95	101	106
CARBOHYDRATES (G)	191	216	251
DIETARY FIBER (G)	26	33	33
CHOLESTEROL (MG)	141	178	190
SODIUM (MG)	2,407	2,693	2,772
CALCIUM (MG)	1,940	2,056	2,171

Fat Buster!

Have fun when you dine with friends and family, but be extra-vigilant about how much you put in your mouth. A study done at Vanderbilt University in Nashville found that, on average, women took in 696 calories when they ate with others and described their mood as "good." Social eating in a "neutral" mood averaged 590 calories, compared with 476 calories when eating alone.

FRIDAY

1,400	1,600

BREAKFAST

CEREAL: 150 calories of high-fiber cereal topped with 1 cup fat-free milk and 1 small sliced banana

TIP Check label for 5 to 8 grams of fiber per 30-gram serving.

CEREAL: 150 calories of high-fiber cereal topped with 1 cup fat-free milk, 1 small sliced banana, and 2 tablespoons trail mix

TIP Check label for 5 to 8 grams of fiber per 30-gram serving.

LUNCH

HAM AND RICE SALAD: Combine ¾ cup cold cooked rice, 2 ounces diced lean ham, ½ cup cooked peas, 1 chopped celery rib, 1 teaspoon lemon juice, salt, and pepper.

HAM AND RICE SALAD: Combine ¾ cup cold cooked rice, 2 ounces diced lean ham, ½ cup cooked peas, 1 chopped celery rib, 1 teaspoon lemon juice, salt, and pepper.

2 PLUMS OR OTHER FRUIT

SNACK

HOT OR COLD CHOCOLATE MILK: 1 cup fat-free milk with 2 teaspoons chocolate syrup

HOT OR COLD CHOCOLATE MILK: 1 cup fat-free milk with 2 teaspoons chocolate syrup

DINNER

VEGETABLE PIZZA: Quick Veggie Pizza (recipe on page 388), 2 slices of a large pizza topped with vegetables but not meat (2 of 8 slices of a 14-inch pizza, such as Domino's Hand-Tossed), or 525 calories' worth of frozen pizza

SALAD: 2 cups mixed greens, ½ cup chopped cucumber or other vegetable, and 1 tablespoon reduced-calorie dressing

VEGETABLE PIZZA: Quick Veggie Pizza (recipe on page 388), 2 slices of a large pizza topped with vegetables but not meat (2 of 8 slices of a 14-inch pizza, such as Domino's Hand-Tossed), or 525 calories' worth of frozen pizza

SALAD: 2 cups mixed greens, ½ cup chopped cucumber or other vegetable, and 1 tablespoon reduced-calorie dressing

TREAT

PRETZELS: 1 ounce, or another 100-calorie treat, such as 12 ounces light beer (see page 254 for more suggestions)

PRETZELS: 1 ounce, or another 100-calorie treat, such as 12 ounces light beer (see page 254 for more suggestions)

1,800

BREAKFAST

CEREAL: 150 calories of high-fiber cereal topped with 1 cup fat-free milk, 1 small sliced banana, and 2 tablespoons trail mix

TIP Check label for 5 to 8 grams of fiber per 30-gram serving.

LUNCH

HAM AND RICE SALAD: Combine ¾ cup cold cooked rice, 2 ounces diced lean ham, ½ cup cooked peas, 1 chopped celery rib, 1 teaspoon lemon juice, salt, and pepper.

2 PLUMS OR OTHER FRUIT

SNACK

HOT OR COLD CHOCOLATE MILK: 1 cup fat-free milk with 2 teaspoons chocolate syrup

GRAHAM CRACKERS: 2 rectangles, each spread with ½ tablespoon peanut butter

DINNER

VEGETABLE PIZZA: Quick Veggie Pizza (recipe on page 388), 2 slices of a large pizza topped with vegetables but not meat (2 of 8 slices of a 14-inch pizza, such as Domino's Hand-Tossed), or 525 calories' worth of frozen pizza

SALAD: 2 cups mixed greens, ½ cup chopped cucumber or other vegetable, and 1 tablespoon regular dressing

TREAT

PRETZELS: 1 ounce, or another 100-calorie treat, such as 12 ounces light beer (see page 254 for more suggestions)

Nutrition Tallies

	1,400	1,600	1,800
CALORIES	1,429	1,589	1,832
FAT (G)	25	31	46
SATURATED FAT (G)	9.2	10.3	13
PROTEIN (G)	67	70	76
CARBOHYDRATES (G)	227	252	277
DIETARY FIBER (G)	23	25	27
CHOLESTEROL (MG)	71	71	71
SODIUM (MG)	2,831	2,874	3,085
CALCIUM (MG)	1,023	1,043	1,054

SATURDAY

1,400	1,600

BREAKFAST

SCRAMBLED TOFU: Crumble ⅓ cup tofu into a nonstick skillet with 1 teaspoon butter, trans-free margarine, or canola or olive oil. Add salt and pepper and scramble until heated through.

ENGLISH MUFFIN: 1 whole wheat or oat bran English muffin, split and toasted, spread with 1 teaspoon butter or trans-free margarine and 1 teaspoon jam or jelly

CANTALOUPE: 1 cup of this or other fruit

FAT-FREE MILK: 1 cup

SCRAMBLED TOFU: Crumble ⅓ cup tofu into a nonstick skillet with 1 teaspoon butter, trans-free margarine, or canola or olive oil. Add salt and pepper and scramble until heated through.

ENGLISH MUFFIN: 1 whole wheat or oat bran English muffin, split and toasted, with 1 teaspoon butter or trans-free margarine and 1 teaspoon jam or jelly

CANTALOUPE: 1 cup of this or other fruit

FAT-FREE MILK: 1 cup

LUNCH

PEANUT BUTTER AND HONEY SANDWICH: Spread 1 slice whole wheat bread with 1 tablespoon peanut butter and 1 teaspoon honey.

PEACH-BANANA SMOOTHIE: In a blender, process until smooth 1 small ripe banana, ½ cup fresh or canned (in juice or light syrup) peaches, ½ cup fat-free milk, ½ cup low-fat plain yogurt, 2 teaspoons honey, and 1 or 2 ice cubes.

PEANUT BUTTER AND HONEY SANDWICH: Spread 2 slices whole wheat bread with 2 tablespoons peanut butter and 2 teaspoons honey.

PEACH-BANANA SMOOTHIE: In a blender, process until smooth 1 small ripe banana, ½ cup fresh or canned (in juice or light syrup) peaches, ½ cup fat-free milk, ½ cup low-fat plain yogurt, 2 teaspoons honey, and 1 or 2 ice cubes.

SNACK

TRAIL MIX: 2 tablespoons

TRAIL MIX: 2 tablespoons

DINNER

SALSA CHICKEN: Place a 4-ounce skinless, boneless chicken breast on a piece of foil and top with 2 to 4 tablespoons salsa. Close foil and bake at 350°F for 30 to 40 minutes, or until the juices run clear when the meat is pierced with a sharp knife.

ROASTED POTATOES AND MUSHROOMS: See recipe on page 404.

SALSA CHICKEN: Place a 4-ounce skinless, boneless chicken breast on a piece of foil and top with 2 to 4 tablespoons salsa. Close foil and bake at 350°F for 30 to 40 minutes, or until the juices run clear when the meat is pierced with a sharp knife.

ROASTED POTATOES AND MUSHROOMS: See recipe on page 404.

TREAT

1 FUDGSICLE: Have this or another 100-calorie treat (see page 254).

1 FUDGSICLE: Have this or another 100-calorie treat (see page 254).

1,800

BREAKFAST

SCRAMBLED TOFU: Crumble ⅓ cup tofu into a nonstick skillet with 1 teaspoon butter, trans-free margarine, or canola or olive oil. Add salt and pepper. Scramble until heated through.

ENGLISH MUFFIN: 1 whole wheat or oat bran English muffin, split and toasted, with 1 teaspoon butter or trans-free margarine and 1 teaspoon jam or jelly

CANTALOUPE: 1 cup of this or other fruit

FAT-FREE MILK: 1 cup

LUNCH

PEANUT BUTTER AND HONEY SAND-WICH: Spread 2 slices whole wheat bread with 2 tablespoons peanut butter and 2 teaspoons honey.

PEACH-BANANA SMOOTHIE: In a blender, process until smooth 1 small ripe banana, ½ cup fresh or canned (in juice or light syrup) peaches, ½ cup fat-free milk, ½ cup low-fat plain yogurt, 2 teaspoons honey, and 1 or 2 ice cubes.

SNACK

TRAIL MIX: 2 tablespoons

DINNER

SALSA CHICKEN: Place a 4-ounce skinless, boneless chicken breast on a piece of foil and top with 2 to 4 tablespoons salsa. Close foil and bake at 350°F for 30 to 40 minutes, or until the juices run clear when the meat is pierced with a sharp knife.

ROASTED POTATOES AND MUSHROOMS: See recipe on page 404.

MIXED GREENS: 2 cups, tossed with 1 tablespoon regular dressing

TREAT

1 DOVE CHOCOLATE BAR: Have this or another 200-calorie treat (see page 255).

Nutrition Tallies

	1,400	1,600	1,800
CALORIES	1,412	1,627	1,766
FAT (G)	41	51	62
SATURATED FAT (G)	9.5	11.3	12.7
PROTEIN (G)	85	92	95
CARBOHYDRATES (G)	192	221	230
DIETARY FIBER (G)	20	23	26
CHOLESTEROL (MG)	89	89	93
SODIUM (MG)	1,426	1,673	1,845
CALCIUM (MG)	1,682	1,721	1,802

Nutrient Booster!

YES, YOU HAD TOFU TWICE THIS WEEK! If you can develop a taste for soy foods, you'll do your body a favor. Soy has been linked to prevention of the bone-thinning disease osteoporosis, and animal research shows it helps prevent cancer (human research isn't conclusive yet). What is certain: 25 grams of soy protein daily can reduce blood cholesterol. A half-cup of tofu has 10 grams of protein. One cup of soy milk contains about 6 grams. And ⅓ cup of roasted soy nuts is loaded with 23 grams.

SUNDAY

1,400	1,600
BREAKFAST	
WAFFLES: 2 whole grain toaster waffles topped with 1 cup berries or chopped fruit, 2 teaspoons butter or trans-free margarine, and 2 teaspoons maple syrup **TIP** Choose waffles with about 170 calories and 4 grams of fiber for 2 waffles.	**WAFFLES:** 2 whole grain toaster waffles topped with 1 cup berries or chopped fruit, 2 teaspoons butter or trans-free margarine, and 2 teaspoons maple syrup **TIP** Choose waffles with about 170 calories and 4 grams of fiber for 2 waffles.
FAT-FREE MILK: 1 cup	**FAT-FREE MILK:** 1 cup
LUNCH	
VEGGIE BURGER: Cook 1 vegetable burger (about 120 calories) according to package directions. Melt 1 slice (1 ounce) reduced-fat cheese on top and place in 1 whole wheat bun with 1 teaspoon low-fat mayo, mustard, tomato slices, and lettuce.	**VEGGIE BURGER:** Cook 1 vegetable burger (about 120 calories) according to package directions. Melt 1 slice (1 ounce) reduced-fat cheese on top and place in 1 whole wheat bun with 1 teaspoon low-fat mayo, mustard, tomato slices, and lettuce.
PEAS: ½ cup with ½ teaspoon butter or trans-free margarine	**PEAS:** ½ cup with ½ teaspoon butter or trans-free margarine
	1 MANGO OR OTHER FRUIT
SNACK	
YOGURT: 8 ounces reduced-calorie flavored yogurt with no more than 120 calories	**YOGURT:** 8 ounces reduced-calorie flavored yogurt with no more than 120 calories
DINNER	
LEMONY PAN-SEARED TUNA: See recipe on page 405.	**LEMONY PAN-SEARED TUNA:** See recipe on page 405.
WHOLE WHEAT COUSCOUS: 1 cup, cooked	**WHOLE WHEAT COUSCOUS:** 1 cup, cooked
CAULIFLOWER OR OTHER VEGETABLE: ½ cup, steamed with a spritz of lemon juice	**CAULIFLOWER OR OTHER VEGETABLE:** ½ cup, steamed with a spritz of lemon juice
TREAT	
1 DOLE FRUIT-N-GEL BOWL: Have this or another 85-calorie treat (see page 254 for more suggestions).	**1 DOLE FRUIT-N-GEL BOWL:** Have this or another 85-calorie treat (see page 254 for more suggestions).

1,800

BREAKFAST

WAFFLES: 2 whole grain toaster waffles topped with 1 cup berries or chopped fruit, 2 teaspoons butter or trans-free margarine, and 2 teaspoons maple syrup

TIP Choose waffles with about 170 calories and 4 grams of fiber for 2 waffles.

FAT-FREE MILK: 1 cup

VEGGIE BURGER: Cook 1 vegetable burger (about 120 calories) according to package directions. Melt 1 slice (1 ounce) reduced-fat cheese on top and place in 1 whole wheat bun with 1 teaspoon low-fat mayo, mustard, tomato slices, and lettuce.

PEAS: ½ cup with ½ teaspoon butter or trans-free margarine

1 MANGO OR OTHER FRUIT

YOGURT: 8 ounces reduced-calorie flavored yogurt with no more than 120 calories

LEMONY PAN-SEARED TUNA: See recipe on page 405.

WHOLE WHEAT COUSCOUS: 1 cup, cooked

CAULIFLOWER OR OTHER VEGETABLE: 1 cup, steamed with a spritz of lemon juice

LIGHT LAUGHING COW CHEESE: 2 wedges, and 1 Dole Fruit-n-Gel Bowl or another 85-calorie treat (see page 254 for suggestions)

Nutrition Tallies

	1,400	1,600	1,800
CALORIES	1,410	1,545	1,776
FAT (G)	40	41	48
SATURATED FAT (G)	12.2	12.3	13.3
PROTEIN (G)	85	86	90
CARBOHYDRATES (G)	173	208	250
DIETARY FIBER (G)	25	29	33
CHOLESTEROL (MG)	123	123	130
SODIUM (MG)	1,792	1,796	2,080
CALCIUM (MG)	1,278	1,299	1,379

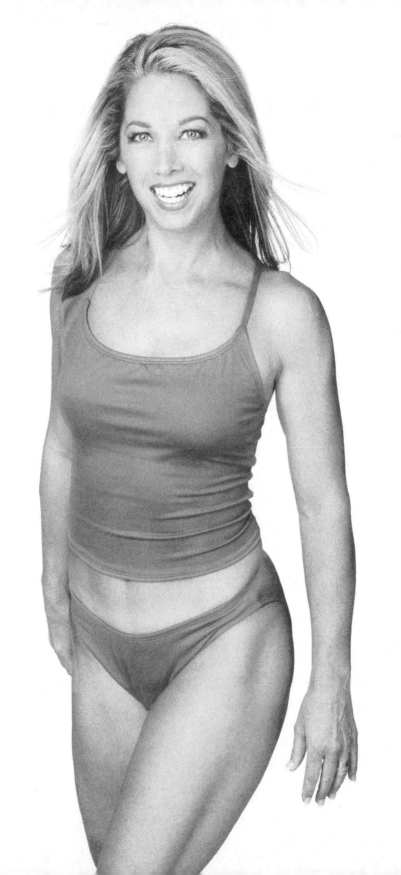

PART 5

The Shrink Your Female Fat Zones Tools

CHAPTER 16

THE SHRINK YOUR FEMALE FAT ZONES TOOLS

Recipes for Success

Meals with my family are very important to me. They're our chance to reconnect, talk about our days, and share silly laughs. But because my days aren't nearly as leisurely, preparing these meals needs to be quick and easy.

Over my years as a working mom, I've collected a bunch of tasty, lean recipes for healthy dishes that keep me and my family fit. The best of these recipes are fast, simple, and—of course!—mouthwateringly good. Here are a few of the key favorites that I've also included in your menu plans.

Most recipes are for two servings—feel free to double the recipes for groups of four, triple them for groups of six, and so on.

I usually make a few batches at a time and freeze what we don't eat that evening. Then, on those busy soccer-practice-and-dance-lessons days, we can still eat healthily. Just a few quick minutes in the microwave is all it takes to stick with my program—and give the girls something I *know* they'll eat.

Dig in and enjoy!

ROASTED CHICKEN

MAKES 4 SERVINGS

Chicken stays moist if you cook it with the skin on, but the skin itself is high in fat. So before eating, remove the skin from your piece and rub it over the meat to transfer the herb flavoring. Then discard that skin.

1 chicken (3½ pounds)

1 tablespoon olive oil

1 clove garlic, crushed

1 teaspoon dried herbes de Provence, other mixed herbs (such as rosemary, thyme, and oregano), or poultry seasoning

Salt and pepper to taste

1 large lemon, cut into wedges

Preheat the oven to 425°F.

Rinse the chicken inside and out with cold water and pat dry with paper towels. Remove any excess fat from the cavity.

In a small bowl, mix the oil, garlic, and herbs. Rub over the chicken. Sprinkle the skin and cavity with salt and pepper. Place the lemon wedges inside the cavity. Tie the legs together with cotton string. Place the chicken on a rack inside a roasting pan.

Roast for 15 minutes. Reduce the oven temperature to 350°F. Roast, basting occasionally, for another 1 to 1¼ hours, or until a meat thermometer inserted in the thickest part of the inner thigh reads 180°F and the juices run clear. Let stand for 15 minutes before carving.

CAESAR SALAD DRESSING

MAKES ½ CUP, ENOUGH FOR A LARGE SALAD (A WHOLE HEAD OF ROMAINE LETTUCE PLUS 1 TO 2 CUPS OF CHOPPED VEGETABLES)

Although this has less than half the calories of regular Caesar dressing and just one-third the fat, it's so flavorful that your family will never know the difference. Turn your salad into a main course by topping each plate with about ½ cup cooked chicken.

- ¼ cup low-fat plain yogurt
- ¼ cup grated Parmesan cheese
- 1 tablespoon olive oil
- 1 teaspoon lemon juice
- 1 teaspoon Dijon mustard
- ½ teaspoon vinegar (preferably balsamic)
- ½ teaspoon Worcestershire sauce
- ½ teaspoon anchovy paste
- ¼ teaspoon mashed garlic
- Salt and pepper to taste

In a small bowl, whisk together the yogurt, cheese, oil, lemon juice, mustard, vinegar, Worcestershire sauce, anchovy paste, and garlic. Season with salt and pepper.

FETTUCCINE WITH TOMATO ALFREDO SAUCE

MAKES 2 SERVINGS

The jarred low-fat Alfredo sauces are great fakes! I always feel like I'm getting something super rich and creamy when I have them.

- 4.8 ounces whole wheat fettuccine (for 1,600- and 1,800-calorie plans, use 5.5 ounces), see note
- ½ cup reduced-fat Alfredo sauce, such as Buitoni (or ¼ cup DiGiorno, which is a little higher in calories and fat)
- ½ cup chopped tomatoes or halved cherry tomatoes

Cook the fettuccine according to the package directions. Drain and return to the pot.

Meanwhile, heat the Alfredo sauce in a small saucepan over medium heat until it starts to simmer. Add the tomatoes. Cover and simmer for about 2 minutes. Pour over the fettuccine and toss to coat.

> **Note:** 4.8 ounces dry fettuccine is a little more than one-quarter of a typical 16-ounce box and makes 1½ cups cooked; 5.5 ounces makes 3 cups cooked. If using fresh pasta, have 250 calories' worth; check the label to determine the amount.

GRILLED FISH

MAKES 2 SERVINGS

If you like garlic, combine equal parts olive oil and lemon juice with a clove of crushed garlic, and brush on fish just before removing from the grill.

2 fish fillets, such as salmon, tuna, or monkfish (5 ounces each)

1 teaspoon olive oil

Salt and pepper to taste

Juice of ½ lemon

Preheat the broiler or outdoor grill. Rub the fillets with the oil. Place under the broiler (about 4" from the heat source) or on the grill. Cook for 4 minutes per side, or until the fish is opaque all the way through or flakes easily. Season with salt, pepper, and lemon juice.

GRILLED HONEY-MUSTARD CHICKEN

MAKES 4 SERVINGS

These boneless, skinless thighs cook quickly and are easy to prepare under the broiler if it's not grilling season.

¾ cup low-fat plain yogurt

2 tablespoons Dijon mustard

2 tablespoons chopped fresh dill

1 teaspoon honey

Salt and pepper to taste

1 pound boneless, skinless chicken thighs

1–2 tablespoons olive oil

Preheat the outdoor grill and lightly brush the rack with oil.

While the coals are heating, mix the yogurt, mustard, dill, and honey in a small bowl. Season with salt and pepper.

Rinse the chicken with cold water and pat dry with paper towels. Place on a plate and brush all sides with the oil. Sprinkle with salt and pepper.

Grill about 5" from the coals for 12 minutes per side, or until a meat thermometer inserted in the thickest part reads 160°F and the juices run clear. (If broiling, place about 3" from heat source and broil 12 minutes per side, or until an internal temperature reads 160°F and the juices run clear.) Serve with the honey-mustard sauce.

BEEF AND BROCCOLI STIR-FRY

MAKES 2 SERVINGS

This basic recipe also works well with chicken, shrimp, or tofu.

1   tablespoon canola oil

6   ounces sirloin, trimmed of fat and cut into strips

1   teaspoon minced garlic

1   teaspoon minced fresh ginger

2   cups chopped broccoli

1   teaspoon reduced-sodium soy sauce

3   drops hot-pepper sauce

2   scallions, chopped

2   tablespoons chopped fresh cilantro (optional)

In a large nonstick skillet, warm ½ tablespoon of the oil over medium-high heat. Add the sirloin, garlic, and ginger. Cook, stirring, for about 5 minutes, or until the meat is cooked through and no longer pink. Transfer to a plate.

Add the remaining ½ tablespoon oil and the broccoli to the skillet. Cook, stirring, for 3 minutes. Add the soy sauce, hot-pepper sauce, and meat mixture. Serve sprinkled with the scallions and cilantro (if using).

TUNA AND BEAN SALAD

MAKES 2 SERVINGS

You can make endless varia-tions of this quick meal, by using different types of beans, trying rice, or substituting whole wheat couscous for the corn, and throwing in whatever vegetables are in your fridge.

1   cup canned chickpeas, rinsed and drained

1   cup fresh, frozen, or low-sodium canned corn

1   cup chopped tomatoes or cherry tomatoes

6   ounces water-packed tuna

½   cup chopped green bell peppers

2   scallions, chopped

4   tablespoons chopped fresh parsley, basil, dill, cilantro, or other herb

4   tablespoons reduced-calorie vinaigrette or Italian salad dressing

In a small bowl, combine the chickpeas, corn, and tomatoes. Add the tuna, peppers, scallion, and parsley or other herb. Toss with the dressing.

QUICK VEGGIE PIZZA

MAKES 4 SERVINGS

You can have a great homemade pizza in the time it takes to order out. Only this one's low in fat and good for you.

1 large zucchini, thinly sliced (about 1½ cups)

2 teaspoons olive oil

1 prebaked pizza crust (14 ounces)

¾ cup pizza sauce

1 clove garlic, minced

1 cup shredded part-skim mozzarella cheese

¼ cup grated Parmesan cheese

Preheat the broiler. Place the zucchini on a large baking sheet and drizzle with the oil. Toss to coat the zucchini and spread in an even layer. Broil about 2" from the heat for 10 minutes, or until the slices begin to turn golden. Set aside.

Change the oven temperature to 450°F. Place the crust on a pizza stone or another baking sheet. In a small bowl, combine the sauce and garlic and then spread evenly over the crust. Top with the mozzarella and then the zucchini. Sprinkle with the Parmesan.

Bake for 12 minutes, or until the cheese melts and begins to bubble. Cut into 8 slices.

Shrimp and Vegetable Kebabs

MAKES 2 SERVINGS

They're so delicious, whether you're using the oven's broiler or your outdoor grill.

6   ounces large raw shrimp (about 14 shrimp), peeled

2   medium onions, cut into wedges

1   cup small whole mushrooms or portobello mushrooms, cut into large wedges

⅔   cup cherry or grape tomatoes

Juice of 1 lemon

1   tablespoon olive oil

1   clove garlic, crushed, or ½ teaspoon garlic powder

Salt and pepper to taste

2   tablespoons chopped fresh dill, parsley, or basil (optional)

If using wooden skewers, soak them in cold water for about 10 minutes. Preheat the broiler or outdoor grill.

Alternate the shrimp and about half of the onions on 2 skewers. Alternate the mushrooms, tomatoes, and the remaining onions on 2 skewers.

In a small bowl, mix the lemon juice, oil, and garlic or garlic powder. Pour half into a cup and set aside. Brush the remainder over the skewers and discard any that's left.

Place the vegetable skewers on a broiler pan or outdoor grill. Broil or grill for about 2 minutes, then turn. Add the shrimp skewers. Cook for 5 to 7 minutes, turning all the skewers after about 3 minutes.

Using a clean brush, brush the skewers with the reserved lemon mixture. (A clean brush prevents possible contamination with bacteria from raw shrimp on first brush.) Season with salt and pepper. Sprinkle with the herbs (if using).

Pasta with Broccoli and Chicken

MAKES 2 SERVINGS

What a timesaver! Although you have only one pot to clean, you have made an entire balanced meal. Feel free to substitute any other pasta strands or shapes.

4 ounces whole wheat spaghetti or 2 cups ziti (for 1,600- and 1,800-calorie plans, use 6 ounces spaghetti or 3 cups ziti)

2 cups broccoli florets, coarsely chopped

1 cup sliced cooked chicken breast (use precooked chicken, if desired)

4 tablespoons grated Parmesan cheese

4 teaspoons olive oil

Pinch of red-pepper flakes (optional)

Prepare the pasta according to package directions. Drain, reserving 1 cup of the liquid. Return the liquid to the pot. Place the pasta in a bowl and cover to keep warm.

Bring the liquid to a boil. Add the broccoli, cover, and cook for 4 to 5 minutes, or until soft, but not soggy. Add the pasta, chicken, cheese, oil, and pepper flakes (if using). Toss well.

Apricot-Glazed Chicken

MAKES 2 SERVINGS, PLUS LEFTOVERS FOR CHICKEN WALDORF SALAD

Here's a different twist on baked chicken breast.

4 boneless, skinless chicken breast halves (4 ounces each)

⅓ cup apricot preserves

2 teaspoons Dijon mustard

5 drops hot-pepper sauce

Preheat the oven to 425°F. Rinse the chicken with cold water and pat dry with paper towels. Place in a single layer in an 11" × 17" baking dish.

In a small bowl, mix the preserves, mustard, and hot-pepper sauce. Spoon over the chicken. Bake for 15 minutes. Baste with any sauce that dripped off the chicken. Bake for another 10 to 20 minutes, or until a meat thermometer inserted in the thickest part reads 160°F and the juices run clear. (Refrigerate 2 pieces for tomorrow's Chicken Waldorf Salad.)

Avocado and White Bean Salad

MAKES 2 SERVINGS

The juiciness of the tomato, creaminess of the avocado, and softness of the beans make for a moist and tender dish without a drop of oil.

1 cup canned white cannellini beans, rinsed and drained

½ Haas (dark-skinned) avocado, chopped (for 1,600- and 1,800-calorie plans, use 1 avocado)

1 cup halved cherry tomatoes

½ cup chopped green bell peppers

2 tablespoons chopped fresh basil

Juice of 1 lemon

In a small bowl, combine the beans with the avocado. Add the tomatoes, peppers, and basil. Toss with the lemon.

Lemon Couscous

MAKES 2 CUPS

Miracle! A whole wheat grain dish that's ready in under 10 minutes.

⅔ cup water

½ teaspoon butter

Dash of salt

½ cup dry whole wheat couscous

2 tablespoons raisins

1 teaspoon grated lemon zest

In a small saucepan, bring the water, butter, and salt to a boil. Add the couscous. Cover, turn off the heat, and let stand for 5 minutes.

Fluff with a fork. Add the raisins and lemon zest. Toss to combine.

CHICKEN WALDORF SALAD

MAKES 2 SERVINGS

This revamped classic has less total fat and more beneficial unsaturated fat than the original. And it's high in protein for a satisfying lunch.

2   cups cooked chicken breast cut into 1" chunks (use the extra Apricot-Glazed Chicken from last night)

4   small apples, chopped

4   tablespoons low-fat plain yogurt

4   tablespoons raisins

4   tablespoons walnut halves or almonds

2   tablespoons low-fat mayonnaise

In a medium bowl, combine the chicken, apples, yogurt, raisins, walnuts or almonds, and mayonnaise.

EASY HOMEMADE CHILI

MAKES 6 SERVINGS

Canned beans make this the fastest homemade chili ever!

1   tablespoon olive oil

4   large cloves garlic, chopped

1   can (19 ounces) diced tomatoes

1   can (15 ounces) black beans, rinsed and drained

1   can (15 ounces) kidney or pinto beans, rinsed and drained

2   tablespoons chili powder

1   tablespoon ground cumin

1–2   teaspoons red wine vinegar

Salt and pepper to taste

In large saucepan, warm the oil over medium heat. Add the garlic and stir for 1 minute, or until fragrant. Add the tomatoes, black beans, kidney or pinto beans, chili powder, and cumin. Bring to a simmer.

Cover, reduce the heat to low, and simmer for 30 minutes. Season with the vinegar, salt, and pepper.

FISH WITH OLIVES AND CAPERS

MAKES 2 SERVINGS

Here's a fish dish that won't make your house smell fishy.

2 teaspoons olive oil

1 clove garlic, chopped

1 can (14 ounces) whole tomatoes

Pepper to taste

2 fish fillets, such as red snapper, tilapia, or other fish (5–6 ounces each)

2½ tablespoons chopped fresh basil

2 tablespoons chopped, pitted black olives (preferably kalamata or Moroccan)

1 teaspoon capers, chopped

In a large nonstick skillet, warm the oil over medium heat. Add the garlic and stir for 30 seconds. Add the tomatoes. Bring to a boil, breaking the tomatoes into coarse chunks with a spoon. Reduce the heat to medium-low and simmer for 10 minutes. Season with pepper.

Add the fish and spoon the sauce over it to cover completely. Cover and simmer for 10 minutes, or until the fish flakes easily. Transfer just the fish to a serving dish.

Stir the basil, olives, and capers into the tomatoes. Simmer for 30 seconds and pour over the fish.

OVEN-BAKED CHICKEN

MAKES 2 SERVINGS

This is a low-fat, high-fiber version of breaded and fried chicken.

2   teaspoons olive oil

2   boneless, skinless chicken breast halves (about 5 ounces)

¼   cup all-purpose flour

3   tablespoons reduced-fat sour cream

⅔   cup bran flakes, coarsely crushed

1   teaspoon dried mixed Italian herbs or 1½ tablespoons chopped fresh basil, parsley, or other herbs

Preheat the oven to 350°F. Brush a small baking dish with the oil.

Rinse the chicken with cold water and pat dry with paper towels. Roll each piece in the flour to coat; shake off the excess.

Place the sour cream in a shallow bowl. Dip each chicken piece into it to coat.

Mix the bran flakes and herbs in another shallow bowl. Dip each chicken piece into it to coat. Transfer to the baking dish. Bake for 35 to 40 minutes, or until a meat thermometer inserted in the thickest part reads 160°F and the juices run clear.

SAUTÉED SPINACH

MAKES 2 SERVINGS

If you're a real garlic lover, mince the garlic and leave it in the spinach.

2   teaspoons olive oil

1   clove garlic, halved

6   cups packed spinach (use washed and bagged spinach for convenience)

Salt to taste

In a large nonstick skillet, warm the oil over medium heat. Add the garlic and cook for about 30 seconds (to avoid burning it). Add the spinach and cook just until wilted. Season with salt. Remove and discard the garlic.

POACHED SALMON WITH HERB SAUCE

**MAKES 2 SERVINGS, PLUS
LEFTOVERS FOR SALMON
BURGERS**

*Easy and elegant. Perfect for
a romantic dinner for two.*

3 cups water

1 cup dry white wine

1 small onion, halved, or 2 scallions, halved

½ teaspoon salt

10 peppercorns

2 cloves garlic

2 whole cloves

1 salmon fillet (1 pound), cut into 4 pieces,
  or 4 fillets (4 ounces each)
  Herb Sauce (below)

In a large skillet, combine the water, wine, onion or scallions,
salt, peppercorns, garlic, and cloves. Bring to a boil over
high heat. Reduce the heat to medium-low and simmer for
10 minutes.

Carefully add the salmon in a single layer. Cover and simmer—
do not boil—for 6 to 8 minutes, or until the fish is opaque
all the way through and tender. Serve with the Herb Sauce.
(Refrigerate 2 fillets for tomorrow's Salmon Burgers.)

HERB SAUCE

MAKES 4 SERVINGS

*Use 2 servings for Poached
Salmon with Herb Sauce
and 2 servings for Salmon
Burgers. For best results,
use reduced-fat sour cream,
not fat-free.*

4 tablespoons reduced-fat sour cream

2 tablespoons chopped fresh herbs, such as dill, parsley,
  or basil
  Juice of ¼ to ½ lemon
  Salt and pepper to taste

In a small bowl, mix the sour cream and herbs. Season with
the lemon juice, salt, and pepper.

SALMON BURGERS

MAKES 2 SERVINGS

A yummy way to use leftover salmon (especially from yesterday's Poached Salmon with Herb Sauce)!

2 salmon fillets (4 ounces each), cooked and flaked (about 1½ cups)

¼ cup crushed whole grain crackers

2 tablespoons chopped fresh dill

2 scallions, chopped

1 large egg white

2 drops hot-pepper sauce

   Pinch of salt

2 teaspoons olive or canola oil

   Lemon wedges

   Herb Sauce (page 395)

In a large bowl, mix the salmon, crackers, dill, scallions, egg white, hot-pepper sauce, and salt. Form into 2 cakes.

In a large nonstick skillet, warm the oil over medium heat. Add the cakes and cook for 4 minutes, or until browned. Turn and cook for 4 minutes. Serve with the lemon wedges and Herb Sauce.

PASTA PRIMAVERA

MAKES 2 SERVINGS

You get a nutritious variety of vegetables in just one dish.

1 tablespoon olive oil

1 clove garlic, halved

1 cup thinly sliced zucchini

1 cup sliced portobello or other mushrooms

3 tablespoons chopped fresh basil or 2 teaspoons dried

4 ounces whole wheat spaghetti or linguine or 3 cups short pasta

8 asparagus spears, cut into 2" lengths

4 tablespoons grated Parmesan cheese

In a large nonstick skillet, warm the oil over medium heat. Add the garlic and cook for 30 seconds. Add the zucchini and mushrooms. Cook, stirring occasionally, for about 7 minutes, or until the vegetables are soft but not mushy. Remove and discard the garlic. Stir in the basil.

Meanwhile, prepare the pasta according to the package directions. Add the asparagus for the last 3 minutes of cooking. Drain and return to the pot. Add the cooked vegetables and toss to mix. Serve topped with the cheese.

EGGPLANT PASTA

MAKES 2 SERVINGS

Grilling eggplant instead of frying it turns this into a nice, lean dish.

1   medium eggplant, cut into ½" chunks (about 3 cups)

2   teaspoons olive oil

2¼ cups whole wheat ziti, penne, or other tubular pasta (for 1,600- and 1,800-calorie plans, use 3¼ cups)

⅔ cup marinara sauce

¼ cup shredded part-skim mozzarella cheese

Preheat the oven to 450°F.

In a medium bowl, toss together the eggplant and oil. In a jelly-roll pan, baking sheet, or large baking dish, spread in an even layer. Bake, stirring once, for about 12 minutes, or until the eggplant is soft (this can be done a day in advance).

Meanwhile, prepare the pasta according to the package directions. Drain and return to the pot. Add the eggplant, sauce, and cheese. Toss to mix.

FENNEL, ORANGE, AND OLIVE SALAD

MAKES 2 SERVINGS

Wow your dinner guests with this gorgeous salad.

1   fennel bulb, sliced (see note)

2   small oranges or tangerines, peeled and sliced crosswise or separated into sections with the membranes removed

10 black olives, pitted (preferably kalamata or Moroccan)

1   teaspoon olive oil

½ teaspoon vinegar (preferably balsamic)

   Salt and pepper to taste

In a medium bowl, mix the fennel, oranges or tangerines, olives, oil, vinegar, salt, and pepper. Let stand for at least 15 minutes (or up to 8 hours in the refrigerator).

Note: To process a fennel bulb, first cut a slice off the bottom to expose the stalk ends. Cut off the tops where the stalks turn thin. Reserve the feathery dill-like ends and chop 2 tablespoons to add to this salad. Slice the bulb crosswise or lengthwise. If cutting it lengthwise, remove the thick core.

Pasta with Shrimp and Broccoli

MAKES 2 SERVINGS

Another one-dish wonder that gives you a completely balanced meal.

2 cups whole wheat ziti, penne, or other tubular pasta (for 1,600- and 1,800-calorie plans, use 3 cups)

1 tablespoon + 1 teaspoon olive oil

1 garlic clove, minced, or 1 teaspoon garlic powder

5 ounces peeled and deveined shrimp (about 15 large or 24 medium shrimp)

1½ cups broccoli florets, cut into small pieces

1 tablespoon chopped fresh basil (optional)

Prepare the pasta according to the package directions. Drain and return to the pot.

Meanwhile, in a large nonstick skillet, warm 1 tablespoon of the oil over medium heat. Add the garlic or garlic powder and cook for 30 seconds. Add the shrimp. Cook, stirring, for 4 to 5 minutes, or until the shrimp turn opaque. Add to the drained pasta.

Add the broccoli and the remaining 1 teaspoon of oil to the skillet. Cook, stirring often, for 3 minutes, or until just tender. Add to the pasta and toss to mix. Sprinkle with the basil (if using).

SPICY ORANGE PORK TENDERLOIN WITH MANGO RICE

MAKES 3 SERVINGS, PLUS LEFTOVERS FOR TOMORROW

This is an interesting way to serve pork tenderloin, a wonderfully tender—but low-fat—meat.

1 tablespoon maple syrup

¼–1 teaspoon Thai red curry paste (see note)
Grated rind and juice of 1 orange

1 pound pork tenderloin, trimmed of fat
Mango Rice (below)

In a large bowl, mix the maple syrup, curry paste, and orange rind and juice. Add the pork and turn to coat all sides. Refrigerate for 1 to 4 hours, turning occasionally.

Preheat the oven to 400°F. Transfer the pork and 2 tablespoons of the marinade to a loaf pan or small glass baking dish. Discard any remaining marinade.

Bake for 30 to 35 minutes, or until a meat thermometer inserted in the thickest part registers 155°F and the juices run clear. Transfer to a cutting board and let rest for 5 minutes before cutting into 4 equal pieces.

Cut 3 of the pieces into 4 to 6 thin slices each. Serve with the rice. (Refrigerate the remaining 1 piece for tomorrow's pork tenderloin sandwich.)

Note: You be the judge of how spicy you want this dish—¼ teaspoon of the curry paste makes it barely spicy; 1 teaspoon makes it moderately spicy.

MANGO RICE

MAKES 3 SERVINGS

Adding mango takes plain rice to a new level.

¾ cup uncooked brown rice

1 ripe mango, peeled and chopped (about ¾ cup)

2 scallions, finely chopped

In a medium saucepan, prepare the rice according to the package directions. Let cool until just warm, not hot. Gently mix in the mango and scallions.

THAI CHICKEN CURRY

MAKES 4 SERVINGS

Surprise! This tastes authentically Thai but has only about a third the fat, thanks to light coconut milk.

1 can (14 ounces) light coconut milk (see note)

1–3 teaspoons red curry paste

1 tablespoon fish sauce

1 tablespoon white or brown sugar

1 pound boneless, skinless chicken breast halves, cut into bite-size pieces

2 cups frozen peas

2 tablespoons chopped fresh basil

In a large skillet, mix the coconut milk and 1 teaspoon of the curry paste. Warm over medium heat. Taste and add more curry paste, if you like it spicier. Simmer for 5 minutes.

Stir in the fish sauce and sugar. Add the chicken and peas. Bring to a simmer and cook for 10 minutes, or until the chicken is opaque throughout. Taste the sauce one more time and add a little more curry paste, if desired. Stir in the basil.

Note: Choose reduced-calorie coconut milk with no more than 50 calories per 2-ounce serving, such as Thai Kitchen or Trader Joe's. Look for the Thai ingredients in the international section of your supermarket.

WILD RICE, PEAS, AND CHICKEN

MAKES 3 TO 4 SERVINGS

You can customize this recipe to your own taste. For instance, you can use dill instead of tarragon, almonds in place of pine nuts, and turkey rather than chicken. If you're following the 1,400- or 1,600-calorie plan, consider one-quarter of the recipe a serving. For 1,800 calories, have one-third of the recipe.

2 tablespoons pine nuts

1 can (14½ ounces) reduced-sodium chicken broth

½ cup uncooked wild rice

2 cups cubed cooked chicken breast

1 package (10 ounces) frozen peas, defrosted

1 scallion, thinly sliced

2 tablespoons minced fresh tarragon or 2 teaspoons dried

2 tablespoons olive oil

1 tablespoon balsamic vinegar

   Salt and pepper to taste

Toast the pine nuts in a toaster oven at 350°F for 5 to 10 minutes, or until fragrant.

Meanwhile, in a medium saucepan, combine the broth and wild rice. Bring to a boil over high heat. Cover, reduce the heat to medium-low, and simmer for 50 minutes, or until the rice is tender and the liquid has been absorbed.

Stir in the chicken, peas, scallion, and tarragon.

In a small bowl, whisk together the oil and vinegar. Season with salt and pepper. Pour over the chicken mixture and toss to combine. Sprinkle with the pine nuts.

Mexican Lasagna

MAKES 6 TO 8 SERVINGS

A crowd pleaser with left-overs you can freeze for another day.

1 tablespoon olive oil

1 large onion, chopped

1 pound ground turkey

2 cans (15 ounces each) low-sodium chili beans (no flavorings added), pinto beans, or other beans

3–5 tablespoons chili powder

12 corn tortillas (6")

1½ cups shredded reduced-fat Cheddar cheese

1 can (14½ ounces) diced tomatoes

1 jar (16 ounces) enchilada sauce

Preheat the oven to 350°F. Coat a 13" × 9" baking dish with olive oil.

In a large nonstick skillet over medium heat, cook the onion in the oil for 3 minutes. Add the turkey. Cook, stirring and breaking up the meat with a spoon, for about 6 minutes, or until the turkey is no longer pink. Add the beans and chili powder. Cook, stirring occasionally, for 4 minutes.

Place 6 tortillas, overlapping, in the bottom of the baking dish. Spoon the turkey mixture evenly over the tortillas. Cover with the remaining 6 tortillas. Sprinkle with the cheese. Spoon on the tomatoes and enchilada sauce. Bake for 1 hour.

Tofu, Mushroom, and Chicken Risotto

MAKES 2 SERVINGS

A good way to get introduced to tofu—you hardly know it's there!

2	teaspoons olive oil
1	small clove garlic, minced
2	cups sliced mushrooms
½	cup sliced tofu, at room temperature
1½	cups hot cooked brown or white rice (basmati or jasmati works well here)
⅔	cup sliced cooked chicken breast (use precooked Perdue or Louis Rich, if desired)
¼	cup grated Parmesan cheese
2	tablespoons chopped fresh herbs, such as basil, parsley, or dill
	Salt and pepper to taste

In a large nonstick skillet, warm the oil over medium heat. Add the garlic and cook for about 2 minutes. Add the mushrooms and cook for 2 minutes.

Add the tofu. Cook for 3 minutes, or until the mushrooms soften.

In a large bowl, mix the rice, chicken, cheese, and herbs. Add the tofu mixture and mix well. Season with salt and pepper.

Roasted Potatoes and Mushrooms

MAKES 2 SERVINGS

Most roasted potatoes are drenched in fat. In this low-fat rendition, the softness of the mushrooms keeps things moist.

1	cup potato wedges
2	teaspoons olive oil
1	teaspoon rosemary or other herbs
	Salt and pepper to taste
1	cup sliced portobello or other mushrooms

Toss the potato wedges with 1 teaspoon of the olive oil, ½ teaspoon of the rosemary or other herbs, and salt and pepper. Spread on a baking sheet and bake at 350°F for 15 minutes. Toss the mushrooms with salt and pepper and the remaining 1 teaspoon olive oil and ½ teaspoon rosemary or other herbs. Add to potatoes. Bake for 30 to 40 minutes, or until the potatoes are tender.

LEMONY PAN-SEARED TUNA

MAKES 2 SERVINGS

Very easy, with a wonderful taste and smell of lemon.

2 tuna steaks (5 ounces each, about ¾" thick)

Salt and pepper to taste

3 lemons

3 tablespoons olive oil

⅓ cup chopped fresh parsley

Lemon wedges

Rinse, dry, then salt and pepper the tuna. Place on a plate. Grate the rind from 1 lemon into a wide, shallow bowl. Squeeze in the juice plus the juice from the remaining 2 lemons. Add 1 tablespoon of the oil and most of the parsley (save 1 tablespoon parsley for garnish).

In a large cast-iron skillet, warm the remaining 2 tablespoons oil over medium-high heat until hot. Carefully place the tuna in the skillet. Cook for 3 minutes per side. (The center will still be a little pink. If you like it really well-done, cook a little longer.) Sprinkle with the remaining parsley and serve with lemon wedges.

CHAPTER 17

THE SHRINK YOUR FEMALE FAT ZONES TOOLS

Your 6-Week Fat Zone Workbook

Studies have shown that the act of keeping a journal is one of the most consistent predictors of permanent weight loss. Can you believe it? The simple process of writing can coax those pounds off more quickly, and keep them off for good!

With that in mind, I've created an at-a-glance workout log and eating journal that will help you follow the program and track your progress, all in one page.

I've included the blueprint for the 6 weeks of the entire Shrink Your Female Fat Zones plan right here. Just photocopy one page per day for each day in that week. You'll find a place to note your stretching, walking, and strengthening workouts. Because you'll be following the menu plans instead of filling in blank spaces to note your food intake, I've created checklists for you to note the ways in which you've reinforced the eating lessons of that week. (Some women find it easier to keep separate food journals—that decision is up to you.)

Every adventure begins with a good map—turn the page to find yours!

DAILY LOG
DAY __

TODAY'S MEASUREMENT: _____ lbs/inches/%body fat

BEGINNING: _____

MY GOAL: _____

STRETCH

This week's stretching goal:
3 times a day

Today, I did my:

Morning wake-up ❑

Tension tamers ❑

Evening wind-down ❑

WALK

This week's walking goal:
4 (25-minute) endurance walks

Today, I walked: _____

_____

How it felt: _____

_____

_____

_____

Fat Zone Walking Moves
I tried: _____

_____

_____

TONE

FAT ZONE: UPPER BODY. This week's workout goals:
3 Upper Body, 1 Lower Body, 1 Midsection

Today, I did a(n):   How did it feel?

❑ Upper Body Workout _____

❑ Midsection Workout _____

❑ Lower Body Workout _____

FAT ZONE: MIDSECTION. This week's workout goals:
3 Midsection, 1 Upper Body, 1 Lower Body

Today, I did a(n):   How did it feel?

❑ Upper Body Workout _____

❑ Midsection Workout _____

❑ Lower Body Workout _____

FAT ZONE: LOWER BODY. This week's workout goals:
3 Lower Body, 1 Upper Body, 1 Midsection

Today, I did a(n):   How did it feel?

❑ Upper Body Workout _____

❑ Midsection Workout _____

❑ Lower Body Workout _____

EAT

This week's eating goal: *Control portion distortion*

MEALS   SNACK   TREAT

❑ ❑ ❑   ❑   ❑

WATER (8 OZ. GLASSES)

❑ ❑ ❑ ❑ ❑ ❑ ❑

MULTIVITAMIN

❑

Today, I controlled portions by: _____

At breakfast, I _____

At lunch, I _____

At dinner, I _____

At snack time, I _____

At treat time, I _____

DAILY LOG
DAY ___

TODAY'S MEASUREMENT: _____ lbs/inches/%body fat

BEGINNING: _____

MY GOAL: _____

STRETCH

This week's stretching goal:
3 times a day

Today, I did my:

Morning wake-up ❏

Tension tamers ❏

Evening wind-down ❏

WALK

This week's walking goal:
4 (25-minute) endurance walks

Today, I walked: _____

_____

How it felt: _____

_____

_____

_____

Fat Zone Walking Moves
I tried: _____

_____

_____

TONE

FAT ZONE: UPPER BODY. This week's workout goals:
3 Upper Body, 1 Lower Body, 1 Midsection

Today, I did a(n):   How did it feel?

❏ Upper Body Workout _____

❏ Midsection Workout _____

❏ Lower Body Workout _____

FAT ZONE: MIDSECTION. This week's workout goals:
3 Midsection, 1 Upper Body, 1 Lower Body

Today, I did a(n):   How did it feel?

❏ Upper Body Workout _____

❏ Midsection Workout _____

❏ Lower Body Workout _____

FAT ZONE: LOWER BODY. This week's workout goals:
3 Lower Body, 1 Upper Body, 1 Midsection

Today, I did a(n):   How did it feel?

❏ Upper Body Workout _____

❏ Midsection Workout _____

❏ Lower Body Workout _____

EAT

This week's eating goal: *Maximize fiber*

MEALS   SNACK   TREAT

❏ ❏ ❏   ❏   ❏

WATER (8 OZ. GLASSES)

❏ ❏ ❏ ❏ ❏ ❏ ❏

MULTIVITAMIN

❏

Today, I maximized fiber by: _____

At breakfast, I _____

At lunch, I _____

At dinner, I _____

At snack time, I _____

At treat time, I _____

DAILY LOG
DAY __

TODAY'S MEASUREMENT: _____ lbs/inches/%body fat

BEGINNING: _____

MY GOAL: _____

STRETCH

This week's stretching goal:
3 times a day

Today, I did my:

Morning wake-up ❑

Tension tamers ❑

Evening wind-down ❑

WALK

This week's walking goal:
2 (35-minute) endurance walks
1 (35-minute) fat zone walk
1 (35-minute) fat-burning walk

Today, I walked:_____

How it felt:_____

_____

_____

Fat Zone Walking Moves
I tried:_____

_____

TONE

FAT ZONE: UPPER BODY. This week's workout goals:
3 Upper Body, 1 Lower Body, 1 Midsection

Today, I did a(n):   How did it feel?

❑ Upper Body Workout _____

❑ Midsection Workout _____

❑ Lower Body Workout _____

FAT ZONE: MIDSECTION. This week's workout goals:
3 Midsection, 1 Upper Body, 1 Lower Body

Today, I did a(n):   How did it feel?

❑ Upper Body Workout _____

❑ Midsection Workout _____

❑ Lower Body Workout _____

FAT ZONE: LOWER BODY. This week's workout goals:
3 Lower Body, 1 Upper Body, 1 Midsection

Today, I did a(n):   How did it feel?

❑ Upper Body Workout _____

❑ Midsection Workout _____

❑ Lower Body Workout _____

EAT

This week's eating goal: *Savor good fats*

MEALS   SNACK   TREAT
❑ ❑ ❑   ❑   ❑

WATER (8 OZ. GLASSES)
❑ ❑ ❑ ❑ ❑ ❑ ❑

MULTIVITAMIN
❑

Today, I savored good fats by:_____

At breakfast, I _____

At lunch, I _____

At dinner, I _____

At snack time, I _____

At treat time, I _____

DAILY LOG
DAY ___

TODAY'S MEASUREMENT: _____ lbs/inches/%body fat

BEGINNING: _____

MY GOAL: _____

STRETCH

This week's stretching goal:
3 times a day

Today, I did my:

Morning wake-up ❑

Tension tamers ❑

Evening wind-down ❑

WALK

This week's walking goal:
2 (35-minute) endurance walks
1 (35-minute) fat zone walk
1 (35-minute) fat-burning walk

Today, I walked: _____

_____

How it felt: _____

_____

_____

Fat Zone Walking Moves
I tried: _____

_____

TONE

FAT ZONE: UPPER BODY. This week's workout goals:
3 Upper Body, 1 Lower Body, 1 Midsection

Today, I did a(n):   How did it feel?

❑ Upper Body Workout _____

❑ Midsection Workout _____

❑ Lower Body Workout _____

FAT ZONE: MIDSECTION. This week's workout goals:
3 Midsection, 1 Upper Body, 1 Lower Body

Today, I did a(n):   How did it feel?

❑ Upper Body Workout _____

❑ Midsection Workout _____

❑ Lower Body Workout _____

FAT ZONE: LOWER BODY. This week's workout goals:
3 Lower Body, 1 Upper Body, 1 Midsection

Today, I did a(n):   How did it feel?

❑ Upper Body Workout _____

❑ Midsection Workout _____

❑ Lower Body Workout _____

EAT

This week's eating goal: *Boost fruits and vegetables*

MEALS   SNACK   TREAT
❑ ❑ ❑   ❑   ❑

WATER (8 OZ. GLASSES)
❑ ❑ ❑ ❑ ❑ ❑ ❑

MULTIVITAMIN
❑

Today, I boosted fruits and vegetables by: _____

At breakfast, I _____

At lunch, I _____

At dinner, I _____

At snack time, I _____

At treat time, I _____

DAILY LOG
DAY __

TODAY'S MEASUREMENT: _____ lbs/inches/%body fat

BEGINNING: _____

MY GOAL: _____

STRETCH

This week's stretching goal:
3 times a day

Today, I did my:

Morning wake-up ☐

Tension tamers ☐

Evening wind-down ☐

WALK

This week's walking goal:
1 (45-minute) endurance walk

2 (45-minute) fat zone fat-burning walks

1 (45-minute) fat-burning walk

Today, I walked: _____

_____

How it felt: _____

_____

_____

Fat Zone Walking Moves
I tried: _____

_____

TONE

FAT ZONE: UPPER BODY. This week's workout goals:
3 Upper Body, 1 Lower Body, 1 Midsection

Today, I did a(n):   How did it feel?

☐ Upper Body Workout _____

☐ Midsection Workout _____

☐ Lower Body Workout _____

FAT ZONE: MIDSECTION. This week's workout goals:
3 Midsection, 1 Upper Body, 1 Lower Body

Today, I did a(n):   How did it feel?

☐ Upper Body Workout _____

☐ Midsection Workout _____

☐ Lower Body Workout _____

FAT ZONE: LOWER BODY. This week's workout goals:
3 Lower Body, 1 Upper Body, 1 Midsection

Today, I did a(n):   How did it feel?

☐ Upper Body Workout _____

☐ Midsection Workout _____

☐ Lower Body Workout _____

EAT

This week's eating goal: *Home in on hunger*

MEALS	SNACK	TREAT
☐ ☐ ☐	☐	☐

WATER (8 OZ. GLASSES)
☐ ☐ ☐ ☐ ☐ ☐ ☐

MULTIVITAMIN
☐

Today, I homed in on hunger by:

_____

_____

_____

_____

_____

Hunger Level (circle one)				
Not Hungry				Ravenous
At breakfast 1	2	3	4	5
At lunch 1	2	3	4	5
At dinner 1	2	3	4	5
At snack 1	2	3	4	5
At treat 1	2	3	4	5

DAILY LOG
DAY ___

TODAY'S MEASUREMENT: _____ lbs/inches/%body fat

BEGINNING: _____

MY GOAL: _____

STRETCH

This week's stretching goal:
3 times a day

Today, I did my:

Morning wake-up ☐

Tension tamers ☐

Evening wind-down ☐

WALK

This week's walking goal:
1 (45-minute) endurance walk

2 (45-minute) fat zone fat-burning walks

1 (45-minute) fat-burning walk

Today, I walked: _____

_____

How it felt: _____

_____

_____

Fat Zone Walking Moves
I tried: _____

_____

TONE

FAT ZONE: UPPER BODY. This week's workout goals:
3 Upper Body, 1 Lower Body, 1 Midsection

Today, I did a(n):   How did it feel?

☐ Upper Body Workout   _____

☐ Midsection Workout   _____

☐ Lower Body Workout   _____

FAT ZONE: MIDSECTION. This week's workout goals:
3 Midsection, 1 Upper Body, 1 Lower Body

Today, I did a(n):   How did it feel?

☐ Upper Body Workout   _____

☐ Midsection Workout   _____

☐ Lower Body Workout   _____

FAT ZONE: LOWER BODY. This week's workout goals:
3 Lower Body, 1 Upper Body, 1 Midsection

Today, I did a(n):   How did it feel?

☐ Upper Body Workout   _____

☐ Midsection Workout   _____

☐ Lower Body Workout   _____

EAT

This week's eating goal: *Change behaviors*

MEALS   SNACK   TREAT
☐ ☐ ☐   ☐   ☐

WATER (8 OZ. GLASSES)
☐ ☐ ☐ ☐ ☐ ☐ ☐

MULTIVITAMIN
☐

	Hunger Level (circle one) Not Hungry — Ravenous	How did I feel?	Where did I eat?
At breakfast	1 2 3 4 5	_____	_____
At lunch	1 2 3 4 5	_____	_____
At dinner	1 2 3 4 5	_____	_____
At snack	1 2 3 4 5	_____	_____
At treat	1 2 3 4 5	_____	_____

INDEX

Underscored page references indicate boxed text and tables. **Boldface** references indicate photographs.

A

Abdominal fat
    health risks from, 11–12
    from stress, 357–59
Abdominal toning
    after age 40, 141
    after pregnancy, 140
Abdominal weakness, causes of, 141
Aerobic capacity, increasing, with walking, 37
Aging
    metabolism slowed by, 258
    muscle loss with, 9, 26
    weight gain with, 8–9
Alpha-linolenic acid, 300
Appetite suppressant
    fiber as, 280–81, 285
    walking as, 38
Apricot-Glazed Chicken, 390
Arches, toning, 41, **41**
Arms, upper body routine for, 97
Avocado, Tomato, and Corn Salad, 304
Avocado and White Bean Salad, 391
Avocados, health benefits from, 305

B

Back, lower, midsection routine for, 144
Bagels, estimating portion of, 262
Ballet, 29, 184, 198
Banana Split, 326
Barbecued Chicken, 332
Beach walking, 42, 45
Bean Burrito, 274
Bean Burrito with Avocado, 304

Beans, health benefits from, 291
Beef and Broccoli Stir-Fry, 387
Belly fat. *See* Abdominal fat
Berries, 252, 287
Biceps, upper body routine for, 97
Bingeing, 371
Blood sugar, controlling, with fiber, 280–81
Blueberries, health benefits from, 252, 287
Body-fat percentage, for tracking progress, 16
Body shape
    changing, 12, 73–74
    identifying, 5, 11
Breakfast, benefits from, 253, 257
Breast cancer, preventing, with phytoestrogens, 252
Breathing
    for lower body routine, 184
    for midsection routine, 145
    for stretches, 77
    for upper body routine, 98
Broccoli, health benefits from, 335
Broccoli and Chicken Stir-Fry, 312
Broccoli and Shrimp Stir-Fry, 312
Brownie Sundae, 366
Buttocks, lower body routine for, 183

C

Caesar Salad Dressing, 385
Calcium
    daily requirement for, 251
    sources of, 251
    for weight loss, 277

Calorie burning
    from mini workouts, <u>43</u>
    from strength training, 27
    from walking, 23, 37, 38, <u>43, 48–49</u>
    after workouts, 26
Calorie levels
    for Shrink-Fat Eating Plan, 248–49
    for weight loss, 257
Calories, in weight loss, 257
Calves, toning, 183
Cancer, preventing, with foods, 252, 281,
    318, <u>333, 335, 369, 377</u>
Carbohydrates, high-fiber, 253, <u>289</u>
Cardiovascular exercise, benefits of, 18, 19,
    22–23
Cellulite, 25, 75, 180, 181, 183
Cereals, high-fiber, 257, <u>285</u>
Cheese and Tomato Sandwich, <u>266</u>
Cheese Tortellini with Marinara Sauce,
    <u>366</u>
Chest, upper body routine for, 97
Chicken Caesar Salad, <u>268</u>
Chicken Enchilada, <u>278</u>
Chicken Waldorf Salad, 392
Children, healthy foods for, <u>247, 329</u>
Chile peppers, health benefits from, <u>355</u>
Cinnamon Oatmeal, <u>290</u>
Clothing
    for stretching routines, <u>78</u>
    for walking workouts, <u>51</u>
Clothing size, for tracking progress,
    <u>16</u>
Coleslaw, health benefits from, <u>333</u>
Colon cancer, preventing, with phytoes-
    trogens, 252
Constipation, preventing, with fiber,
    281
Cookies, estimating portion of, <u>262</u>
Cool Cucumber Salad, <u>342</u>
Cravings
    foods to satisfy, <u>358</u>
    overcoming, 336–39, 361–63
Curried Tuna Salad, <u>314</u>
Curry, health benefits from, <u>315</u>

D

Dairy products
    calcium in, <u>277</u>
    in Shrink-Fat Eating Plan, 251
Deltoid muscles, upper body routine for,
    97
Depression, preventing, with walking,
    39
Diabetes, preventing, with walking, 39
Dieting
    fad, problem with, 246
    slowing metabolism and, 13, 15, 27
Digestion, improving, with walking, 39
Dumbbells, <u>29,</u> 98

E

Easy Homemade Chili, 392
Eating journal, 406, <u>407–12</u>
Eating Plan, Shrink-Fat
    breakfast in, 253, 257
    calorie levels for, 248–49
    cheating on, 245–46
    lack of hunger from, 248
    as lifestyle change, 246, 259
    moderation in, 245
    nutrient sources in
        dairy foods, 251
        fish, 253
        fruits and vegetables, 251–52
        whole grains, 252
    overview of, 30–31, 33
    slimming strategies in, 246–48
        eating good fats, 31, 247, 298–301
        increasing fiber intake, 30–31, 247,
            280–81
        increasing fruit and vegetable intake,
            31, 248, 318–19
        portion control, 30, 246, 260–63
        recognizing hunger signals, 31, 248,
            336–39, <u>343, 349</u>
        stopping overeating, 31, 248,
            356–63
    treats in, <u>254–55</u>

week 1, 30
  calories in, <u>263</u>
  charting progress of, 263
  menus for, <u>266–79</u>
  portion control guidelines, 260–63
  shopping list for, <u>264–65</u>
week 2, 30–31
  calories in, <u>281</u>
  charting progress of, <u>281</u>
  fiber guidelines in, 280–81
  menus for, <u>284–97</u>
  shopping list for, <u>282–83</u>
week 3, 31
  calories in, <u>301</u>
  charting progress of, <u>299</u>
  eating good fats in, 298–301
  menus for, <u>304–17</u>
  shopping list for, <u>302–3</u>
week 4, 31
  calories in, <u>319</u>
  charting progress of, <u>319</u>
  increasing fruit and vegetable intake in, 318–19
  menus for, <u>322–35</u>
  shopping list for, <u>320–21</u>
week 5, 31
  calories in, <u>339</u>
  charting progress of, <u>337</u>
  hunger eating in, 336–39
  menus for, <u>342–55</u>
  shopping list for, <u>340–41</u>
week 6, 31
  calories in, <u>362</u>
  charting progress of, <u>357</u>
  menus for, <u>366–79</u>
  shopping list for, <u>364–65</u>
  stopping overeating in, 356–63
Egg Burrito, <u>354</u>
Eggplant Pasta, 398
Equipment, exercise, <u>29</u>, <u>51</u>, <u>127</u>, <u>198</u>, <u>224</u>
Evening stretches. *See* Stretches, Evening Wind-Down
Excuses for skipping exercise, 222, 223

F
Fad diets, problem with, 246
Family
  dinnertime with, 258–59
  exercising with, 223
Fast food, <u>275</u>
Fast Guacamole, <u>292</u>
Fat loss, from strength training, 27
Fats, dietary
  bad, 301
  fiber, for removing, 281
  good, 299–301
  in peanut butter, <u>273</u>
  in Shrink-Fat Eating Plan, 31, 247, 298–301
  trans fats, <u>254</u>, <u>267</u>, 301
Fat zones, female
  aging and, 8–9
  identifying, <u>5</u>
  location of, 4, 11
  reducing, personal stories on, <u>10</u>, <u>14</u>, <u>24</u>, <u>32</u>, <u>142</u>, <u>182</u>, <u>250</u>, <u>256</u>
  role of hormones in, 7–8, 11
  science of, 6–7
Fat Zone Walking Moves
  ab tightener, <u>68</u>, **68**
  ab twist, <u>67</u>, **67**
  arm circles, <u>64</u>, **64**
  back-of-arm scissors, <u>63</u>, **63**
  biceps curl, <u>66</u>, **66**
  punches, <u>65</u>, **65**
  rear leg press, <u>72</u>, **72**
  scissors, <u>62</u>, **62**
  triceps toner, <u>60–61</u>, **60–61**
  tush tightener, <u>69</u>, **69**
  walking kickout, <u>71</u>, **71**
  walking lunge, <u>70</u>, **70**
  when to do, <u>60</u>
Feelings Log, for stopping overeating, 357, 359–60, <u>360</u>
Fennel, Orange, and Olive Salad, 398
Fettuccine with Tomato Alfredo Sauce, 385

Fiber
  in carbohydrates, 253, <u>289</u>
  in cereals, 257, <u>285</u>
  in Shrink-Fat Eating Plan, 30–31, 247,
    280–81
  sources of, <u>293</u>
Fidgeting, as exercise, <u>43</u>, 223
Fish, in Shrink-Fat Eating Plan, 253
Fish oils, 300
Fish with Olives and Capers, 393
Flax, phytoestrogens in, 252
Folate, health benefits from, 252, <u>369</u>
Food choices, for weight loss, 257–58
Food labels
  checking, <u>267</u>
  for portion control, 261
French Toast and Berries, <u>314</u>
Friends, exercising with, 223
Fruits
  bone strength from, <u>325</u>
  frozen, <u>331</u>
  phytonutrients in, 251–52, 318
  serving sizes of, <u>327</u>
  in Shrink-Fat Eating Plan, 31, 248,
    251–52, 318–19
  for weight loss, <u>323</u>

G

Garlic Bread, <u>347</u>
Gluteals, 183
Grilled Fish, 386
Grilled Honey-Mustard Chicken, 386

H

Ham and Cheese Sub, <u>366</u>
Ham and Rice Salad, <u>374</u>
Hamstrings, 183
Hats, for walkers, <u>51</u>
Heart disease
  preventing, with foods, 253, <u>291</u>, 318,
    <u>369</u>
  reducing, with walking, 39

Hearty Salad, <u>312</u>
Herb Sauce, 395
Hip flexors, lower body routine for, 183
Hips, toning, 181
Hormones, in fat storage, 7–8, 11
Hummus and Pita Sandwich, <u>308</u>
Hummus and Spinach Sandwich, <u>328</u>
Hunger Record, 337–39, <u>338</u>
Hunger signals, recognizing, in Shrink-Fat
    Eating Plan, 31, 248, 336–39, <u>343</u>,
    <u>349</u>
Hydrogenated oils, <u>254</u>, <u>267</u>, 301

I

Insulin, lowering, with fiber, 281
Insulin resistance, preventing, with
    walking, 39

J

Journal, for recording workouts and
    eating, <u>281</u>, <u>299</u>, <u>319</u>, <u>337</u>, <u>357</u>,
    359–60, <u>359</u>, <u>407–12</u>

K

Kickboxing, <u>210</u>

L

Labels, food
  checking, <u>267</u>
  for portion control, 261
Lemon Couscous, 391
Lemony Pan-Seared Tuna, 405
Lipoprotein lipase (LPL), lowering, with
    walking, 7, 8, 13, 37–38
Love handles, 141, 143, 144
Lower body, fat stored in, 180–81
Lower-Body Fat Zone routine
  areas targeted by, 181, 183
  do's and don'ts for, 184–85
  repetitions in, <u>185</u>

sample schedules for, 21
for weeks 1 and 2, 186
    butt lift, 190, **190**
    butt toner, 193, **193**
    down dog, 194, **194**
    front/back, 187, **187**
    inner thigh firmer, 188, **188**
    leg circles, 191, **191**
    leg circles with band, 192, **192**
    outer thigh and hip lift, 186, **186**
    outer thigh and hip stretch, 189,
      189
    pigeon, 197, **197**
    thigh blaster, 196, **196**
    thigh toner, 195, **195**
for weeks 3 and 4, 198
    ballet lift, 198, **198**
    butt-tap squat, 207, **207**
    half-forward bend, 209, **209**
    inner thigh beats, 202, **202**
    lunge with chair, 203–4, **203–4**
    plié, 206, **206**
    ronde de jambe, 199, **199**
    standing front/back, 200, **200**
    standing hamstring curl, 208, **208**
    standing hip opener, 205, **205**
    thigh stretch, 201, **201**
for weeks 5 and 6, 210
    back kick, 218, **218**
    diagonal lunge, 213, **213**
    forward bend, 219, **219**
    front kick, 217, **217**
    standing hip opener, 220, **220**
    standing quad stretch, 212, **212**
    wall sit, 210, **210**
    wall sit with ball, 211, **211**
    warrior, 215–16, **215–16**
    wide-angle forward bend, 214, **214**
Low-fat diet, moderately, 298–99
Lox, health benefits from, 317
LPL. *See* Lipoprotein lipase
Lycopene
  sources of, 252
  in tomatoes, 279

M

Mall walking, 42
Mango Rice, 400
Maple Milk, 296
Measurements, body, for tracking progress,
    16
Measurements, food, for portion control, 261
Melon Smoothie, 306
Menopause, fat storage after, 8–9, 11, 141
Menus for Shrink-Fat Eating Plan
  week 1, 266–79
  week 2, 284–97
  week 3, 304–17
  week 4, 322–35
  week 5, 342–55
  week 6, 366–79
Metabolism
  affected by
    aging, 258
    chronic dieting, 13, 15, 27
    exercise, 19, 22
    starvation, 249, 258
    stress, 15–16
  boosting, 17, 26, 27, 253
Mexican Lasagna, 403
Midday stretches. *See* Stretches, Midday
    Tension-Relieving
Midsection Fat Zone routine
  do's and don'ts for, 144–46
  muscles targeted by, 143–44
  repetitions in, 146
  results from, 141, 143
  sample schedules for, 21
  for weeks 1 and 2, 147
    child's pose, 156, **156**
    full-body reach, 152, **152**
    lower back strengthener, 155, **155**
    modified T-stand, 153, **153**
    plank, 154, **154**
    pulsing crunch 1, 148, **148**
    roll-down 1, 147, **147**
    single-leg stretch, 149, **149**
    twisting crunch, 150, **150**
    twisting crunch on ball, 151, **151**

Midsection Fat Zone routine *(cont.)*
    for weeks 3 and 4, <u>157</u>
        full-body reach, <u>162,</u> **162**
        plank with leg tuck, <u>165,</u> **165**
        pulsing crunch 2, <u>158,</u> **158**
        pulsing crunch 2 on ball, <u>159,</u> **159**
        roll-down 2, <u>157,</u> **157**
        single straight-leg stretch, <u>160,</u> **160**
        spinal twist, <u>167,</u> **167**
        superwoman, <u>166,</u> **166**
        T-stand, <u>164,</u> **164**
        twisting crunch with straight legs,
           <u>161,</u> **161**
        ultimate tummy trimmer, <u>163,</u> **163**
    for weeks 5 and 6, <u>168</u>
        bent-arm plank with knee kiss, <u>177,</u>
           177
        bicycle, <u>171,</u> **171**
        child's pose, <u>179,</u> **179**
        double crunch, <u>170,</u> **170**
        roll-down with arms overhead,
           <u>168–69,</u> **168–69**
        spinal twist, <u>176,</u> **176**
        swimming, <u>178,</u> **178**
        T-stand with twist, <u>174–75,</u> **174–75**
        ultimate tummy trimmer 2, <u>172,</u>
           172
        ultimate tummy trimmer 2
           (variation), <u>173,</u> **173**
Mini Peach Smoothie, <u>316</u>
Mini workouts, <u>43</u>
Monounsaturated fat, 301
Morning stretches. *See* Stretches, Morning
    Wake-Up
Mozzarella and Tomato Sandwich, <u>326</u>
Muffins, estimating portion of, <u>262</u>
Multivitamins, 251
Muscle loss, with aging, 9, 26

N

Neighborhood walks, 45
New Potatoes, <u>352</u>
Nutrition Facts panel, for portion control,
    261

O

Obliques, midsection routine for, 143
Omega-3 fatty acids, in fish, 253, 300,
    301
Osteoporosis, 28, 251, <u>377</u>
Oven-Baked Chicken, 394
Overeating
    nighttime, <u>367</u>
    reasons for, 356–57, 360–61, <u>371,</u> <u>373</u>
    recovering from, <u>371</u>
    stopping
        with Feelings Log, 357, 359–60,
           <u>360</u>
        in Shrink-Fat Eating Plan, 31, 248,
           356–63

P

Pasta, estimating portion of, <u>262</u>
Pasta Primavera, 397
Pasta with Broccoli and Cheese, <u>334</u>
Pasta with Broccoli and Chicken, 390
Pasta with Shrimp and Broccoli, 399
Pasta with Zucchini Sauce, <u>346</u>
Peach-Banana Smoothie, <u>288</u>
Peanut butter, health benefits from, <u>273</u>
Peanut Butter and Honey Sandwich,
    <u>376</u>
Peanut Butter and Jelly Sandwich, <u>272</u>
Pectoralis major, upper body routine for,
    97
Pedometers, <u>51</u>
Phytoestrogens, sources of, 252
Phytonutrients, sources of, 251–52, 318
Pilates, 29, 144, <u>147,</u> 184, <u>186</u>
Poached Salmon with Herb Sauce, 395
Pork Tenderloin Sandwich, <u>344</u>
Portion control, in Shrink-Fat Eating Plan,
    30, 246, 260–63
Power Yoga, 29, 184
Pregnancy
    abdominal toning after, 140
    weight loss after, <u>14,</u> <u>142,</u> <u>250</u>
Progress, tracking, <u>16.</u> *See also* Journal, for
    recording workouts and eating

Q

Quadriceps, 181, 183
Quick Veggie Pizza, 388

R

Recipes, 383
  week 1
    Bean Burrito, 274
    Beef and Broccoli Stir-Fry, 387
    Caesar Salad Dressing, 385
    Cheese and Tomato Sandwich, 266
    Chicken Caesar Salad, 268
    Chicken Enchilada, 278
    Fettuccine with Tomato Alfredo
      Sauce, 385
    Grilled Fish, 386
    Grilled Honey-Mustard Chicken, 386
    Peanut Butter and Jelly Sandwich,
      272
    Quick Veggie Pizza, 388
    Roasted Chicken, 384
    Sautéed Greens, 274
    Strawberry-Banana Smoothie, 266
    Tuna and Bean Salad, 387
  week 2
    Apricot-Glazed Chicken, 390
    Avocado and White Bean Salad, 391
    Chicken Waldorf Salad, 392
    Cinnamon Oatmeal, 290
    Easy Homemade Chili, 392
    Fast Guacamole, 292
    Fish with Olives and Capers, 393
    Lemon Couscous, 391
    Maple Milk, 296
    Pasta with Broccoli and Chicken, 390
    Peach-Banana Smoothie, 288
    Satisfying Veggie Salad, 286
    Scrambled Eggs, 294
    Shrimp and Vegetable Kebabs, 389
    Spaghetti, 294
    Tuna Sandwich, 288
    Turkey and Cheese Sandwich, 284
    Veggie Cheeseburger, 296
    Waffles, 296
  week 3
    Avocado, Tomato, and Corn Salad,
      304
    Bean Burrito with Avocado, 304
    Broccoli and Chicken Stir-Fry, 312
    Broccoli and Shrimp Stir-Fry, 312
    Curried Tuna Salad, 314
    French Toast and Berries, 314
    Hearty Salad, 312
    Herb Sauce, 395
    Hummus and Pita Sandwich, 308
    Melon Smoothie, 306
    Mini Peach Smoothie, 316
    Oven-Baked Chicken, 394
    Pasta Primavera, 397
    Poached Salmon with Herb Sauce,
      395
    Salmon Burgers, 396
    Salsa Omelet, 310
    Sautéed Spinach, 394
    Southwestern Salad, 316
    Strawberries Dipped in Chocolate,
      316
    Tomato and Green Pepper Salad, 308
    Turkey and Chutney Roll-Up, 316
  week 4
    Banana Split, 326
    Barbecued Chicken, 332
    Eggplant Pasta, 398
    Fennel, Orange, and Olive Salad, 398
    Hummus and Spinach Sandwich, 328
    Mozzarella and Tomato Sandwich,
      326
    Pasta with Broccoli and Cheese, 334
    Pasta with Shrimp and Broccoli, 399
    Salsa Scramble, 330
    Sautéed Veggies, 330
    Tuna and Chickpea Salad, 334
    Veggie Sandwich with Cheese, 332
  week 5
    Cool Cucumber Salad, 342
    Egg Burrito, 354
    Garlic Bread, 347
    Mango Rice, 400
    New Potatoes, 352

Recipes *(cont.)*
  week 5 *(cont.)*
    Pasta with Zucchini Sauce, <u>346</u>
    Pork Tenderloin Sandwich, <u>344</u>
    Spicy Orange Pork Tenderloin with
      Mango Rice, 400
    Spinach Salad, <u>348</u>
    Strawberry Shortcake, <u>352</u>
    Thai Chicken Curry, 401
    Veggie Burger, <u>352</u>
    Veggie Roll-Up, <u>350</u>
  week 6
    Brownie Sundae, <u>366</u>
    Cheese Tortellini with Marinara
      Sauce, <u>366</u>
    Ham and Cheese Sub, <u>366</u>
    Ham and Rice Salad, <u>374</u>
    Lemony Pan-Seared Tuna, 405
    Mexican Lasagna, 403
    Peanut Butter and Honey Sandwich,
      <u>376</u>
    Roasted Potatoes and Mushrooms,
      404
    Salsa Chicken, <u>376</u>
    Scrambled Tofu, <u>376</u>
    Super Spinach Salad, <u>368</u>
    Tofu, Mushroom, and Chicken
      Risotto, 404
    Turkey and Cheese Sub, <u>366</u>
    Wild Rice, Peas, and Chicken, 402
Rectus abdominis, midsection routine for,
  143
Roasted Chicken, 384
Roasted Potatoes and Mushrooms, 404
Running, injuries from, 38

S

Salmon Burgers, 396
Salsa Chicken, <u>376</u>
Salsa Omelet, <u>310</u>
Salsa Scramble, <u>330</u>
Satisfying Veggie Salad, <u>286</u>
Saturated fat, 301
Sautéed Spinach, 394

Sautéed Veggies, <u>330</u>
Scrambled Eggs, <u>294</u>
Scrambled Tofu, <u>376</u>
Shinsplints, preventing, <u>38</u>, <u>41</u>, **41**
Shoes, walking, <u>29</u>, <u>44</u>, **44**, <u>51</u>
Shopping lists, for Shrink-Fat Eating Plan,
  <u>264–65</u>, <u>282–83</u>, <u>302–3</u>, <u>320–21</u>,
  <u>340–41</u>, <u>364–65</u>
Shoulders, upper body routine for, 97
Shrimp and Vegetable Kebabs, 389
Shrink-Fat Eating Plan. *See* Eating Plan,
  Shrink-Fat
Shrink Your Female Fat Zones program
  charting progress in, <u>16</u>
  components of
    cardiovascular exercise, 18, 19, 22–23
    eating plan, 30–31, 33
    strength training, 25–28
    stretching, 23, 25
  effects of, 18
  equipment for, <u>29</u>
  metabolism boosters in, 17
  overview of, 3–5, 33
  for redesigning body, 28–29
  sample schedules for, <u>20–21</u>
  workbook for, <u>407–12</u>
Sleep, stretching before, 76, <u>87</u>
Socks, for walkers, <u>51</u>
Southwestern Salad, <u>316</u>
Soy foods, health benefits from, <u>377</u>
Spaghetti, <u>294</u>
Spicy Orange Pork Tenderloin with
  Mango Rice, 400
Spinach, health benefits from, 252, <u>351</u>
Spinach Salad, <u>348</u>
Stability ball, for upper body exercises, <u>127</u>
Step, aerobics, for 10-Minute Total-Body
  Blast, <u>224</u>
Strawberries, health benefits from, <u>287</u>
Strawberries Dipped in Chocolate, <u>316</u>
Strawberry-Banana Smoothie, <u>266</u>
Strawberry Shortcake, <u>352</u>
Strength training
  benefits of, 26–28
  frequency of, 25–26

Stress
    abdominal fat from, 15, 357–59
    affecting metabolism, 15–16
    reducing, 23, 362–63
Stretches
    benefits of, 23, 25, 73–76, 223
    do's and don'ts for, 76–77
    Evening Wind-Down
        hip opener on wall, 89, **89**
        leg circulation series, 90–91, **90–91**
        purpose of, 87
        wall hang, 87–88, **87–88**
    lower body
        down dog, 194, **194**
        forward bend, 219, **219**
        half-forward bend, 209, **209**
        outer thigh and hip stretch, 189, **189**
        pigeon, 197, **197**
        standing hip opener, 220, **220**
        standing quad stretch, 212, **212**
        thigh stretch, 201, **201**
        wide-angle forward bend, 214, **214**
    Midday Tension-Relieving
        hip opener, 86, **86**
        neck and shoulder release, 83, **83**
        one-arm reach, 85, **85**
        purpose of, 83
        shoulder and chest relaxer, 84, **84**
    midsection
        child's pose, 156, **156**, 179, **179**
        full-body reach, 152, **152**, 162, **162**
        importance of, 146
        spinal twist, 167, **167**, 176, **176**
    Morning Wake-Up
        benefits of, 78
        forward bend, 82, **82**
        healthy back stretch, 79, **79**
        reach-for-the-sky stretch, 78, **78**
        shoulder roll, 80, **80**
        standing cat stretch, 81, **81**
    pre-walk
        Achilles stretch, 53, **53**
        benefits of, 52
        butt and thigh stretch, 56, **56**
        calf stretch, 52, **52**

        hamstring stretch, 58, **58**
        leg and back stretch, 57, **57**
        quad stretch, 54, **54**
        waist twist, 55, **55**
    10-Minute Total-Body Blast
        child's pose, 238, **238**
        circular hip opener, 240–41, **240–41**
        cobra stretch, 236, **236**
        forward bend, 231, **231**
    upper body
        bear hug, 120, **120**
        chest expansion, 103, **103**
        chest opener, 117, **117**
        seated arm stretch, 139, **139**
        seated chest expansion, 130, **130**
        seated triceps stretch, 126, **126**
        triceps stretch, 110, **110**
        upper back and shoulder stretch, 114,
        114
Success stories, 10, 14, 24, 32, 142, 182,
    250, 256
Sunglasses, for walkers, 51
Sunscreen, for walkers, 51
Super Spinach Salad, 368
Syndrome W, 12

T

Tahini, health benefits from, 309
10-Minute Total-Body Blast exercises
    back extension, 239, **239**
    biceps curl with off-the-back lunge,
        224–25, **224–25**
    bicycle, 232, **232**
    child's pose, 238, **238**
    circular hip opener, 240–41, **240–41**
    cobra stretch, 236, **236**
    description of, 224
    do's and don'ts for, 222–23
    double-leg stretch, 233, **233**
    forward bend, 231, **231**
    lunge with upper back fly, 230, **230**
    overhead raise with side lift, 228–29,
        228–29
    plank with leg lift, 235, **235**

10-Minute Total-Body Blast exercises *(cont.)*
  pushup, <u>237</u>, **237**
  rollover, <u>234</u>, **234**
  triceps kickback with rear leg lift,
    <u>226–27</u>, **226–27**
  when to use, 221–22
Tension-relieving stretches. *See* Stretches,
  Midday Tension-Relieving
Thai Chicken Curry, 401
Thighs, lower body routine for, 181, 183
Time management, 222
Tofu, Mushroom, and Chicken Risotto,
  404
Tomato and Green Pepper Salad, <u>308</u>
Tomatoes, lycopene in, 252
Tomato sauce, as vegetable serving, <u>279</u>
Track walking, 45
Trail walking, 45
Trans fats, <u>254</u>, <u>267</u>, 301
Transverse abdominis, midsection routine
  for, 143
Treadmill walking, 42, <u>60</u>
Treats, in Shrink-Fat Eating Plan, <u>254–55</u>
Triceps, upper body routine for, 97
Tuna and Bean Salad, 387
Tuna and Chickpea Salad, <u>334</u>
Tuna Sandwich, <u>288</u>
Turkey and Cheese Sandwich, <u>284</u>
Turkey and Cheese Sub, <u>366</u>
Turkey and Chutney Roll-Up, <u>316</u>

U

Upper-Body Fat Zone exercises
  areas targeted by, 96–97
  do's and don'ts for, 97–99
  repetitions in, <u>99</u>
  sample schedules for, <u>20</u>
  for weeks 1 and 2, <u>100</u>
    chest expansion, <u>103</u>, **103**
    chest fly, <u>100</u>, **100**
    lat pullover, <u>101</u>, **101**
    modified beginner pushup, <u>102</u>, **102**
    one-arm row, <u>106</u>, **106**
    one-arm row with chair, <u>107</u>, **107**

    seated biceps curl, <u>105</u>, **105**
    standing biceps curl, <u>104</u>, **104**
    standing front raise, <u>111–12</u>, **111–12**
    standing overhead press, <u>113</u>, **113**
    standing triceps kickback, <u>108</u>, **108**
    standing triceps toner, <u>109</u>, **109**
    triceps stretch, <u>110</u>, **110**
    upper back and shoulder stretch, <u>114</u>,
      114
  for weeks 3 and 4, <u>115</u>
    bear hug, <u>120</u>, **120**
    bilateral kickback, <u>122</u>, **122**
    bilateral row, <u>118</u>, **118**
    chest opener, <u>117</u>, **117**
    chest press, <u>115</u>, **115**
    double-arm fly, <u>119</u>, **119**
    lat pulldown 1, <u>125</u>, **125**
    low hover, <u>123</u>, **123**
    low hover on knees, <u>124</u>, **124**
    pushup on knees, <u>116</u>, **116**
    seated triceps stretch, <u>126</u>, **126**
    standing lateral raise, <u>121</u>, **121**
  for weeks 5 and 6, <u>127</u>
    chest press incline, <u>127</u>, **127**
    lat pulldown 2, <u>131</u>, **131**
    pushup, <u>128</u>, **128**
    pushup on ball, <u>129</u>, **129**
    seated arm stretch, <u>139</u>, **139**
    seated back fly, <u>133</u>, **133**
    seated chest expansion, <u>130</u>, **130**
    seated combined front and lateral
      raise, <u>135–36</u>, **135–36**
    seated double-arm row, <u>132</u>, **132**
    seated overhead press, <u>134</u>, **134**
    triceps chair dip, <u>137</u>, **137**
    triceps chair dip on one leg, <u>138</u>, **138**
Upper body toning, benefits of, 95–96

V

Varicose veins, 25, 75
Vegetables
  encouraging children to eat, <u>329</u>
  frozen, <u>331</u>
  phytonutrients in, 251–52, 318

serving sizes of, <u>327</u>
in Shrink-Fat Eating Plan, 31, 248,
    251–52, 318–19
for weight loss, <u>323</u>
Veggie Burger, <u>352</u>
Veggie Cheeseburger, <u>296</u>
Veggie Roll-Up, <u>350</u>
Veggie Sandwich with Cheese, <u>332</u>
Visors, for walkers, <u>51</u>

W

Waffles, <u>296</u>
Walking
    benefits of, 19, 22–23
    calorie burning from, <u>48–49</u>
    clothing and equipment for, <u>51</u>
    finding opportunities for, 40–41, <u>43</u>
    health benefits from, 37–40
    locations for, 41–42, 45
    shoes for, <u>29</u>, <u>44</u>, **44**, <u>51</u>
    stretches for (*see* Stretches, pre-walk)
    technique for, <u>59</u>, **59**
    time spent on, 40
    uphill, <u>38</u>
    workouts for (*see* Walking workouts)
Walking workouts
    combined fat zone and fat-burning
        walk, 40, <u>47</u>, 50
    endurance walk, 40, <u>46</u>, 47, <u>47</u>, 50

fat-burning walk, 40, <u>46</u>, <u>47</u>, 50
fat zone walk, 40, <u>46</u>, 50
    exercises for (*see* Fat Zone Walking
        Moves)
schedule for, <u>46–47</u>
starting, 47
Watches, for walkers, <u>51</u>
Water drinking, for walkers, <u>51</u>
Watermelon, lycopene in, 252
Weight gain, with aging, 8–9
Weight loss
    calories and, 257
    food choices for, 257–58
    journal for, 406, <u>407–12</u>
    personal stories on, <u>24</u>, <u>32</u>
    postpregnancy, <u>14</u>, <u>142</u>, <u>250</u>
    from walking, 37
Weight maintenance, personal stories of,
    <u>182</u>, <u>256</u>
Whole grains, in Shrink-Fat Eating Plan,
    252
Wild Rice, Peas, and Chicken, 402
Willpower, <u>349</u>
Workout logs, <u>281</u>, <u>299</u>, <u>319</u>, <u>337</u>, <u>357</u>,
    <u>407–12</u>

Y

Yoga, <u>210</u>
    Power, 29, 184